THE McDOUGALL PROGRAM
FOR A HEALTHY HEART

The McDOUGALL

A Life-Saving Approach to Preventing and Treating Heart Disease

PROGRAM *for a*
HEALTHY HEART

John A. McDougall, M.D.
Recipes by Mary McDougall

A DUTTON BOOK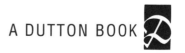

A NOTE TO THE READER

The ideas, procedures, and suggestions contained in this book are not intended as a substitute for consulting with your physician. All matters regarding your health require medical supervision.

DUTTON
Published by the Penguin Group
Penguin Books USA Inc., 375 Hudson Street, New York, New York 10014, U.S.A.
Penguin Books Ltd, 27 Wrights Lane, London W8 5TZ, England
Penguin Books Australia Ltd, Ringwood, Victoria, Australia
Penguin Books Canada Ltd, 10 Alcorn Avenue, Toronto, Ontario, Canada M4V 3B2
Penguin Books (N.Z.) Ltd, 182–190 Wairau Road, Auckland 10, New Zealand

Penguin Books Ltd, Registered Offices: Harmondsworth, Middlesex, England

First published by Dutton, an imprint of Dutton Signet,
a division of Penguin Books USA Inc.
Distributed in Canada by McClelland & Stewart Inc.

First Printing, February, 1996
2 4 6 8 10 9 7 5 3

 REGISTERED TRADEMARK—MARCA REGISTRADA

LIBRARY OF CONGRESS CATALOGING-IN-PUBLICATION DATA:
McDougall, John A.
The McDougall program for a healthy heart : a life-saving approach to preventing and treating heart disease / John A. McDougall ; recipes by Mary McDougall.
p.   cm.
Includes bibliographical references.
ISBN 0-525-93868-0
1. Coronary heart disease—Popular works.   I. McDougall, Mary A. (Mary Ann)
II. Title.
RC685.C6M36   1996
616.1'2306—dc20   95-31121
CIP

Printed in the United States of America
Set in Times New Roman
Designed by Eve L. Kirch

This book is printed on acid-free paper.

To my father, John McDougall Sr., who has lived the story of heart disease—in good times and bad—both of us learning from his experiences.

CONTENTS

Part III.   The Best Medical Care You Can Get

Part IV.   Shopping Help, Cooking Tips, and the Recipes

ACKNOWLEDGMENTS

Our gratitude and thanks to:

Tom Monte, who took my knowledge and beliefs, and wove them into an indispensable guide for the prevention and treatment of artery disease, especially epidemic heart disease. Santa Rosa Community Hospital Library and its librarian, Joan Chilton, for help gathering information and providing the supporting scientific studies. BRS Colleague for on-line computer research services. Word processing was done on Amipro and the charts and graphs were done on Freelance Graphics, both by Lotus. Illustrations were made by Mary Albury-Noyes of Medical Arts Services, Burnsville, Minnesota.

A very special thanks to the people who volunteered to share their stories.

Mary and I are indebted to all the people we have become personally involved with over the years. Friends, patients, radio show listeners, and readers of our books and newsletter have taught us valuable lessons. Our most important education has come from those who have attended my twelve-day live-in program at St. Helena Hospital in the Napa Valley, California; for information, phone (800) 358-9195.

If you have any questions, or ideas you would like to share, please write or call:

> The McDougalls
> P.O. Box 14039
> Santa Rosa, CA 95402
> (800) 570-1654
> fax: (707) 576-3313

AUTHOR'S NOTE

Read Carefully

Heart disease can be life-threatening. You must obtain the help of a competent, caring physician when you suffer from this disease. These days more doctors are paying attention to their patients' diet and lifestyle—often offering advice that includes a recommendation to follow *The McDougall Program for a Healthy Heart.*

Diet is powerful medicine. Do not change your diet if you are seriously ill or on medication unless you are under the care of a physician knowledgeable in nutrition and its effects on cardiovascular (heart and blood vessel) disease. Do not change medications without professional advice. The information in this book is general and not to be taken as specific medical advice for your special health problems. Share this book with your doctor. Then together you will be able to work out the best possible route for your recovery.

The people in this book are real. If you do as they have done, you should expect similar remarkable results. Although no treatment gives ideal outcomes for everyone, in most cases this approach offers you the best chance of regaining your lost health.

The McDougall Program for a Healthy Heart uses a pure vegetarian diet based around starches with the addition of vegetables and limited amounts of fruit. If you follow the diet strictly for more than three years, or if you are pregnant or nursing, then take a minimum of 5 micrograms (mcg) of supplemental B_{12} each day.

COMMON PROBLEMS AND SOLUTIONS

Diet and Lifestyle Concerns
IF . . .

you want to prevent heart disease . . .

THEN follow the basic *McDougall Program* diet based on starches, vegetables, and fruits, stay physically active, avoid destructive habits such as smoking and drinking coffee (even decaf) and excess alcohol.

you need to recover from heart disease and other forms of atherosclerosis . . .

THEN follow the more restrictive diet in *The McDougall Program for a Healthy Heart*—the diet is also starch-based with the addition of vegetables. Fruits, fruit juice, and all simple sugars are limited (often eliminated), because they elevate cholesterol and triglycerides in sensitive people. Exercise daily. Stop all destructive habits—smoking and drinking coffee, including decaffeinated coffee.

you must use salt . . .

THEN sprinkle lightly on the surface of the food where the tongue directly contacts this flavorful substance. Do not use it in cooking. Seasonings will help flavor a low-sodium meal plan. Salt substitutes (potassium salt) are usually not recommended because they can lead to other health problems in some people. However, some people may find them helpful and tolerable.

you must have a sweetener . . .

THEN sprinkle sugar lightly on the surface of the food where the tongue directly contacts it. Do not use in cooking. Artificial sweeteners are usually not recommended because they can lead to other health problems in some people. However, some people may find them helpful and tolerable.

you desire a hot beverage . . .

THEN choose tea, especially green tea, because of its beneficial effects on your cholesterol and triglyceride levels.

you must drink alcohol . . .

THEN choose red wine because of its known benefits on heart disease. However, alcohol raises triglycerides in sensitive people and has many other very serious drawbacks.

you are overweight . . .

THEN eat plenty of healthy food and exercise within your physical limits. This is the only way you will permanently regain lost health and appearance. Eliminate flour products, including breads, bagels, and pasta, and increase intake of green and yellow vegetables. Increase exercise. Read *The McDougall Program for Maximum Weight Loss* for further help in understanding how starches make you thin.

you don't like to cook . . .

THEN keep it simple by making a few favorite starches—potatoes, rice, beans, spaghetti—and adding convenience products, such as prepared soups and sauces found in the list of canned and packaged products on pages 266–285.

you don't like the food . . .

THEN be patient! It may take you a week to find a few dishes you enjoy and for your taste buds to finally adjust. Eat frequently (six or more times a day). Use familiar ingredients, especially favorite spices and prepared sauces. People who have the most difficult time learning to like the foods usually are the ones who get the most dramatic benefits from the McDougall Program for a Healthy Heart (because they are the ones who started with the worst diets and lifestyles).

you want to take supplements . . .

THEN take vitamins A (beta carotene), C, and E (in a dry form), because they have been associated with healthier arteries (less heart disease). Mineral supplements, especially magnesium, zinc, and iron, should be avoided—they have been linked to more artery disease.

you don't like to exercise . . .

THEN make the effort. Try to find an exercise partner, join a cardiac rehabilitation program, hire a personal trainer from your local health club, and/or find something you like to do.

Medical Concerns
IF . . .

you have sudden onset of chest pains, shortness of breath, or in any other way feel seriously ill . . .

THEN obtain medical attention immediately—this may mean calling an ambulance and a visit to the nearest emergency room.

you are asked to start a medication . . .

THEN ask the doctor to explain the necessity of each medication. How long will I have to take it? How will I know it is working properly? What are the adverse side effects? Are there alternatives? Can I do without it?

you are on medication . . .

THEN ask the doctor to explain the necessity of each medication. Are there any safer substitutes? What would be the consequences of quitting it? How do I safely reduce or stop the medication. Can we experiment a little by seeing how I do with less medication or none at all?

your cholesterol fails to come down to ideal (less than 150 mg/dl) . . .

THEN after following the diet strictly for all its cholesterol-lowering benefits, begin the "natural" cholesterol-lowering medications on page 188. If you need more help, then start on the doctor-prescribed medications on page 186.

your triglycerides fail to come down to ideal (less than 150 mg/dl) . . .

THEN after following the diet strictly (with no fruit, fruit juice, or other simple sugars) and exercising for all their triglyceride-lowering benefits, begin the "natural" cholesterol-lowering medications on page 183, like garlic and gugulipid, which are known to lower triglycerides. Under doctor's supervision try niacin (vitamin B_3). If you need more help, then start on the doctor-prescribed medications on page 186.

your blood pressure fails to fall to ideal (110/70 mm Hg without medication) . . .

THEN after following the diet strictly and exercising daily for all of their blood pressure–lowering benefits, remove all added salt from your diet. Loss of excess body fat may help lower blood pressure in time. Check your blood pressure at home for the most meaningful readings. Readings in the doctor's office often represent the level of fear of your doctor. If the diastolic remains over 100 mm Hg for months then you may need to start on doctor-prescribed medications. Don't overtreat (keep the diastolic above 85 mm Hg while on medication).

you are asked to have a test . . .

THEN ask the doctor to explain how the test will change the way he cares for you. Will this test lead to other tests or treatments? What are the costs, adverse effects, alternatives to the recommended test(s)?

you have symptoms of heart disease, like chest pain or shortness of breath . . .

THEN see your doctor. Heart disease is diagnosed by a thorough history and an EKG in almost all cases—not by "high-tech" tests.

you are diagnosed with heart disease by a thorough history and an EKG . . .

THEN the next step is a treadmill stress test. If this is normal, further testing is unnecessary. (Many doctors will try to rush you from the initial doctor's visit to the angiogram, which is the test that usually leads to heart surgery.)

the treadmill stress test is abnormal . . .

THEN the next step is a radionuclide test, like a thallium scan. If this test is normal, further testing is unnecessary. (Many doctors will try to rush you from the initial doctor's visit to the angiogram, which is the test that usually leads to heart surgery.)

the radionuclide test shows a large amount of heart muscle is at risk . . .

THEN the next step is an angiogram. Heart surgery usually follows this invasive test.

you are asked to have heart surgery . . .

THEN ask the doctor for a clear explanation for the necessity for the surgery. Insist on the evidence that supports the belief that this surgery will prolong your life based on the findings in your specific case. Seek a second opinion. Investigate your options, including the option of doing nothing. Find a doctor and a hospital with lots of experience with heart surgery and a great record for successful outcomes.

you have to have heart surgery . . .

THEN choose angioplasty over bypass surgery because of reduced pain, side effects, complications, and costs (assuming you have a choice of either operation).

you have had heart surgery . . .

THEN take every effort to make sure you regain your lost health and prevent any repeat heart surgery through the McDougall Program for a Healthy Heart.

Part I

THE CAUSE AND THE CURE

1. The Surest Path to Health

- *Heart disease struck my life many times.*
- *Getting well is accomplished by stopping the cause.*
- *Don't be a helpless victim. The right information will restore your lost health.*

Warning: Compromises Can Be Dangerous to Your Health

Not too long ago, one of my patients presented me with an age-old dilemma. He wanted to know how he could avoid sickness and dying with the least amount of effort. "I'm tired of this chronic cough and I want to avoid lung cancer," he said. "How many cigarettes can I smoke and still be on the safe side?" As his physician, I could only give him one answer. "None," I said.

I confront the same dilemma whenever someone asks me how they can avoid heart disease. Invariably, a patient will ask me how many steaks, eggs, and pieces of cheese he can eat and still be on the safe side. I have no other choice but to provide him with the only correct and accurate answer I know. "None." If you want to prevent or cure heart disease, you have to avoid the poisons that create the disease in the first place. That, in its essence, is the McDougall Program for a Healthy Heart. Everyone else will offer you a compromise, much like telling a smoker that he can smoke ten cigarettes per day and still have his health.

In the course of this book, I will spell out my program and the reasons it works in great detail. But the first thing you should understand is that because I make no compromises with your health, my program is the fastest and most efficient program for combating heart disease. People who adopt the McDougall Program for a Healthy Heart experience a dramatic improvement, and they see it quickly. They also have very little trouble following my advice, because the program is clear and powerful. As I often say, "Big changes beget big results." And your unequivocal results will keep you on the program.

I am not going to fool you with half-truths, sleights of hand, or sales pitches that say you can go on eating the same old way and still beat heart disease. It's not going to happen. There are lots of programs and medical doctors out there who will tell you that you can eat "a certain amount" of unhealthy foods and still have a reasonable chance at avoiding heart disease. The fact is that everyone who eats food rich in fat and cholesterol is playing Russian roulette. Eventually, the bullet will go off and it's going to hit you in the heart, or the breast, or the prostate, or the colon, or the brain, or some other vulnerable place in your body. The rich American diet—high in fat and cholesterol, deficient in dietary fiber and unbalanced in vitamins and minerals—is responsible for most of the heart disease, high blood pressure, stroke, cancer, and diabetes we experience today. These illnesses are actually different manifestations of the same underlying disease. That underlying causal disease is essentially the poisoning of the body through the consumption of excessive amounts of rich foods.

Most of the people who adopt the McDougall Program adjust to the dietary changes quickly. In fact, as soon as you learn how to prepare the McDougall foods, you'll be amazed at how delicious your meals are, and how easy it is to eat this way. You will not be chained to your kitchen, either. I'll show you how to cook foods in no time at all, to eat healthfully in restaurants, when you travel and socialize with your friends—*and* enjoy good health. In a way, you're almost getting something for nothing. You go about the business of enjoying life, eating delicious foods, while your body's busy repairing itself. That sounds like too good a deal to pass up.

The Biggest Killer Known to Humankind

This book is for everyone concerned about illnesses of the heart and arteries, including heart disease, high blood pressure, angina pectoris, and various forms of peripheral vascular disease, such as claudication—which, based on statistics, is almost every man, woman, and child in

Western civilization. This book will show you how to overcome and prevent the most widespread killer in human history.

Sixty-nine million Americans suffer from cardiovascular disease, and so the odds are pretty good that you, my reader, are already one of them. Those of you who are coping with heart disease—and especially those who have recently had a heart attack—are probably worried, and perhaps even terrified. Time seems short and running out. Let me assure you—even those of you who have just suffered a heart attack—that there is time to recover in almost every case. Or to put it more accurately, there is time to choose.

You can choose health. Your decision does not require any words. Your behavior from this moment onward will reveal the choice you have made. It will also determine the outcome.

Before you undergo any kind of invasive treatment such as a coronary angiogram, angioplasty, or bypass surgery, you should read this book and discuss the information with your doctor. However, even if you decide that surgery is your best answer, your long-term health and survival still depend primarily on adopting a healthful way of eating and living. And in this book, I'm going to provide you with a program that is the best available treatment for heart disease.

I'm not going to speak to you like some know-it-all doctor who has a bunch of facts and no real understanding of your fears and concerns. I'm going to talk to you as someone who has been right where many of you are right now: in the hospital and fighting for your life. At the age of 18, I suffered a stroke that left me completely paralyzed on the left side of my body. Recovery was slow but incomplete. Even to this day, I walk with a limp, which reminds me of my vulnerability.

My family has also suffered from this terrible disease. More than a dozen years ago, both my father and father-in-law suffered heart attacks and were encouraged to have coronary bypass surgery before I intervened and put them on the McDougall Program for a Healthy Heart, which kept them in good health for many years.

But like anyone with a family member facing a grave health crisis, I agonized over the right course of treatment. And as I will discuss later in this book, I continue to wrestle with the right decisions. What I am telling you is that I know just about every angle of this disease. I know the illness from firsthand knowledge; I know it as a loved one who wants desperately to save a relative's life; and I know it as a doctor who sees hundreds of patients each year who suffer from an illness that kills nearly a million people annually. I know the fear this disease causes; I know how health can be restored; and I know the reluctance people have to changing deeply ingrained behaviors. I, too, was reluctant to change.

Part of the solution to heart disease is to be honest with yourself. We have to face the facts squarely and act accordingly. Heart disease is caused by eating rich foods like meat, chicken, cheese, milk, eggs, oils, cakes, and candies as well as refined and processed foods. These foods will surely cause you further misery and even premature death, like they have hundreds of millions of others. There is no way to soft-pedal the facts.

Even if you have had a coronary bypass operation, in which one or more of the blocked arteries leading to your heart have been replaced by another vessel, you're still at risk of having another heart attack because your new vessels will be damaged, just like the old ones, if you continue to eat rich foods and live an unhealthy lifestyle. Surgery and medication may buy you some time, but they will not save you from this illness because they do not address the underlying cause of the disease. There's only one way to deal with this disease effectively, and I'm going to show you how to do it.

This book is a guide to getting well. It's a user's manual for those who have heart disease; for those who want to prevent a heart attack, stroke, or some form of peripheral vascular disease; and for those who want to help someone recover from cardiovascular disease.

If right now you are lying in your sick bed recovering from a heart attack or stroke, I want you to know that this program can work for you. It can help you recover your strength and allow you to go back to enjoying your life. Indeed, it can even give you greater health and vitality than you had before you were struck down. I will tell you what I tell all my patients: Those of you who are most ill have the greatest potential to be the stars of this program.

Let me tell you about one of my biggest stars, my father. For more than thirty years, he was a design engineer for the Ford Motor Company. In March 1980, Ford sent him to Brazil as a consultant to supervise body design for South American automobile manufacturers. My father was 58 years old at the time, and as he likes to say, "I felt indestructible. I could eat anything. Nothing could hurt me, I thought." My father enjoyed life. He and my mother traveled. He was a pilot, owned two airplanes, and did a lot of flying. But flying wasn't nearly as risky as the way he ate during most of his adult life, especially while he was in Brazil. There he indulged in a lot of high-fat foods—lots of beef, deep-fried chicken, eggs, dairy products, and fish. "They fed me so well down there that I weighed 200 pounds when I returned home to Michigan in December 1980. And I'm only five feet nine inches tall."

I had been trying to get my father to change his diet for years without success. I even went so far as to give a lecture on diet and health to the doctors at the hospital where he would later be treated. Surely, I believed, my father, who sat in the audience, would now recognize the value of my program. But I was wrong. Actually, what he was thinking, he later confided to me, was "If this program is go good, why don't all the other doctors use it to treat heart disease?" And then he had a heart attack.

One morning in March 1981, he was hurrying to work. Michigan winters can be long, and there was still snow on the ground that March morning. He parked, hurried out of his car, and "it hit me," he would say later. "It felt like an elephant sat on my chest. I never felt a pain like that before in my life. I wanted to lie down, but I couldn't lie in the snow. Somehow, I made it into the office." He collapsed there and coworkers called an ambulance.

He was immediately taken to a local hospital and diagnosed as having had a heart attack. At first, there wasn't much the hospital could do for him except give him drugs and oxygen, and schedule him for a coronary bypass operation. His condition was stable and because of his reluctance to have immediate bypass surgery, he was sent home. What most people do not realize is that they have time after a heart attack to delay surgery and consider their options.

At that time, I was living in Hawaii. I telephoned my father's doctors and told them that he was going to wait to see the effects of diet and lifestyle on his illness.

The heart attack had changed my father's attitudes toward his diet and lifestyle. "It really turned me around quick," he recalled. "I was glad to see each day come and go. I started to think about life in a whole new way. Having something like that happen makes quite a difference in your thinking, let me tell you."

Fortunately for all of us, my sister, Linda—a registered nurse—lived in Michigan and was already eating a healthy diet. She was a good cook and could prepare the foods so that my parents could enjoy them. I gave her instructions on exactly what my father should eat and she cooked for both my parents. I also described an exercise program that he could begin as soon as he was able to get out of bed. This time, my father followed the program to the letter.

"The change was so dramatic, I could hardly believe it," he said. "After one week, I said, 'It's working!' I felt it. In three weeks' time, I could briskly walk a mile. And three weeks after that, I could briskly walk three miles. I felt like a new person."

My father adapted well to the program. Before his heart attack, he resisted the changes I suggested because he was afraid he'd miss his old ways of eating. Also, he believed that he could eat those foods with impunity. But shortly after adopting the program, he found that he really enjoyed the foods I recommended. And the benefits more than outweighed those early sacrifices.

Without this program, my father probably would have been dead years ago. But my father didn't realize that his battle with heart disease wasn't over. We both had much more to learn about his illness, as I will reveal in later chapters of this book.

Obviously, my father isn't alone in his reluctance to change, and suffer the consequences. Illnesses of the heart and arteries, collectively known as cardiovascular disease, kill approximately 1 million people each year. That's nearly as many deaths as from all other causes combined, including cancer and accidents.

The Killer We Take for Granted

Currently, 69 million Americans suffer from diseases of the heart and blood vessels, known as cardiovascular disease, more than a quarter of the population, according to the American Heart Association. One and a half million Americans will have heart attacks this year, and 500,000 of them will die. There are more than 6 million people alive today who have suffered a heart attack, or have angina pectoris (chest pain), or both. And these are not just old men, as many people commonly believe. Approximately 675,000 of those who have heart attacks each year are under the age of 65. My father was only 59 when his heart attack struck. Walk through a coronary care unit in any hospital today and you'll find young adults. In fact, more and more teenagers are suffering heart attacks, high blood pressure, and strokes. Neither are women immune from heart disease. It is true that men suffer more heart attacks than women *prior to the time women experience menopause*. Once they emerge from menopause, however, women experience just as many heart attacks as men do. In 1995 cardiovascular disease caused more than 500,000 deaths among women, according to the American Heart Association.

When we examine the landscape of this disease and then look below the surface, we find that the vast majority of adult Americans are either sick with cardiovascular disease, or at risk of getting it soon. Some 63 million Americans have high blood pressure, which means that one out of every three Americans has hypertension, a major risk factor for heart attack, stroke, kidney disease, and other serious illnesses. More than 102 million Americans have unsafe blood cholesterol levels, which are the underlying cause of heart disease. What do you think could happen to those 102 million if they don't change their diets?

Each year diseases of the heart and blood vessels kill approximately 1 million people in the United States. When you compare this death and disability toll of heart disease to that of any other illness we face today, you realize that there is no comparison. Each year, cancer kills nearly 500,000 Americans, which is approximately half the number killed by cardiovascular disease. AIDS kills about 30,000 Americans, which is about 3 percent of cardiovascular disease deaths. Compare the actual numbers (1 million versus 30,000) and the relative degrees of public outcry about cardiovascular disease versus AIDS, and you realize that we've come to accept cardiovascular disease as a natural consequence of living. That's not only a false belief, but a dangerous one. In fact, most cases of cardiovascular disease are unnecessary. Moreover, most of the people who currently suffer with the illness can overcome it—usually without surgery.

Heart disease is a relatively recent epidemic. Through the nineteenth century, and the early part of the twentieth, most people avoided heart disease. In 1900 pneumonia and influenza were the leading killers. Heart disease was way back in the number four position. Pneumonia and influenza killed 202 people per 100,000 population; heart disease killed only 137 people per 100,000. But by 1930 heart disease had become number one, and it stayed there. By the late 1970s, it was killing 337 people per 100,000, and by the early eighties that number was even higher.

There are people in the world who don't even think about heart disease because the cholesterol levels in their blood are so low that heart disease doesn't touch them. The reason they avoid heart disease is because they do not eat the quantities of red meat, poultry, eggs, cheese, milk, and other high-fat foods, but instead live on a diet of starches, vegetables, and fruits.

To give you a little more perspective on how different things are in other parts of the world, I worked for a Chinese-trained medical oncologist in 1977 as part of my residency. He told me that when he was a medical student in Hong Kong, heart attacks were so rare that whenever one occurred doctors all over the city rushed to the autopsy lab to see this medical curiosity.

Things haven't changed that much in China. People there eat a diet composed mostly of grains, vegetables, beans, and fruits. They eat twice the starchy vegetables and only one-third as much animal fat and protein as Americans do. Consequently, they have extremely low rates of heart disease, high blood pressure, cancer, and osteoporosis. The average blood cholesterol level among Chinese living on their traditional diet is 127 milligrams of cholesterol per deciliter of blood. The average American's is about 100 points higher than that. Blood cholesterol rises as you eat more fat- and cholesterol-rich foods.

T. Colin Campbell, Ph.D., of Cornell University, the man who supervised a study of 6,500 Chinese, their diets, and disease patterns, said that the clearest indicator of health among the Chinese is their cholesterol levels.

"We've seen that plasma cholesterol is a good predictor of the kinds of diseases people are going to get," Dr. Campbell told the *New York Times* in May of 1990. "Those with higher cholesterol levels are prone to diseases of affluence—cancer, heart disease, and diabetes."

Based on this and other research, Dr. Campbell made this assessment: "We're basically a vegetarian species and should be eating a wide variety of plant foods."

This is borne out by research the world over.

The Japanese are the longest-living people on earth. Although their diets are becoming more like our own in the West, they are still eating diets comparatively lower in fat and cholesterol. The office worker in Osaka, for example, gets only 23 percent of his total calories from fat, while people living in rural Kochi, Japan, get only 11 percent of their calories from fat. Not only do the Japanese live longer, but their rates of heart disease are much lower than ours. Compare them to Americans who get more than 40 percent of their total calories from fat and you see why we have far more heart disease than Asians.

You may be thinking that Asians are genetically protected against heart disease, cancer, and other illnesses that we suffer from, but that isn't so. When Asians come to the United States and adopt a more Western-style diet, they have the same rates of heart disease and cancer that we have.

I saw this same phenomenon demonstrated in my own medical practice. In the early 1970s, I provided medical care to Chinese, Japanese, and Filipinos who worked on plantations in Hawaii. I had the opportunity to care for as many as five generations of people within the same family. What I saw was that the older generation who had continued to follow their traditional eating patterns had none of the heart disease, high blood pressure, cancer, arthritis, and intestinal disorders that their children had. At first, this baffled me, until I began to ask family members what they were eating. These first-generation Asian-Americans, who migrated from their native lands to Hawaii, never developed the habit of eating meat or dairy products. Their diets were made up primarily of rice and vegetables. Their children and grandchildren, who were raised in Hawaii, ate the standard American fare—hamburgers, cheese, milk, eggs, chicken, and oils. It didn't take me long to put two and two together: The younger generations were being poisoned by fat and cholesterol.

Thanks to fast food and our emphasis upon convenience items, our children are consuming these rich foods in quantities never before realized. And, not surprisingly, they are sicker than ever. In fact, most American youths are having their arteries clogged by atherosclerotic plaque to some degree, according to many studies published in the scientific literature. By the time our children reach the teenage years, they already suffer from the early stages of heart disease.

Researchers performed 1,532 autopsies on teenagers and young adults who died of accidents in big cities across the country. They discovered that by the age of 19, 100 percent of these young adults had significant cholesterol blockage of the aorta, the body's main oxygen-carrying artery.

"Aortic fatty streaks are universal by age 15 and increase rapidly in extent during the following decade," the researchers reported. In fact, this study demonstrates that our children today are actually sicker than they were more than forty years ago, when autopsies were done on the young men killed in the Korean War.

In fact, cholesterol plaque has been detected in children as young as eight months. Babies fed high-fat infant formula and cow's milk are already on their way to heart disease.

I am living proof of this. I grew up eating eggs, white bread that was layered with butter, roast beef, ring bologna sandwiches, steaks, ham, pizza, fried chicken, and chocolate ice cream. And to top it off, I drank what I thought was the healthiest food Mother Nature created: milk. I drank milk by the gallons. I had to have four to six glasses of milk each day because I wanted to grow up to be big and strong.

One day, when I was 18 and a freshman at Michigan State University, I woke up feeling anxious, confused, and exhausted. My anxiety and confusion increased throughout the morning. I had been told by an up-perclassman that if I attended all my classes, I would pass. So I was committed to going to class, no matter what. This time it wasn't easy, but I managed to get to my English class in a daze. Once there, I put my head down on the desk and slept through the class. Afterward, I stag-gered back to my dormitory room. On the way to the dorm, I was hit twice by slow-moving cars. Neither I nor the cars were injured. Upon re-turning to my dormitory, I tried to sleep. When I woke up, I found that I had lost the use of the left side of my body. Friends took me to Michigan State University's campus health center, where I was put in isolation. From there, I was taken to Grace Hospital in Detroit, Michigan, where I underwent a spinal tap (an experience I would wish on no one), skull X rays, and, finally, an angiogram of the blood vessels that supplied the essential nutrients to my brain. The angiogram determined that I had had a stroke, a phenomenon commonly seen only in the elderly.

When my doctors entered the room, I asked them, "What's wrong with me? What are you going to do for me? When am I going home?" They just shook their heads at me in bewilderment. Eventually, my doc-tors discovered that a small artery located deep inside my brain had been closed by a blood clot. Part of a cholesterol plaque had ruptured, causing blood platelets and clotting proteins to form a clot, also called a throm-bus, within the artery. That clot became large enough to cut off blood supply and oxygen to a section of the brain that controlled the muscle function of the entire left side of my body. Parts of my brain suffocated and died, an event known as a stroke.

I was fully paralyzed on the left side of my body, from my forehead to my toes. However, within two weeks I could move my left thumb a quarter of an inch and hop on my right leg. I literally dragged myself from place to place. "Heck, that's good enough to make it to class," I said to myself. Making it to class and passing on the basis of good atten-dance was still my central motivational force. So I checked myself out of the hospital and never went back.

It took years before I managed to regain the limited physical coordi-nation that I have today. Naturally, these events changed my life forever.

I had been studying hotel, restaurant, and institutional management at school, but I lacked any real direction in my life. My experience in the hospital convinced me that I could be a doctor. (I could nod in bewilderment as well as the next guy.) The stroke had also been a confrontation with mortality, and that straightens out even the most hardened or insensitive of people. Now I wanted to make something of my life, and from that point on I was an "A" student with a passion for learning and succeeding. As my father would say many years after he suffered his heart attack, I saw life in a whole new light, and I wanted to make the most of it.

This experience did not change my eating habits, however. No one told me that diet and health were connected until years later when my older sister, Kay—the original McDougall vegetarian—insisted that my high-fat and cholesterol-laden diet was going to land me back in the hospital, if not the morgue. At that time, my cholesterol level was 335 mg/dl. I was 22 years old. It wasn't until I became a doctor and started practicing medicine in Hawaii that I began to put two and two together. The differing health patterns among my older and younger Asian patients gave me the initial insight into the relationship between diet and health. As I said earlier, I watched the older generation of Asian patients gently grow older, without suffering from the terribly debilitating diseases that their children endured. It was obvious that the older Asians were eating little meat and no dairy products. I went to the medical library to see if the scientific literature supported such a connection. Indeed it did. There was an abundance of research pointing to the fact that those people who eat a low-fat, low-cholesterol diet enjoy relative freedom from heart disease, high blood pressure, cancer, diabetes, arthritis, and other so-called degenerative illnesses.

All of this information came to me over about a four-year period. I'd examine my older patients and ask about their lifestyles and diets. Shortly thereafter I'd go to the library to research the conclusions I had drawn from my interviews with patients. Pretty soon, however, I was asking my wife, Mary, to change the way we were eating at home.

Today, when Mary and I give seminars around the country, Mary likes to recall how we changed our diets. "John would come home and say, 'Gee, I think red meat is unhealthy. We've got to give it up.' So I'd learn to cook more chicken and fish dishes. Then he confronted me with the fact that chicken and fish had as much cholesterol as beef and pork. Not too long afterward, he came home and said dairy products are essentially 'liquid meat.' Cheese has the same amount of fat and cholesterol as beef. Finally, he said, the vegetable oil has to go because it promotes cancer, gall bladder disease, and obesity. At that point, he stressed me out so much that I felt like telling him that he had to go. Pretty soon, he had eliminated everything that we were used to eating. So I started to collect vegetarian cookbooks and found that they were still full of dairy, eggs, and oil. Eventually, I had to write my own recipes, based on the ways I learned to cook grains, beans, and vegetables so that they tasted good and were satisfying to our family. And that's how we got started doing what we're doing today."

While Mary was experimenting in the kitchen. I was trying to introduce better eating habits to my patients.

This change in our lives came at a critical time in my medical practice. I had become disenchanted with the results I had been seeing in my patients who were taking the drugs I had been prescribing. The symptoms would disappear for a while and then return. Some of my patients seemed to get sicker on the medication. I started to believe that I was just a bad doctor. Maybe I wasn't cut out to do this in life, because I was not seeing people get well, which is why I went to medical school in the first place. In fact, this is a very depressing experience for many physicians, especially because most doctors are very conscientious. Despite what you may have read or believe about doctors, most of them really do care about their patients and are personally involved in their patients' well-being.

But as I began to see the relationship between diet and health, and recognized that this relationship was supported by the medical literature, I underwent a personal and professional transformation that led me to use diet and lifestyle as my principal methods of therapy. Since then, I have seen literally thousands of my patients undergo remarkable recoveries from virtually every kind of chronic illness. And I trace all of this back to a tragedy in my life, and the education I received from my plantation patients.

I wish that I had not suffered the stroke and had to endure this limp the rest of my life. But I realize, too, that a lot of good can come of bad things. In all likelihood, I would not have become a doctor. Nor would I have changed my diet and lifestyle, and I might well have suffered a premature stroke or heart attack that could have been fatal in my early thirties. Looking back, I have never regretted changing my eating habits, nor the way I practice medicine.

The Way Out of Your Dilemma

You can make changes, too. You must realize that there are two primary causes of heart disease. The first and most common is a rich diet, high in fat and cholesterol. The second is heredity, or your genes. You can control only one of those factors, your diet. In addition, you can add exercise to strengthen your cardiovascular health. By doing this, you can avoid your first health tragedy, or you can save yourself from suffering another heart attack or stroke.

My program consists of a diet composed of starch-based meals. I will describe the diet completely in Chapter 5 and again in Part IV. I'll also give you more than 100 recipes for heart-healthy meals. In general, the diet is composed of the following:

- Whole grains and whole grain flour products, such as pasta, whole grain breads, bagels, and tortillas
- A wide assortment of root vegetables, such as potatoes, sweet potatoes, yams, turnips, and rutabagas
- Legumes, such as beans, peas, and lentils
- Green and yellow vegetables
- Limited amounts of fruit
- Low-fat dressings and sauces

The diet avoids all foods high in cholesterol, fat, and vegetable oil, including:

- All meat, poultry, and fish
- All eggs and products containing eggs
- All dairy products, including milk, cheese, butter, and products containing milk products
- All vegetable oils, such as olive oil, corn oil, and safflower oil
- All margarine and shortenings
- Refined and simple sugars

I'll discuss each of these foods and show you how to use the McDougall Program for a Healthy Heart to create a wide variety of tastes, textures, and gastronomic satisfaction. I'll also show you why it's essential to avoid animal foods and oils. These foods create heart disease. Even in small amounts, they will slow or even prevent your recovery.

In the chapters that follow, I will show you how heart disease and other cardiovascular illnesses are caused and cured. I will lead you through every step of the McDougall Program for a Healthy Heart, a program that can save your life. Part II explores diet, exercise, and lifestyle. I provide a full exercise program for those who have heart disease in Chapter 6. And in Chapter 7, we'll talk about how you can effectively deal with stress and achieve a more health-promoting lifestyle. In Part III, I will show you how your doctor diagnoses heart disease. I will describe the medical tests used to diagnose the severity of the illness; what the possible results of each test mean, and how you can make decisions based on those results. I'll tell you which tests are necessary and meaningful, and which ones are dangerous and should be avoided. I will provide you with a full discussion of all the standard medications used in the treatment of heart disease and other cardiovascular illnesses, including their side effects. I'll show you how to use natural herbs and supplements to bring down cholesterol and lower blood pressure. These natural remedies can be alternatives to standard medications. I'll also help you establish a program with your physician to wean yourself from your medication. This will be necessary because as you progress on the McDougall Program for a Healthy Heart, you'll likely need to lower your medication doses, and may eventually need to stop them altogether.

In Chapter 13, I'll provide you with all the pros and cons of bypass surgery; I'll show you how you can avoid a bypass, and, in the event that it is essential, how you can select a surgeon and a hospital that will mitigate its risks and side effects.

In Chapter 15, I'll try to answer the questions facing women who must decide whether or not to take hormone replacement therapy, especially as a way to prevent heart disease and osteoporosis.

Part IV contains shopping help, cooking tips, and more than 100 mouth-watering recipes for heart-healthy meals.

The McDougall Program for a Healthy Heart is a program to keep you from being a victim of heart and artery diseases. You have a great deal more control over your health and future than perhaps you currently know or believe. I want to give you the keys to youthful vitality and robust health. I want to help you gain control of your life.

2. The Inner You

- *The heart is "the little engine that could."*
- *Blood is the ocean of life within you.*
- *Hearts get broken by the tiniest things.*
- *The poisonous effects of fat and cholesterol on your heart.*

Let Me Introduce You to Your Heart

You can gaze through telescopes or peer way down into the microscopic world; you can travel in the heavens or around the earth. But in all your explorations you will not find a single wonder more miraculous than your own heart. This amazing organ is the archetypal "little engine that could." It is courageous and mighty and, as you will see, long-suffering beyond your imagination. Our intuitive appreciation for the attributes of the heart is revealed in our language. Indeed, the heart stands as a metaphor for all that is good within us. A brave person is said to be "lionhearted" or "stout-hearted"; his action "shows a lot of heart." The heart is said to be the truest part of our being—"he spoke from his heart," we like to say when a person expresses his deepest feelings, or those things "closest to his heart." And in the end, the heart is a symbol of our greatest love: "I give you my heart," one lover says to another.

All of these expressions reveal our deep appreciation for this miraculous organ, but ironically our appreciation is small in comparison to the heart's heroic struggle, especially in the face of all that we Westerners put it through. I'd like you to get to know your heart a little better so that you can make wiser choices in your diet and lifestyle from this moment on. So let's begin this chapter by describing some of the basics about this wondrous organ.

Dwarfing the Labors of Hercules

In adults, the heart is no bigger than a man's fist. In most people, it beats between 60 and 80 times per minute. That adds up to about 100,000 beats per day, or 2.5 billion beats in your lifetime, assuming you live to be 65 or 70. While you're resting, the heart pumps about one-sixth of a pint of blood per beat. But if you take a brisk walk around the block, or even run a little bit, your heart automatically triples its efficiency, thus pumping three times the volume per beat in order to meet the body's increased demands for oxygen. Again, if we add up those numbers, we find that your heart pumps about 2,000 gallons of blood per day, or about 50 million gallons in a lifetime. For most of us, that's inconceivable. But it gives you a vague idea of how hard your heart works. And it does it without much attention (or gratitude) from you or me.

There are many misconceptions about the heart. Some of them are harmless; others can be fatal. Part of the reason we abuse our heart is we don't think much about it. Despite its elevated status in science, art, and mythology, the heart is pretty abstract for most of us. We know some vague facts, such as its location in the center of our chest, and the fact that the heart pumps blood, but how many of us know what the heart needs to survive and even thrive? Even fewer of us live in ways that support the health of the heart. That's why 1 million of us die each year from heart disease. We neglect our hearts until it is too late. You do not need a heart attack in order to start appreciating your heart, however. Just place your ear against someone's chest and listen to the sound of life itself.

Four Rooms Shaped in a Valentine

Though less exaggerated than it's often portrayed, the heart is shaped pretty much as those Valentine cards describe it, like an inverted cone. Inside the heart are four chambers, which are arranged like four adjoining rooms. The upper rooms—located in the wider part of the cone—are called the *atria* (each one is an *atrium*); the lower rooms are called the *ventricles*. The heart is divided into left and right sides, which are separated by a thick, muscular wall called the *septum*. Each side of the heart has an atrium and a ventricle. And all four chambers beat simultaneously.

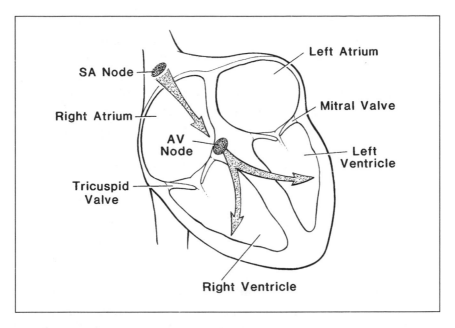

The heart is made of four chambers—two on each side. The right side of the heart pumps blood to the lungs and the left side pumps blood to the rest of the body. The pumping action is coordinated by electricity that flows from the top chambers to the lower chambers. Thus, the top chambers contract first, pushing blood into the lower chambers, then the lower chambers contract, pushing blood out of the heart.

The Primordial Dancer

How the heart manages to beat at all is a miracle that researchers still do not fully understand. As far as scientists can tell, there are four primary factors that combine to create the heart's pumping action.

1. The heart is composed of muscle called the *myocardium*, which contracts rhythmically and automatically without any outside assistance—as long as it is provided with enough oxygen and nutrition. If you place the heart of a frog or a turtle in a saline solution, it will continue to beat, even though it is no longer joined to the body. Indeed, even the cells of the myocardium expand and contract on their own, as if they were dancing to their own primordial beat.

2. Electrical stimulation arises from two electrical nodes that exist within the heart. The first, called the *sinoatrial node* (SA), is found above the right atrium; the second, called the *atrioventrical node* (AV), is located in the septum. These nodes fire electrical current along fibers that are embedded in the heart muscle. The nodes set off these bursts of electricity at precise moments, so that the heart's expansion and contraction is rhythmic and coordinated. An electrocardiogram (EKG) measures these electrical currents and can determine a great deal about the health of your heart based on the electrical bursts alone.

3. Your nervous system speeds up or slows down heart rate, depending on whether or not your nervous system is aroused or relaxed.

4. Various hormones, such as epinephrine (adrenaline), norepinephrine, and thyroxin, also affect heart rate. These hormones are secreted when we are afraid, or under stress, or when the flight or fight syndrome is aroused.

Most people think that a heartbeat has two phases—expansion and contraction. In fact, it has three. During the first phase, the heart relaxes and fills with blood. This is called *diastole*. In the second phase, called *atrial systole*, the two atria contract simultaneously, thus pumping blood into the ventricles. The third phase, called *ventricular systole*, occurs when the two ventricles pump blood out of the heart to their respective destinations—the right ventricle to the lungs, the left to the aorta and the general circulation.

Not One Pump, But Two

Most people think of the heart as a pump, but in fact it is two pumps within the same organ, both working in perfect harmony. Each side of the heart receives blood from different parts of the body and then pumps it in different directions. Blood that already has made its rounds throughout the body and is now filled with carbon dioxide enters the right side of the heart, through the right atrium. From there, it is pumped into the right ventricle—and then pumped again into the lungs via the pulmonary artery. Once inside the lungs, the blood gives up its carbon dioxide load and receives a fresh supply of oxygen. Meanwhile, the heart is pumping more blood into the lungs, which moves the existing blood out and back to the heart. Four pulmonary veins bring the blood from the lungs to the left atrium of the heart. From there, the oxygenated blood is pumped into the left ventricle and then pumped again into the general circulation via the aorta, or the main highway of the body.

The old axiom that life isn't fair has fallen on the heart, too. As you can see, the right and left sides of the heart have very different jobs, and one of them is a lot tougher than the other. Both, however, are essential to life. The right side has the easier job because it pumps blood to the lungs, which in a healthy person offer little resistance against the heart's pumping action.

The left side has to pump blood to the general circulation—the seemingly endless pathways of arteries, veins, and capillaries. This job is considerably more difficult because muscle tension, contraction of vessels, and atherosclerosis (which narrows the vessel's opening) all create resistance against the pumping action of the heart. The more these problems accumulate, the harder the heart must work. The result is that all this extra work requires the left side of the heart to be a larger and more powerful muscle.

Despite this disparity in size and strength, the two sides must work together in precise coordination. Each side expands to fill with blood and then contracts simultaneously to pump blood along its rounds.

Arteries: Tunnels of Life

One of the reasons people are so confused about how to take care of their health is because the information dispensed by the so-called experts is often based on the latest up-to-the-minute study, which sometimes seems to contradict yesterday's study. What we often forget is that health is dependent upon rather inflexible needs that are as old as human life on the planet. By meeting these needs, we are kept alive and in good health. Fail to meet them and you become sick. It's that simple. The first need of the body is oxygen and nutrition to survive and function. Deprive cells of oxygen for several minutes and they suffocate and die. Two of the food components that create the conditions in which cells suffocate are fat and cholesterol. They do it by changing the health of your arteries, which are literally tunnels of life.

Arteries carry oxygen-enriched blood from the heart to cells throughout the body. Veins, on the other hand, carry blood containing carbon dioxide and other waste products from the cells back to the heart and lungs, where the blood will be reinfused with oxygen.

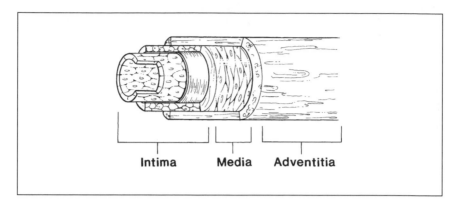

Intima   Media   Adventitia

The artery wall is made of three layers. The inner layer, called the intima, consists of a cobblestone arrangement of cells, providing a smooth surface for the blood cells to flow against. The middle layer, the media, is made of muscle. This muscle relaxes and contracts, changing the flow of blood to the tissues. The outer layer, the adventitia, provides a strong covering for the artery.

Your arteries are tough elastic tubes composed of three layers. The innermost layer, called the *intima*, is covered by a thin layer of cells that are as smooth as lacquered tile. The blood flows easily over this tiled surface. Below the intima is the next layer of cells, called the *media*, composed of muscle cells and elastic fibers of protein, called *collagen*. The outermost layer of the artery is the *adventitia*, which is also composed of thick elastic collagen fibers. The construction of the artery gives it the capacity to expand with increased blood pressure and contract as blood pressure lowers.

Two Coronary Arteries—and Their Many Tributaries— Sustain the Heart's Life

Like any muscle, the heart needs blood and oxygen to survive. You might think that the heart gets its blood and oxygen supply from the blood it pumps, but that would be incorrect. The heart's situation is analogous to that of the person who works at a grocery store: Though he is working around food all day, he doesn't spend his day eating off the racks. Similarly, the heart gets little oxygen from the blood it pumps. Instead, it relies on two arteries that flow to the heart muscle from the

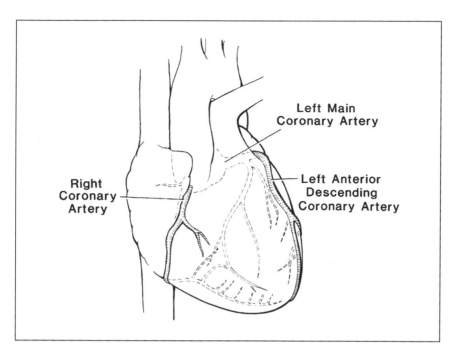

The blood pumped through the heart itself is not used by the heart muscle. Blood for the heart muscle is supplied by arteries that course its surface. There are two main artery branches called the left and right coronary arteries. The beginning of the left coronary artery is so large it is called the left main coronary artery. These arteries are prone to artherosclerosis, and interruption of their blood supply can be fatal.

aorta—the body's main artery carrying oxygen-enriched blood—to provide the heart with blood and oxygen.

The two vessels that give oxygenated blood to the heart muscle are called the *coronary arteries*. Like the trunks of two great trees, the coronary arteries have numerous branches that spread out over the surface of the heart, bringing blood to all the heart cells. The smaller branches are called *arterioles*. Studies have shown that people who exercise regularly have more arterioles than those who are sedentary. Even if you are currently sedentary, however, you can grow more arterioles by increasing your exercise. Exercise increases the demands for oxygen throughout the body, including from the heart muscle itself. The body responds to these demands by growing additional vessels so that more blood and oxygen can be transported to tissues. (The McDougall exercise program outlined in Chapter 6 will help you do that.)

The condition of the blood determines the health of the arteries. Virtually everything that you put into your mouth—indeed, most of the things that you breathe into your lungs—winds up in your blood. Consequently, you have tremendous control over the health of your blood, simply by making healthful food choices and avoiding unhealthy habits (for example, smoking).

Blood: The Foundation of Life and Health

The next time you feel like being awed, take a walk on the shoreline of any ocean and look out upon the vastness of that green and blue universe and know that you are looking at a living womb. Beneath its undulating surface exists such varieties of life that even human imagination cannot conceive. Indeed, the intimation of all those extraordinary life forms that exist beneath its swells, thrills, and intimidates. It awakens us to the primal forces that are the foundation of life.

Though few of us realize it, our blood is like the ocean—a sea of life, varied, complex, and bustling with activity. Red blood cells, like so many bucket-brigaders, carry oxygen to tissues. Armies of white blood cells and other immune constituents fight diseases and infections that would otherwise kill you. Cells communicate with one another across relatively great distances within the body, always adjusting to the changing conditions within and without. A constant flow of nutrition is ferried to hardworking and hungry cells. Waste produced by those cells is whisked away via the blood and brought to the blood-cleansing organs (the liver, kidneys, lungs, and spleen) to be removed from the body. Temperature is regulated; blood volume is controlled. Cells die and others are born. The cycle of life, as rich and as varied as that in the ocean itself, goes on each day within the living sea that courses through your veins. The conditions within that sea inside of you determine not only your health, but how long you live.

What Lies in This Ocean Inside of Me?

The blood can be divided into two general categories: the plasma—the liquid portion—and the many formed elements, such as red and white blood cells, all of which are suspended in the plasma.

Most of the plasma is water (about 91 to 92 percent), with a salt content very similar to that of seawater. That salt content makes the blood slightly alkaline, with a pH of about 7.4. The red color of most of the blood cells makes the color of blood run from red to purple. When these cells are removed, the remaining liquid, known as plasma, is yellow.

There are five general categories of elements that exist within the plasma: blood cells, nutrients, proteins, hormones, and waste products. The two types of blood cells are *red* blood cells, which contain hemoglobin and carry oxygen to tissues, and *white* blood cells, which are part of the immune system that fights disease. Along with these cells flows nutrition. The blood carries nutrition in the form of glucose (which is derived from carbohydrates in food), proteins, fats, vitamins, and minerals.

Meals rich in fat immediately turn the plasma milky white because fat globules pour into the bloodstream in great quantities. If you were to eat a meal consisting of, say, steak, buttered vegetables, and a potato with sour cream (a fairly standard American meal), and then removed some of your blood, you would be able to see a milky white substance running through your blood. If you let the blood sit a little while, the plasma and the milky white globules of fat would separate from each other, just as cream rises to the top of a milk container. These fats are called *triglycerides*. (I'll talk more about triglycerides in Chapter 3.)

In addition to cells and nutrients, the blood carries proteins in the form of amino acids (the building blocks of tissues), fibrinogen (a protein involved in the blood-clotting process), albumin (a protein that binds with minerals and other substances and keeps them in the circulation), and antibodies (which fight viruses and bacteria). The blood also circulates hormones, which regulate the functions of organs and muscles throughout the body. Finally, it contains many waste products.

One of the ways you can think of your blood is as a transportation system that brings life-giving elements to cells, and takes harmful substances away. The waste products—carbon dioxide, lactic acid, urea, cellular debris, and hormones—are delivered to the blood-cleansing organs—the liver and kidneys—which in turn will assist in their elimination. The blood also transports disease-causing agents, such as viruses and bacteria, to be neutralized and eliminated by the liver, kidneys, and spleen.

The blood helps to regulate the body's temperature by moving heat to the lungs and skin. The circulation distributes heat by increasing blood flow to certain areas of the body. An adult of average height has about

10 pints of blood. When filled with oxygen, blood is bright red; when carrying carbon dioxide, it is brownish red (like clay) or purple.

Blood moves fast in the body, especially on the body's main highway, the aorta, where it scoots along about 15 inches a second. It slows down considerably in the capillaries—the tiny vessels of the body—many of which are actually smaller than red blood cells. That forces the red cells to bend and squeeze through these tiny alleyways in order to bring oxygen to cells.

Fat and Cholesterol: A Delicate Balance That Often Goes Awry

Many tissues produce cholesterol, but the liver makes most of it. Cholesterol is not a nutrient, but a waxy, steroidlike substance. The body uses cholesterol to make cell parts (most notably cell membranes); to produce hormones (everything from adrenaline to estrogen and testosterone); to synthesize vitamin D, derived from the action of sunlight on plant sterols; and to make bile acids (a substance made by the liver to help digest fats).

Cholesterol is essential for life, but your body produces all it needs. That means, of course, that all additional cholesterol obtained through your diet will have to be utilized, eliminated from the body, carried in the blood, or deposited in the tissues, where it can create artery disease.

Once inside your body, dietary cholesterol becomes blood cholesterol. Hence, the more cholesterol you eat, the more cholesterol you will have in your bloodstream. There are numerous things that we eat that can lower blood cholesterol. Among them are dietary fiber and plant-derived vitamins.

Cholesterol and fat are often referred to as lipids. Blood cholesterol is carried around on conglomerates of fat and protein called lipoproteins. These lipoproteins determine where the cholesterol goes. One type of lipoprotein, called *low-density lipoproteins* (LDL), brings the cholesterol to the artery walls. LDL is often referred to as the "bad cholesterol" because, by bringing cholesterol to the walls of arteries, it helps to create atherosclerosis. Another type of lipoprotein, called *high-density lipoproteins* (HDL), brings the cholesterol from the arteries to the liver for elimination or acts to prevent deposition of cholesterol into the arteries. Relatively higher HDL is associated with a lower risk of heart disease in many studies, and for this reason is referred to as "good cholesterol."

Once inside your blood, these tiny globules of LDL cholesterol can undergo a chemical change called *oxidation*. In essence, they break down or decay. LDL particles become rancid inside your blood the same way butter becomes rancid if allowed to sit out at room temperature. Your immune system recognizes these decaying particles as a threat to your health. Macrophages and other immune cells gobble up these decaying cholesterol particles, and in the process become engorged with oxidized LDL cholesterol. These swollen immune cells become embedded in the artery wall, where they begin the formation of an atherosclerotic plaque. At this stage, these swollen immune cells are called *foam cells*. As more and more foam cells accumulate within the artery wall, they form a *fatty streak*—the first stage of atherosclerosis.

Infants whose mothers ate a high-fat and cholesterol-rich Western diet while pregnant have been shown to have foam cells and fatty streaks at birth. It is common for such fatty streaks to appear in children as young as eight months. The fatty streak will disappear and the artery will heal—even in adults—if the cholesterol level drops sufficiently. However, if more and more cholesterol and fat are consumed, the process continues. The fatty streaks grow. Muscle cells that are part of the media section of the artery proliferate into the intima, and cause the fatty streak to become larger and thicker, thus becoming a full-blown atherosclerotic plaque. The body attempts to form a cap over the plaque with tough fibrous scar tissue, a process called *fibrosis*.

As the plaques grow larger, they cause the arteries to narrow, and thus reduce the blood supply to the heart, a condition called *ischemia*. Eventually, the ischemia can progress to cause *angina pectoris*, literally a "strangling" pain in the center of the chest due to the diminished blood flow to the heart. If the ischemia becomes so advanced that one of the coronary arteries is entirely blocked, part of the heart muscle can die and one experiences a *myocardial infarction*, or a heart attack.

Exploring the Inner Landscape with the Mind's Eye

In order to visualize the conditions inside your arteries, let's imagine for a few moments that you could shrink yourself to the size of a cell, and that

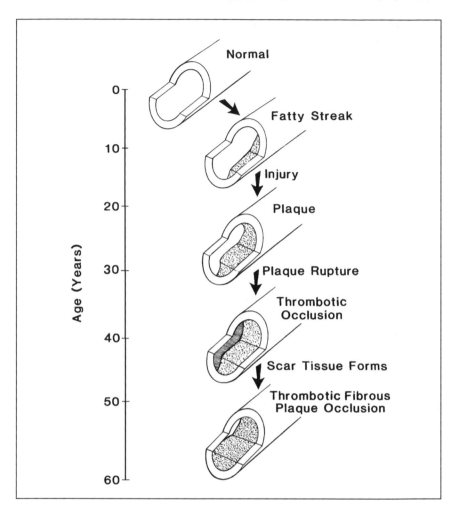

Atherosclerosis develops over a lifetime, beginning in early childhood. Damage from the foods we eat and products of cigarette smoke injure the inside linings of the artery. The resulting sores are known as plaques. The disease generally progresses because the healing processes cannot catch up with the daily injury. Unstable plaques often rupture, causing the formation of a blood clot which partially or completely occludes an artery. Eventually, scar tissue will replace the thrombus, resulting in a fibrous plaque, which may also completely occlude the artery.

you could travel safely inside the walls of an artery. You would see an awe-inspiring world of living cells, proteins, nutrients, and bubbles of cholesterol and fat—all of which float in the living ocean that is your blood. You would see artery walls that were smooth and healthy, and others that were in various stages of atherosclerosis, caused by those very same balls of fat and cholesterol that you see floating through the bloodstream.

From your imaginary vantage inside the artery, you recognize this process as both destructive and disgusting. The courageous immune cells are literally killing themselves by consuming these bubbles of LDL. Not only that, but the beautiful artery wall—once a mosaic of perfectly arranged tiles—has become contoured and bulbous, as if it were afflicted with horrible boils.

Heart Attacks: The True Story

As I mentioned earlier, there are many misconceptions about heart disease, but one of the most widespread is the notion that most heart attacks occur when a cholesterol plaque grows so large that it blocks off an artery entirely. It's true that sometimes a plaque can become large enough to block off a vessel, and thus cause a heart attack, but most heart attacks are not caused this way. Moreover, this belief is actually dangerous because it lulls people into a false sense of security. Those who think that arteries are closed by a slow-growing plaque often comfort themselves by saying, "I've got time to change my diet because my arteries must be at least partially open so that blood can get to my heart." What these people don't realize is that almost all heart attacks occur in people whose arteries are significantly open. The fact is that *small* plaques cause the most deadly heart attacks and strokes.

The atherosclerotic lesions contain cholesterol and fat that collect in pools and make the plaque highly *unstable*. These unstable plaques can—and often do—burst open, or rupture, thus forming an open wound within the artery wall. Blood platelets and clotting proteins rush to the wound and form a blood clot—called a *thrombus*—over the open plaque. That clot can enlarge instantaneously, becoming so big that it causes blood flow to the heart or brain to be completely shut off. The result is a heart attack or a stroke. Ninety-five percent of heart attacks are caused by this process, called *coronary thrombosis*. Ironically, thrombosis occurs most often in the smaller plaques, those that are not, by themselves, large enough to block the artery entirely or cause any symptoms.

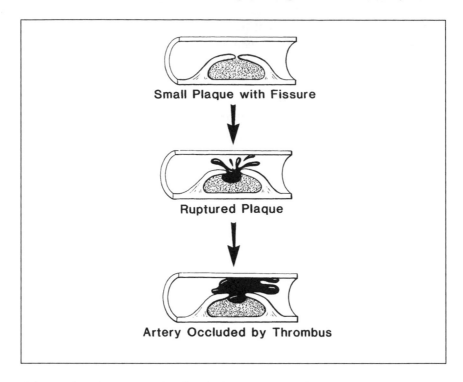

Small Plaque with Fissure

Ruptured Plaque

Artery Occluded by Thrombus

Atherosclerotic plaques are filled with semiliquid, fatty, and necrotic material. An unstable plaque can develop a tear (fissure) in the surface, allowing the contents to rupture into the flowing blood. This rupture acts as a catalyst for the blood to clot, forming a thrombus that partially or completely occludes the artery, causing a heart attack or a stroke. The highest risk of rupture is with tiny fat-filled plaques. Small, but lethal, plaques usually cause no symptoms, thus offering no warning of the impending disaster.

Thus, the key events that lead to a heart attack are:

- The presence of high total cholesterol and LDL cholesterol in the blood
- The initial injury to the lining of the artery wall
- The formation of unstable, cholesterol-filled, fat-filled plaques
- The rupture of the plaque
- The formation of a clot over the open plaque
- The clot closing off blood flow to the heart or brain, causing a heart attack or stroke

Developing Backup Circulation

Sometimes people have stable plaques that gradually grow large enough to close off an artery, but they do not damage the heart muscle because there has been adequate time for backup circulation to grow to that area of the heart muscle, thus taking over the circulation that was lost when the original vessel closed. Arteries can be 100 percent closed, yet the presence of these backup arteries—called *collateral* circulation, or simply collaterals—provides enough blood and oxygen to sustain the life of the muscle.

Whether or not a plaque forms in the first place, and creates a thrombus in the second, depends to a great extent on a person's diet. The most important factors are what you eat, the level of cholesterol in your blood, whether or not you smoke, and whether or not you have indications of heart disease such as angina pectoris (chest pain). As we will see in the next chapter, fat—especially saturated fat derived from animal foods—accelerates the creation of these clots, or thrombi.

A Disease of All Ages

As I said in Chapter 1, this is not a disease of old people. Rather, it begins very early in life, usually in infancy. That's why the National Heart Lung and Blood Institute (NHLBI) now recommends that all children two years of age and older adopt a diet low in fat and cholesterol.

Anyone who suffers a heart attack or stroke and winds up in the hospital is urged to adopt the diet of the American Heart Association (AHA), which is lower in fat and cholesterol than the typical American diet. Unfortunately, as we will see later on, the AHA's diet is still too high in fat and cholesterol to protect you against the disease. If you have already suffered a heart attack or stroke, that diet may insure that you suffer another one.

As grotesque and lethal as atherosclerosis is, it is nevertheless reversible. If followed properly, the McDougall Program for a Healthy Heart can cure heart and artery disease at its source.

Just Ask My Father-in-Law

Cardiovascular disease has hit my life like mortar shells. My father and I have suffered from it, and so has my father-in-law, Marinus "Pat"

Luyk, who today is 84 years old. In 1984 Pat had a cholesterol level of 320 mg/dl and was suffering from intermittent chest pain. The pain became severe in the summer of 1984, after Pat spent an afternoon cutting the grass. He went to his doctor and was told that he had angina pectoris.

He was given a prescription and sent home. A month later, the pain struck again, but this time it was so bad that he had to check himself into the hospital. There doctors X-rayed his chest, performed an EKG and other tests, and informed him that he had had a heart attack. His doctor suggested that Pat have a bypass operation. "Well," said Pat, "let me make a phone call." With that, he telephoned me in Hawaii and told me his condition. "No way," I told him. He put his doctor on the phone and I was told that he did not have the kind of coronary artery disease that would be helped by surgery, so I suggested that we give diet and lifestyle a chance. Then Pat got back on the phone with me. "We'll change your diet and you'll be as good as new, Dad," I told him. (I do not give the same advice to everyone. See Chapter 13 for guidelines on when to avoid a bypass operation, and when to have one.)

Pat recalled his eating habits just before having the heart attack. "At the time, I was eating lots of hamburgers, steak, ham, and cheese. I didn't go in much for milk, but I ate lots of ice cream."

I gave my father-in-law very detailed instructions on what to eat and how to exercise. My mother-in-law also went on the diet and together they followed the program to the letter. As he recalls, changing his diet required some adaptation. "It was hard at first," said Pat recently. "But in the condition that I was in, I just had to accept it. But after a couple of weeks on John's diet, I started to feel better, and in two months I felt wonderful."

He continues to follow the diet at least 95 percent of the time—"Rarely I cheat on something, but not much," he says. And he still follows the simple exercises I recommended years ago. "I walk two miles and I do it in about 30 minutes," he says. "That's brisk enough to get my heart rate up a little bit."

After following the program for two months, my father-in-law was ready to take on the world again, so he decided to go back to work.

Pat's a wonderful carpenter. After he retired from his business a few years ago, he wanted to stay active so he worked a couple of days each week in a floral shop.

"I feel great and I like to keep busy," said Pat.

Today his cholesterol level runs between 138 and 178 mg/dl. His blood pressure is 120/60 mm Hg. He also takes cholesterol-lowering medication (colestipol and lovastatin). "Basically, I eat grains and vegetables every day," he said. "I don't feel deprived. I enjoy my diet."

Pat has come back from the brink, and at 84 years of age he shows no signs of slowing up.

Before you can legally drive a car, you must be trained in safe operation and how to follow the rules of the road. That's only natural, though. After all, cars are dangerous. Approximately 50,000 Americans are killed each year on U.S. highways.

Unfortunately, no one applies the same sound judgment to the necessity of learning to safely care for and operate your body. No one says to you when you're, say, 17 that it's time you learned something about how your body works and how to care for it with proper diet and exercise. Your whole future depends on such knowledge. In the absence of appropriate training, most of us end up killing ourselves. The great majority of us die from an underlying disease called ignorance: We simply don't know how to take care of our hearts.

This book is your owner's manual to a healthy heart. I want you to understand how your heart becomes sick and what you need to do to make yourself well.

3. Following the Fat and Cholesterol Trail

- *Vegetable fat is a serious health hazard.*
- *There are good, bad, and ugly fats.*
- *Chicken and fish are also high in cholesterol.*

Dangerous Misconceptions

There's an old Hungarian tradition of cutting off pieces of fat from recently slaughtered animals and then melting the fat over a fire until it becomes a liquid. The liquid fat is then dripped onto bread and eaten. I'm told by Hungarian friends that this is quite delicious and very popular in Hungary, though to many non-Hungarians—myself included—this food seems rather unpleasant. However, before we non-Hungarians become too inflated by our lofty sensibilities, let me remind my readers that to a Japanese or Chinese person, our practice of spreading milk fat—otherwise known as butter—on bread is equally revolting.

My point is that habits that we take for granted often make us blind to our own behaviors that are not only unhealthful, but downright unattractive. Our consumption of fat is a good example. Whenever I'm out lecturing, I pass around a 5-pound slab of fat to the people in my audience and let them see what fat looks like. When people actually look at and handle this mass of fat, which looks like a soft yellow club, they are revolted. When I tell them that they are eating stuff just like this each day, they become nauseated. I'm fond of challenging people who say they like olive oil to drink a bottle of it—*plain!* I haven't found one person yet who would take me up on that challenge.

You see, this is the problem I face whenever I talk about diet and nutrition. As soon as I mention fat and cholesterol, carbohydrates and protein, I have to remind people that these are not intellectual concepts, but real substances that we eat each day. Fat is the stuff that's taken from animals, either from their tissues or milked from their breast. Fat is that yellow club and the bottle of olive oil that I pass around during my lectures. And fat—as part of beef, chicken, eggs, butter, milk, and salad dressings—is the component of the rich American diet that is killing most people in the Western world today.

The Foods We Eat

Though fat is eaten by itself, it usually appears in foods containing other nutrients. Foods can be broken down into five major nutritional categories: *carbohydrates,* which are used for energy; *proteins,* for cell replacement and repair; *fats,* used primarily as a reserve fuel; and *vitamins* and *minerals*, both essential for metabolism and the healthy function of cells. Another important part of one's diet is *fiber*, which is an indigestible carbohydrate that greatly enhances your ability to digest and eliminate waste from your body. It also influences your blood cholesterol level, because fiber binds with cholesterol and holds onto it while it is eliminated from the intestinal tract. Fiber, therefore, is a very important part of any health-promoting program.

There's nothing wrong with fat per se. In fact, your body needs some fat to metabolize vitamins A, D, E and K, and maintain other cell functions. The problem with fat is that we eat too much of it. In fact, it's impossible to avoid fat entirely because it's present in all natural foods. Not only do animal foods contain fat, but so do whole grains, vegetables, beans, and fruit. The difference is that most animal foods contain a lot more fat than most vegetable foods do.

Since all foods contain fat, you cannot create a diet composed of whole foods that's inadequate in fat. It can't be done. Even a regimen made up entirely of potatoes—which are only 1 percent fat—will give you all the essential fats your body needs because the requirements are so small.

Fats are packaged with energy. In fact, they're the most calorically dense food in the food chain. A gram of fat contains nine calories, while a gram of carbohydrate or protein contains about four. Despite the fact that fat contains so much energy, your body will not accept fat as its primary fuel. Your body's preferred fuel is carbohydrates, found in grains, vegetables, and fruit. As long as you eat sufficient carbohydrates to meet your energy needs, your body will store most of the fat you eat in your tissues (which makes you put on weight). Animal fats will also cause your liver to produce more cholesterol, which winds up in your blood. Excess body weight and cholesterol can cause serious health problems.

What Are Fats?

Fats are compounds composed of carbon, hydrogen, and small amounts of oxygen. Chemically, these compounds are known as fatty acids. They are usually attached to a molecule called glycerol. With three fatty acids and a glycerol, you have *triglycerides*—the word we commonly use to describe fats in the blood.

Fats are divided into three main groups: *saturated,* found in animal foods and a few vegetables; *polyunsaturated,* found in vegetables, vegetable oils, and cold-water fish; and *monounsaturated*, found mostly in olive oil.

The differing chemical structures of these fats make them look different when we use them, and each has a slightly different effect on your body. Saturated fats are molecules that are completely stuffed, or saturated, with hydrogen atoms. This makes the fat more dense. Butter is a saturated fat, and therefore is solid at room temperature.

Polyunsaturated and monounsaturated fats are composed of the same elements—carbon, oxygen, and hydrogen—but they do not have as many hydrogen atoms packed into their molecules, and consequently they are liquid at room temperature, or oils. All oils are fats—they're just the liquid form of fat. Polyunsaturated and monosaturated fats are safe, *as long as you get them as part of the grains and vegetables you eat.* In fact, as part of grains and vegetables, these fats are essential for your health. However, once these fats are separated from their food sources and used as oils, they have many negative side effects.

Sometimes food manufacturers turn oils into saturated fats by adding more hydrogen to the fat molecule. This is how they turn corn oil into margarine. On the labels of such foods you will notice the words, "partially hydrogenated," which means hydrogen atoms have been added to the polyunsaturated oil, making it a more saturated fat.

THERE IS NO SUCH THING AS AN INNOCENT
FAT, *or Half-truths That Can Kill*

When fat hits your stomach—and I'm talking now about all types of fat—your liver secretes bile acids into the first part of your small intestine, called the *duodenum*. These bile acids are the body's detergent; they break down fats into smaller, more digestible particles. Once these particles clear the duodenum, they are absorbed by your small intestine and wind up in your bloodstream as tiny balls of fat called *chylomicrons*.

These balls of fat give your plasma a sticky, milky consistency. The fat also causes your red blood cells to stick together, or sludge, and to become rigid. Some of your capillaries are so small that red blood cells can only pass through by bending in half. When the red blood cells become rigid or clump together, they are unable to bend and twist their way into these tiny vessels. The net effect is a very dense traffic jam, created by your sludged blood.

Because of this reduction in circulation, the oxygen content of the blood drops by as much as 20 percent. Consequently, cells are suffocating. One of the many areas of your body that suffers is your brain, which is now getting diminished supplies of oxygen. You may experience this deprivation of oxygen as sleepiness. You know the feeling, I'm sure. All you can think of is taking a nap. This is just the first sign that things are going wrong inside of you. For many people, this reduction in circulation can be life-threatening.

High-Fat Foods: A Formula for Chest Pain

A meal containing rich quantities of all types of fats—saturated, polyunsaturated, and monounsaturated—is especially dangerous to those who have been diagnosed with heart disease. Studies have shown that a single high-fat meal dramatically increases the incidence of angina pectoris. This occurs as a direct result of the sludging of the blood and the consequent decline in the amount of oxygen being carried by the blood. Less oxygen in the blood means less oxygen getting to your tissues, including your heart. The result is chest pain. (As we will see in the next chapter, your health improves within hours of eating a low-fat, low-cholesterol meal.)

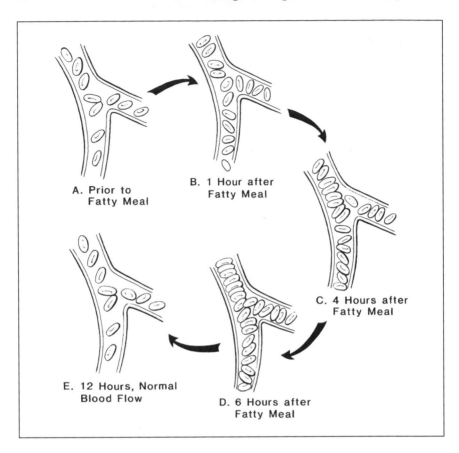

A. Prior to Fatty Meal

B. 1 Hour after Fatty Meal

C. 4 Hours after Fatty Meal

D. 6 Hours after Fatty Meal

E. 12 Hours, Normal Blood Flow

Blood cells within the blood vessels flow freely and bounce off one another prior to a high-fat meal. Approximately one hour after a fatty meal, the cells begin to stick together upon contact and form clumps. As this clump forma-tion progresses, the flow of blood slows. Six hours after the meal, the clumping becomes so severe that blood flow actually stops in many small vessels. Several hours later the clumps break up and the blood flow returns to the tissues. As a result of these changes, the oxygen content of the blood decreases by 20 percent. The consequence of this impaired circulation can be angina, impaired brain function, high blood pressure, fatigue, as well as compromise of the function of any other body part.

On the other hand, chest pain can be relieved by a low-fat diet. Within three weeks of adopting a diet low in fat, a person can experience a 90 percent reduction in the frequency of angina attacks. Since most coro-nary bypass operations that are performed for appropriate reasons are done to relieve chest pain, a low-fat, low-cholesterol diet eliminates the need for most of these surgeries.

There's a lot of loose reporting about the effects of each of these fats on your body, and the misconceptions that come out of such reports can be lethal. You should know the facts about fat before you eat any more of it.

Let's have a closer look at how each of the three types of fat affect your health.

Saturated Fat

Saturated fat is found in large amounts in animal foods—especially in red meat, dairy products, eggs, and poultry—and in a few vegetable foods, such as coconuts and cocoa (as well as its derivative, chocolate). Certain vegetable oils—palm oil, palm kernel oil, coconut oil, and margarines—contain large amounts of saturated fat, too.

Once inside the bloodstream, saturated fat is transformed by your liver into very-low-density lipoprotein, or VLDL, which is transformed next into LDL, or low-density lipoprotein, the so-called "bad cholesterol" that creates atherosclerosis and leads to heart disease.

There is no doubt among scientists that saturated fat raises blood cholesterol, particularly LDL cholesterol. Consequently, every authoritative health body—from the American Heart Association to the National Heart Lung and Blood Institute—recommends that we limit saturated fat. But the truth is, there's no reason to eat foods that contain saturated fat. It makes you sick and fat.

Polyunsaturated and Monounsaturated Fats

The picture concerning polyunsaturated and monounsaturated fats can be a bit more confusing because the information is mixed. If you stand back and look at all the evidence, you may conclude that you are better off consuming these fats only as part of your food. Unfortunately, most people—including many scientists—look at only a fraction of the picture, the part that suggests that these fats may have a health-promoting effect. Yet, even the benefits of such fats are small in comparison to their overall negative impact on health. So let me start out my discussion by saying that polyunsaturated and monounsaturated fats are not the panacea they've been made out to be.

Let's look at the facts—*The Good, The Bad,* and *The Ugly.*

The Good

There are five reasons why some scientists and doctors recommend polyunsaturated and monounsaturated fats:

1. Lower cholesterol. Polyunsaturated fats (found in vegetables, nuts, and fish) and monounsaturated fats (found in olive oil) do lower LDL cholesterol somewhat. Some scientists theorize that polyunsaturated and monounsaturated fats may improve the efficiency of certain LDL receptors in the liver to remove LDL cholesterol from the blood. In other words, poly- and monounsaturated fats may slightly improve the liver's ability to sift out LDL from your bloodstream.

2. Reduce saturated fat intake. The second reason some scientists recommend poly- and monounsaturated fats is that by eating more of these fats, people are eating less saturated fats, which means they consume the lesser of the evils. Many people, for example, have switched from, say, lard to corn oil for cooking, and in the process dropped a saturated fat (lard) for a polyunsaturated fat (corn oil). In reality, this is like choosing hanging over a firing squad.

3. Raise "good" HDL cholesterol. The third reason is that some studies have shown that these fats raise HDL cholesterol—the "good cholesterol"—which takes LDL out of the bloodstream and reduces the likelihood of a heart attack. This is another reason some scientists and doctors recommend vegetable oils.

4. Lower triglycerides. One form of polyunsaturated fat is found in fish oils, which are commonly referred to as *omega-3 polyunsaturated fats,* or simply n-3. These have been shown to lower blood triglyceride levels. Vegetable oils, on the other hand, do not have this effect on the blood. Vegetable oils tend to raise blood triglycerides.

5. Thin the blood. Finally, the fish oils contain a particularly fatty acid, called *eicosapentaenoic acid*, which prevents the blood from forming clots within the arteries. As I've said, clots are the last important step in the process that leads to a heart attack or stroke. While saturated fats make blood platelets sticky—and therefore promote clot forming—fish oils do just the opposite: they "thin" the blood and prevent it from clotting. For this reason, some doctors encourage people with heart disease to eat fish oils.

Let's deal with these claims one by one.

The Bad

People have exaggerated the cholesterol-lowering effects of poly- and monounsaturated fats, claiming that if you eat a diet that contains all three types of fats, you can protect yourself against the effects of saturated fats. But that just isn't true. If you eat saturated fats along with poly- and monounsaturated fats, there will be no lowering of cholesterol. The effects of corn oil and olive oil do not offset the effects of animal fats.

In a study published in 1992 in the *American Journal of Clinical Nutrition*, 48 young men were divided into three groups: one-third of them ate the standard American diet, with 37 percent of calories coming from fat, of which 16 percent came from saturated fat. A second group of men ate a diet composed of 30 percent fat, of which 14 percent was from saturated fat. The third group ate a diet of 30 percent total calories in fat, with only 9 percent coming from saturated fat. Only this last group achieved any significant reduction in blood cholesterol levels. The researchers concluded that ". . . reduction of dietary fat intake from 37 percent to 30 percent of calories did not lower plasma total [cholesterol] and LDL cholesterol concentrations unless the reduction in total fat was achieved by decreasing saturated fatty acids." In English, blood cholesterol levels could not be lowered in the men unless saturated fats were reduced. The cholesterol-lowering effects of polyunsaturated fats alone could not offset the effects of saturated fats.

Hence, eating more vegetable and olive oils will not protect you against the harmful effects of saturated fats from animal foods. Only by decreasing or eliminating saturated fats will your blood cholesterol decline.

But Olive Oil Also Raises HDLs, Right?

It's true that poly- and monounsaturated fats boost HDL levels somewhat, but the fact is that *all fats boost HDL levels*—even saturated fats. Moreover, having a high HDL level is not predictive of cardiovascular health by itself. This was demonstrated in a study published in *The New England Journal of Medicine* (December 12, 1991) that examined the effects of a high-fat diet on a group of native people living in Mexico.

In the Sierra Madre mountains of central Mexico is a tribe of native Americans called the Tarahumara Indians. These people eat a low-fat, low-cholesterol diet composed chiefly of corn, beans, other vegetables, and fruit. They have virtually no history of heart disease, cancer, and other diseases that commonly afflict affluent nations.

Apart from their striking good health, the Tarahumara are among the most physically fit people on earth. The tribe plays a kind of kickball game in which the men run an average of 200 miles in the course of the game. The women also play, but they run only 100 miles. As might be expected on such a low-fat diet, these people have exceedingly low blood cholesterol levels, and as I said they have little or no experience with degenerative diseases. Yet, they also have low levels of HDL. Scientists recommend that your HDL level be 45 mg/dl or higher, but the Tarahumara have an average HDL level of 32 mg/dl. Their average cholesterol level, however, is only 125 mg/dl.

HDL levels are increased by several factors, including exercise. So you would think that given the Tarahumara's incredible fitness, they would have exceedingly high HDL levels. But they don't—that is, until researchers fed them a high-fat diet, and then their HDL levels shot up.

The scientists placed a group of Tarahumara Indians on a typical American diet. After five weeks on the diet, the Tarahumara Indians experienced a 39 percent increase in LDL cholesterol and a 31 percent increase in HDL cholesterol. Overall cholesterol levels went up 31 percent. The researchers noted in the study's conclusions that when these people with "virtually no coronary risk factors" consumed a high-fat diet, "they had dramatic increases in plasma lipid [fats] and lipoprotein levels [cholesterol]," including HDL levels. These increases made the Tarahumaras more likely to suffer from heart disease—despite their increase in HDLs.

The Tarahumara are not unique in their low levels of both LDL and HDL. Worldwide, the people with the lowest HDL levels have the lowest incidence of heart disease and also the lowest blood cholesterol levels. This is because HDL is only one fraction of total cholesterol. People experience declines in both LDL and HDL on a low-fat, low-cholesterol diet that lowers total cholesterol. But those declines are associated with an improvement in cardiovascular health, not the reverse.

Polyunsaturated Versus Monounsaturated Fats: Which One Boosts HDL Levels More?

So much has been made of late about olive oil that people have begun to see it as a cholesterol-lowering miracle food. But when researchers compared the cholesterol-lowering effects of olive oil (a monounsaturated fat) with three different polyunsaturates—peanut, safflower, and corn oils—they found no significant difference in cholesterol-lowering effects. The study, published in the *Journal of the American Medical Association* (May 1990), reported that LDL cholesterol and HDL cholesterol levels did not change substantially while the study participants consumed each of these oils over a twelve-week period. As for olive oil's ability to raise HDL levels, the authors concluded: "We find no advantage with respect to plasma HDL concentrations in using predominately monounsaturated [olive oil] rather than polyunsaturated fats in subjects who consumed reduced-fat, solid-food diets." So much for the hype about boosting HDLs.

But Does It Improve Health?

Let's cut to the chase. The burning question in all of this is simple: Do these fats improve overall health, or positively affect the underlying atherosclerosis? I acknowledge that there is some cholesterol-lowering by poly- and monounsaturated fats, but what I am really interested in is whether that cholesterol-lowering is enough to make a difference in your health? So far, the research says no. A study conducted by David Blankenhorn, M.D., and his associates compared the effects of different types of fats on the growth of atherosclerotic lesions inside the coronary arteries of people by studying the results of angiograms taken one year apart. The study demonstrated that all three types of fat were associated with a significant increase in new atherosclerotic lesions. Most importantly, the growth of these lesions did not stop when polyunsaturated fats or olive oil was substituted for saturated fats. Only by decreasing all fat intake—including poly- and monounsaturated fats—did the lesions stop growing. Dietary polyunsaturated fats are incorporated into human atherosclerotic plaques, thereby promoting damage to the arteries and the progression of atherosclerosis.

And therein lies the secret to curing heart disease. All excess fats must be eliminated in order to improve health and cure the disease.

That's a Lot of Fish—Without a Lot of Proof

As for the protective effects of fish oils, the picture is also mixed. What most people do not realize is how much fish oil you have to eat in order to have a positive effect on cholesterol levels. Researchers had to feed study participants 2.5 to 3.5 ounces (75 to 100 grams) to see a significant cholesterol-lowering effect. That's a lot of fish oils.

It's also a lot of extra calories—675 to 900 extra calories to be exact. All those extra calories of fat can wind up on your body as excess weight. And overweight contributes to heart disease, high blood pressure, and stroke.

Keep in mind that there are still significant amounts of cholesterol in fish, too. Thus, you're constantly working at cross purposes: You're eating fat and cholesterol in order to lower blood cholesterol. Does that make sense? Even for you lovers of fish oils, it's easy to get the formula wrong and have the whole thing backfire on you, simply by not taking enough fish oils, or taking too much.

Many studies have shown that MaxEPA (a popular fish oil product) raises LDL levels. Researchers speculated that this effect might have been due to the high amounts of cholesterol in the oil (600 mg/3.5 oz.). To test this hypothesis, researchers used a purified fish oil that contained no cholesterol to see whether the fish oil itself—without the cholesterol—raised LDL cholesterol. The study found that the purified fish oil did indeed raise LDL cholesterol, too, when given in the doses commonly consumed (twelve 1-gram capsules).

A recent study in the *Journal of the American College of Cardiology* fed patients with heart disease capsules containing either 12 grams of fish oil or olive oil daily for 28 months. In both groups atherosclerotic closure of the coronary arteries increased by similar amounts (about 2.5 percent). The authors concluded, "Fish oil treatment for 2 years does not promote favorable changes in the diameter of atherosclerotic coronary arteries."

Whether or not fish or fish oils have a significant benefit for the prevention of heart disease is hotly debated in the medical world. Unquestionably, heart disease is not due to fish or fish oil deficiency, but rather to too much rich food and an unhealthy lifestyle.

Thinning the Blood with Unintended Consequences

Fish oils do indeed "thin" the blood, which makes clots less likely to form. I also acknowledge this as a benefit of fish oils. However, there are significant negative side effects to that benefit: Thinning stops clots from forming in places where you want them to form, such as over wounds. Preventing your body from doing what it's supposed to do can result in excessive bleeding and loss of life, such as in the case of an automobile accident.

It's not worth it. People who have been diagnosed with heart disease or have already had a heart attack should not be taking fish oils. The only true solution is to eat a diet that is exceedingly low in all fats. That diet, which will "thin" your blood naturally and safely, is the foundation of the McDougall Program for a Healthy Heart.

The Ugly

The Fat You Eat Is the Fat You Wear

When scientists placed the Tarahumara on a high-fat diet, they noted that in the five weeks on that diet, "All the subjects gained weight, with a mean increase of 3.8 kilograms," or 8.3 pounds.

This is a key to understanding the negative effects of fat intake. Fat, no matter whether it's saturated, polyunsaturated, or monounsaturated, adds excessive calories to the body that are easily stored and hard to remove. The Tarahumara—with a physical fitness level that is unprecedented— could not burn those excess calories, and consequently they gained weight.

Overweight is a major risk factor for heart disease, high blood pressure, diabetes, and cancer. Weight is associated with higher cholesterol levels, higher blood pressure, higher LDL, higher triglycerides, and lower HDL. Overweight forces the heart to work harder to pump blood, and new research suggests that overweight may be harder on younger hearts than it is on older ones. One study found that obese men, 45 and younger, had three times more hypertension than older men who were also overweight. By creating hypertension, overweight raises your chances of having a heart attack or stroke. Modest weight gains in women within the range considered "normal" result in a significant increase in the risk of dying from heart disease. In our population, such weight gain contributes as much to death from heart disease in women as does cigarette smoking, according to a recent study in the *Journal of the American Medical Association* (February 1995).

Cancer and Bad Skin to Boot

Many kinds of polyunsaturated fats have been linked to human cancers through various mechanisms. They suppress the immune system, making us vulnerable to illnesses, including infectious diseases and cancer. Fish and vegetable oils deregulate diabetes, causing the blood sugar to rise. Oils make our skin and hair oily, contributing to acne and other skin problems, and promote the development of gallbladder disease.

Looking at only part of the picture and then making an overall judgment or sweeping recommendations is sometimes a problem in science and medicine. Often, we focus only on fragments of the picture, to the exclusion of other, contradictory facts. It's something like saying that steak is good for you because it's loaded with iron and protein, but let's face it: When you add up all the good things about steak and place them against all the bad things, you don't think of a steak as a health food. That's the same situation polyunsaturated and monounsaturated fats are in.

For all of these reasons, I do not recommend the use of polyunsaturated and monounsaturated fats, except as part of a natural food. The McDougall Program for a Healthy Heart is exceedingly low in fat, which provides the surest—and the quickest—road to recovery. The greatest improvements in health come from big improvements in diet. As I am fond of saying, big changes beget big results. To me it is unethical to offer patients anything less than the best opportunity to heal themselves and to stay healthy. To offer less is like recommending a dose of penicillin that is inadequate to cure pneumonia. In the case of diet and medication, half a dose won't work.

I am not one to take risks when it comes to life-and-death conditions. I tell people to get their health back before they start experimenting with foods that have been clearly shown to contribute to heart disease.

Dietary Cholesterol: The Other Evil Twin

You'll be happy to know that the evidence paints a decisive picture when it comes to dietary cholesterol. Like saturated fat, dietary cholesterol directly increases blood cholesterol levels by elevating LDL cholesterol. Cholesterol is found only in the tissues of animals and animal by-products, such as milk. Plants and plant foods do not contain cholesterol.

Cholesterol in Meats

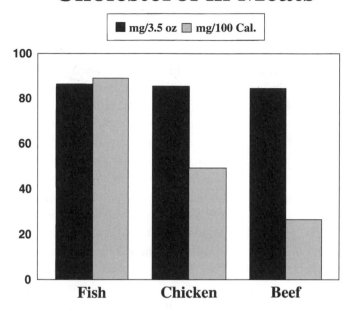

A muscle is a muscle. White meat is no better for you than red meat. All of these meats are high in fat and/or protein, have no carbohydrate or dietary fiber, and are heavily contaminated by environmental contaminants and microorganisms. Based on portion size (3.5 ounces) their cholesterol content is the same. Based on a portion of 100 calories, fish provides three times more cholesterol than beef. Most important, blood cholesterol levels remain essentially the same when people are switched from red to white meat. Comparisons are between T-bone steak, sockeye salmon, and light-meat chicken without the skin. (Source: Pennington, J. Food Values of Portions Commonly Used, *15th ed. Harper & Row, New York, 1989).*

The cholesterol content within most animal foods is similar. For example, 3.5 ounces of beef contains 85 mg of cholesterol, while the skinned white meat of chicken also contains 85 mg. Fish contains anywhere from 50 to 115 mg, depending, of course, on the fish in question.

Because animal foods contain similar cholesterol content, it usually doesn't make much difference in your blood cholesterol when you switch from, say, red meat to chicken. They've both got about the same amount of cholesterol and both contain saturated fat.

About 40 percent of the cholesterol we eat is absorbed through the intestinal wall and into our bloodstream. The human body has great difficulty eliminating cholesterol. Excess cholesterol is excreted, to some extent, through the liver into the intestines as bile acids. We eliminate cholesterol each day as part of our stools.

Unlike dogs and cats, humans do not have the capacity to excrete large amounts of cholesterol through their livers. When you feed carnivores cholesterol-rich foods, their livers increase metabolism and they secrete all the cholesterol. Even if you feed them pure egg yolks, they never develop atherosclerosis because of their unlimited capacity to remove cholesterol from the blood. People have no such ability, however. We retain excess cholesterol and deposit it in our arteries and elsewhere in the body, where it causes disease. Our limited capacity to excrete cholesterol points to the fact that we are primarily vegetarians.

Excess cholesterol that is not excreted from the body accumulates in various tissues, including the skin, muscles, tendons, fat cells, and artery walls. Once inside the artery walls, cholesterol acts like an irritating foreign substance—almost like a sliver of wood stuck under the skin—creating that injury to the artery wall that begins the atherosclerotic process.

Even though cholesterol is a significant and ongoing threat to your arteries, because it is found only in animal foods, it is easy to avoid. Just cut out red meat, eggs, poultry, shellfish, fish, dairy products, and foods made from these animal foods and you will not consume any cholesterol.

Dire Consequences of Diseased Arteries

For those who consume a high-fat and cholesterol-rich diet, atherosclerosis occurs not only in the coronary arteries, but in arteries throughout the body. That means that vessels are narrowing in, say, the neck, legs, and the trunk of the body, depriving cells and organs of needed blood and oxygen. Such deprivation results in a wide variety of symptoms that collectively are known as *peripheral vascular disease.*

Atherosclerosis in the carotid artery—a large vessel that brings oxygenated blood to the brain—can cause stroke. Even before a stroke occurs, however, blocked vessels in the neck and head can give rise to temporary losses of brain function, called *transient ischemic attacks*, or TIAs. Blocked blood flow to the brain also causes senility.

Other serious disorders also arise from blocked arteries. Among the most common are angina pectoris, claudication, high blood pressure (Chapter 14 deals with the cause and cure of hypertension), impotence, hearing loss, vertigo, loss of mental clarity, and even senility. The principle is the same in all cases: Blocked blood vessels prevent adequate blood and oxygen from flowing to specific organs and systems. The result is that those organs are impaired, oftentimes significantly.

Virtually all forms of peripheral vascular disease can be reversed by adopting the McDougall Program for a Healthy Heart. But before we look at the cure, let's have a closer look at the most widespread forms of the disorder.

Angina

Angina pectoris is literally a "strangling" pain in the chest—the grip of death. It occurs when the heart muscle is partially deprived of sufficient oxygen because one or more of the coronary arteries are significantly blocked with plaque. Angina pain, which afflicts 3 million Americans, arises most often when a person with artery disease is forced to increase his or her heart rate, such as during exercise, when excited or under stress (both of which trigger the secretion of adrenaline, which in turn increases heart rate), or when the body is exposed to colder than normal temperatures. An increase in the heart rate forces the muscle to work harder and require more oxygen. However, since the coronary arteries are partially blocked, the heart is prevented from getting the oxygen it needs. The result is a searing or constricting pain in the chest that often spreads to the neck, jaw, and left arm. Usually, the pain lasts about five to ten minutes. It can also arise after a big meal, or after smoking a cigarette. A fat-laden meal can sludge the blood, thus further diminishing the flow of oxygen to the heart. Cigarette smoking deprives the blood of oxygen, which suffocates the heart even more. The pain is relieved with rest, which reduces the demand for oxygen from the body and thus slows the heart.

Curing angina requires improving circulation and opening the coronary arteries. Eating a low-fat, low-cholesterol diet will do both. Moderate exercise will also promote the growth of collateral circulation to the heart muscle, improving circulation.

Claudication

Claudication was named for the Roman Emperor Claudius, who was lame. Like so many modern Americans, Claudius was fond of feasting. The illness is characterized by cramping pain in the legs and buttocks after one has walked a short distance. As with other forms of peripheral vascular disease, claudication is caused by partially blocked arteries. In this case, atherosclerosis prevents the muscles in the legs from getting adequate blood and oxygen during exercise. The principle is the same as with angina: Atherosclerosis prevents sufficient blood and oxygen from reaching muscles, especially during those times when the demand for oxygen has increased. The result of such oxygen deprivation is pain and fatigue. Usually, the pain disappears after the person has rested for a few minutes. For this reason, the disorder is called *intermittent claudication,* meaning it comes and goes, depending upon the level of exertion one is engaged in.

As with angina, curing claudication involves immediately improving circulation and eventually opening the arteries that provide blood to the lower part of the body, along with increasing exercise, which will promote the growth of new blood vessels—both to the legs and buttocks, as well as to the heart. This will increase the blood and oxygen to the affected muscles. The McDougall Program for a Healthy Heart will lower the blood cholesterol, reverse atherosclerosis, improve blood flow, thin the blood, and overall restore the circulation to the legs. The duration people with claudication can walk before experiencing pain increases within days on my program.

Impotence

For most men, the problem is not between their ears. Atherosclerotic lesions can prevent adequate amounts of blood from flowing to the penis and nerves that control erection during sexual arousal, thus causing impotence. Today, as many as 34 percent of middle-aged men suffer from impotence, and a great many of them have no other problem except significant peripheral vascular disease.

By adopting the McDougall Program for a Healthy Heart, you can reverse virtually all forms of peripheral vascular disease, including the obstructions that may be causing impotence.

Hearing Loss

Hearing gradually deteriorates with age in the United States and much of the Western world. We have come to accept this as a "natural" part of aging, but that is a cultural bias rather than a scientific truth. In fact, when researchers examine the hearing capabilities of Third World cultures subsisting on their traditional diets—composed mostly of grains, vegetables, and fruits—they find that no comparable hearing loss occurs. African tribesmen, for example, have better hearing at the age of 70 than the average American has at 20. Scientists surveyed the hearing capabilities of a random sampling of Wisconsin residents between the ages of 30 and 35, and then compared them to African tribespeople called Maabans. Wisconsin, of course, is the dairy capital of the United States. And not surprisingly, researchers could find no Maaban, *at any age*, with hearing losses comparable to those of the Wisconsin sampling.

Similar studies have repeatedly confirmed these findings. When Finnish people, who eat a high-fat and high-cholesterol diet, were compared to people living in what was then called Yugoslavia, researchers found a dramatic difference in hearing. The Finns had an average cholesterol level of 290 mg/dl; the Yugoslavs had an average cholesterol level of 180 mg/dl. Finnish children were found to suffer hearing losses at the age of 10 and by the age of 19 had distinct impairment, with a marked inability to hear sounds in the normal upper ranges. Yugoslavs showed no such impairment, however, and no comparable hearing loss. As in other peripheral vascular diseases, vessels that supply the inner ear become clogged with atherosclerosis, causing the inner ear to lose sensitivity to sound.

Today, there is a growing concern about the fact that we are polluting our ocean and destroying its creatures. But there isn't much emotion expended over the fact that we are polluting our internal seas as well. The living ocean inside of you—the blood that keeps us alive—is being polluted each day by toxins as destructive as any of those being poured into the Pacific. The poisons in your internal environment will kill you long before those of the external world.

4. Curing Heart Disease in Two Stages

- *Hearts can be healed.*
- *Experience lifesaving effects sooner than you think.*
- *Make your arteries cleaner than an adolescent's.*
- *The healing cholesterol level is 150 mg/dl.*

In 1986, Charles Schaefer was only 46 years old and far too young, he believed, to have heart disease. However, in December of that year Charles had a heart attack. A blood clot formed in the left anterior descending artery, closing off the vessel and suffocating the heart. Following the heart attack, Charles underwent balloon angioplasty, in which an inflatable device is inserted into the artery and expanded to open the vessel and allow blood to flow again. His doctors informed him that he would likely need bypass surgery to prevent another heart attack. At the time, Schaefer's cholesterol level was 220 mg/dl—about the average for Americans. He was not particularly overweight and his blood pressure was well within the normal ranges.

After being released from the hospital, he heard me talk about heart disease on my daily radio show in Santa Rosa, California. "I went on the McDougall Program right away," Schaefer recalled. "My cholesterol dropped from 220 to 180 milligrams. After I started the program, I saw Dr. McDougall. He put me on a cholesterol-lowering drug for a while to get my cholesterol level down even lower to 150 milligrams. And that's about where I've been since."

Charles also began exercising. He walked or bicycled three to four times a week for at least a half hour per session. Meanwhile, his family, which was very supportive of the diet and lifestyle changes, also adopted the program. All the family meals centered around the McDougall diet. As a result, Charles's health improved dramatically. Within the last four years, he's had four radionuclide stress treadmill tests, all of which have shown that his coronary arteries are wide open. His heart is healthy and he feels in better shape today than he did when he was a much younger man.

"If I had stayed on the rich American diet, I would not be alive today," said Charles. "If I could go back to my old diet right now, I wouldn't. I wouldn't eat any other way."

What Charles Schaefer and many thousands of others have done is the surest and best way to cure heart disease. That is not a statement of personal bias—though I believe it with all my heart—but one that is grounded in the best scientific evidence to date.

When you adopt the McDougall Program for a Healthy Heart, you are curing heart disease in two stages. The first is the short-term phase, which takes you out of immediate danger and starts you on the road to reversal of the underlying plaque. The second is the long-term effect, which is the actual reversal—or shrinkage—of the cholesterol-laden plaques in your arteries. Actually, reversal of atherosclerosis is accomplished slowly and in small increments. It takes about a year for a low-fat, low-cholesterol diet to create significant reversal of atherosclerosis that can be seen with today's high-tech imaging techniques.

Many people mistakenly believe that they do not derive much benefit from my program until after their plaques have visibly shrunk. In fact, just the opposite is true. Many scientists believe that the initial effects of a cholesterol-lowering program are the most powerful, because they reverse the conditions that create the clots (thrombi) that cause most heart attacks. The McDougall Program for a Healthy Heart is the fastest way for you to prevent clots and keep you far from danger.

So, in this chapter I want to talk to you about these two levels of healing that take place on the McDougall Program: the reduction of the clotting and the reversal of atherosclerosis. Let's begin with the short-term effects.

The First Stage: Reduce Clotting

Stabilize Your Plaques

Heart disease is so terrifying to most of us that when we are diagnosed with the illness, or even worse, when we suffer a heart attack, our first thought is to do whatever it takes to get out of immediate danger and stay alive. It's as if we just experienced an earthquake and all we want now is some sense of stability. Unfortunately, our fear and our lack of knowledge often cause us to rush into the operating room for bypass surgery. As I will show in Chapter 13, that's a big mistake for most people. Most people do not need the operation; even worse, they don't need the side effects of the surgery, which I will document later on. Even those who have just had a heart attack must realize that hearts are healed in stages, and for the vast majority of people, there is time to heal the heart without surgery—even after a heart attack.

As I described in Chapters 2 and 3, cholesterol-laden plaque is not a single unified mass, but a volatile blockage. Inside the typical plaque is a pool of semiliquid necrotic material that includes both liquid and crystalline cholesterol. As I said, the plaque is highly unstable and even volatile. You can think of that pool of lipids as the volcanic lava that erupts from a volcano.

When the blood is loaded with cholesterol and fat, these lipids are actually fed into the plaque, thus making it more unstable and more likely to rupture. Eventually, such a rupture can give rise to a clot that totally closes the flow of blood and brings on a heart attack.

However, when you lower the cholesterol significantly, the process reverses. You are now draining the lipids out of the plaque, and taking the tension off its surface, which dramatically reduces the risk of rupture—as if you've drained the lava from a volcano. It not only makes the plaque more stable, but shrinks the plaque somewhat. This initial stage of the healing process accounts for most of the protection against heart attacks, scientists now believe.

Because the McDougall Program for a Healthy Heart is the healthiest diet for the arteries, containing little saturated fat and no cholesterol, this initial stage of the healing process begins within hours of adopting the program.

Unstick the Platelets

When the plaque breaks open, blood platelets and clotting proteins move quickly to patch over the rupture. Unfortunately, when you eat a diet rich in fat and cholesterol, these platelets become excessively sticky and more reactive than healthy platelets to ruptures in the plaque. They clump together, or adhere to one another in what doctors refer to as "aggregates." Also, sticky platelets overreact to the rupture, sending more platelets than necessary to the site to close it off. The resulting clot, or thrombus, is therefore larger than necessary, which increases the risk of closing off blood flow in the artery entirely. The tendency of platelets to overreact and form larger clots is caused primarily by high levels of animal fat in the blood. Hence, animal foods—meats, dairy foods, and eggs—are powerful creators of dangerous clots, and the primary causes of heart attacks.

Meals rich in animal foods also cause blood-clotting proteins, such as factor VII, to coagulate excessively. Like platelets, these clotting proteins aggregate to form larger blood clots, which close off the arteries and lead to heart attacks and strokes. Most heart attacks occur in the early morning, perhaps because a high-fat dinner the previous night has caused excessive coagulation of blood-clotting proteins to form clots while the person slept.

Polyunsaturated fats, like vegetable oils, do just the opposite: They "thin" the blood by making both platelets and blood-clotting proteins less reactive to plaque ruptures and less likely to form clots, thereby reducing the risk of heart attacks. However, polyunsaturated fats also have significant side effects, including the fact that they depress immune function and increase the likelihood of cancer, obesity, and gallbladder disease. The McDougall Program for a Healthy Heart makes platelets and blood-clotting proteins less reactive without the negative side effects.

Reducing Prostaglandins

When platelets clump, they release groups of fatty acids called *prostaglandins*, hormones that, among other things, cause arteries to spasm, or suddenly constrict, for short periods of time. They can cause so much contraction of an artery, in fact, that blood flow to the heart muscle can be severely reduced and cause angina. Picture the person who has plaque rupturing, platelets clumping, and large clots forming. At the same time,

prostaglandins are released by those platelets, causing the artery to contract. In rare situations, all these factors can combine to cause a heart attack
or stroke. On the McDougall Program, prostaglandins are not produced
in such dangerous quantities, simply because my diet does not cause
platelets to clump.

Thus, in just the first stage of healing on the McDougall Program for a
Healthy Heart, you've accomplished the following:

    1. You've taken the tension off the surface of the plaques by drain-
ing them of some of their lipid pools. This greatly diminishes the likelihood of their rupturing.
    2. You've reduced the tendency for your blood platelets to stick
together, thus making them less hyperreactive, and less likely to form
the clots that cause heart attacks and strokes.
    3. You've lowered the levels of prostaglandins produced by your
platelets, which keeps your arteries from going into spasm.

These are the immediate benefits of the McDougall Program for a
Healthy Heart, which you start to derive the very day you begin the
program.

All the available evidence supports this approach over any other, including surgery. During the past decade, the rate of heart attacks has declined. The evidence emerging from a number of studies suggests that
this decline cannot be attributed so much to reversal of atherosclerosis as
to lowering blood cholesterol enough to reduce the rate of plaque rupture and thrombus formation. It's the first stage of the healing process
that is causing the drop in heart attacks. Probably, most people have not
reduced their cholesterol levels enough to show actual shrinkage of their
cholesterol plaques on angiographic studies. Yet, even short of this, they
have increased their protection against heart attacks.

Walter's Story

In 1977 when Walter Zolezzi, the owner of the Fly Trap Restaurant,
an old and popular eatery in San Francisco, was 50, he suffered his first
heart attack. A year later, he had another one. Two angioplasties were
performed, which temporarily opened his arteries somewhat. But the net

effect of both heart attacks was to leave Walter a near-invalid. His cholesterol level hovered above 290 mg/dl. He was overweight and could no longer perform any type of exertion or exercise. In fact, Walter was in such poor health that his doctors refused to perform a coronary bypass operation, for fear that he would not survive the surgery. He had gout (a form of arthritis), angina, terrible fatigue, and shortness of breath. "Walter couldn't walk up the hill to our house," recalled his wife, Elaine. A lover of sailing and other outdoor activities, Walter had to give up anything and everything that might strain his heart. That included his work. At the age of 50, Walter was watching his life shrink. And it would be that way for the next decade. "For more than ten years, he had to put his life on hold," said Elaine.

In 1990 Elaine purchased my book *The McDougall Plan*, and began to see that perhaps there was hope after all. A few months later, they came to my program at St. Helena Hospital in the Napa Valley of California. Walter's cholesterol had already begun to drop as a result of following the program haphazardly for several months before coming to St. Helena. But at the clinic, Walter and Elaine both saw some remarkable results. Walter's cholesterol went from 260 mg/dl to 180 mg/dl in two weeks. Within a month, he lost 20 pounds, and began to feel his old vitality coming back.

Walter and Elaine were fully committed to the McDougall Program for a Healthy Heart, which was the reason they continued to see such dramatic improvements in his health. His cholesterol level fell even further to 160 mg/dl, and he lost another 15 pounds, bringing his total weight loss to 35 pounds. He's been at about 150 pounds ever since. His angina disappeared and he no longer feels any pressure in his chest— *unless he strays from the diet,* he says.

"The McDougall Program gave Walter back his life," said Elaine. "He's back to working long days at the restaurant. Sometimes he works 14 hours a day. He's got energy and he's very active again. He sails. And he looks great. His physique looks like that of a young man."

Like so many other people, Walter and Elaine Zolezzi found that the power to restore their health was in their own hands. All they needed was someone to show them how to eat healthfully and do some mild exercises. But what I tell people who adopt the program is that they are, essentially, living proof of the scientific evidence. Everything that I am saying is based on the science. I am simply implementing that evidence in people's lives.

Yet, despite the evidence, I am amazed at how many scientists and cardiologists avoid the subject of diet and rely exclusively upon drugs and surgery to treat this disease.

A couple of years ago, I attended a conference in Santa Rosa in which a doctor from the University of San Francisco was lecturing on reversal of atherosclerosis. She argued correctly that we should halt the creation of atherosclerotic plaque right after a person suffers a heart attack and is still in the intensive care unit of a hospital. I agreed with her wholeheartedly. After all, as long as you eat a moderate- to high-fat diet you're increasing the likelihood of suffering a second heart attack, one that could be fatal. Unfortunately, I stopped agreeing with her when she got around to telling us how she planned to protect patients in the coronary care unit (CCU). Her approach, which she called the "triple whammy," was to give patients niacin (which reduces cholesterol) and two other cholesterol-lowering drugs, colestipol (Colestid) and lovastatin (Mevacor). She offered no significant dietary advice.

"How does the high-fat, clot-producing diet that is routinely served to patients in the CCU fit into your approach to save dying patients?" I asked her.

She had no answer. And that, of course, is the problem. You have to significantly reduce dietary fat and cholesterol to prevent the whole constellation of events that create ruptures and clots. And drugs will not do that as effectively as diet will, especially the elimination of saturated fat.

The Second Stage: Reverse Atherosclerosis

Since the 1920s, scientists have been examining the question of whether atherosclerosis can be reversed by lowering blood cholesterol through dietary means, drug treatment, or both. Most of these studies have been done on animals, including monkeys, but many have been done on humans, too. Consequently, there is a vast body of evidence accumulated and much of it has shown that you can reverse atherosclerosis, even in the coronary arteries of humans.

Not all of what we know has occurred in the laboratory, or under scientifically controlled conditions, however. In fact, scientists believe that a good example of reversal of atherosclerosis occurred among large numbers of people who were *forced* to eat a low-fat, low-cholesterol diet.

During World War II, high-fat foods were rationed in order to send them to the soldiers at the fronts. Many Flemish, French, and Dutch people, for example, were forced to eat their traditional "peasant diets," composed chiefly of grains, potatoes, and garden vegetables. Autopsies done after the war on people who experienced such rationing showed significantly less atherosclerosis than in those who ate the affluent diet after the hostilities ceased. Dr. William Castelli, who was a practicing physician in Europe after the war, remembers the period well. "There wasn't enough atherosclerosis in those people to show medical school students what atherosclerosis looked like," said Dr. Castelli. Consistent with that reversal of atherosclerosis was the sharp decline in deaths from heart disease in all age groups, even among people in their sixties and seventies.

Following the war, studies done at the University of Chicago repeatedly showed reversal in rhesus monkeys with the use of a low-fat, low-cholesterol diet. In fact, reversal in monkeys was demonstrated so consistently that it prompted William Castelli to lament at the time that "the only ones that are getting the right treatment for heart disease are the monkeys."

Later, scientists at the University of Southern California Medical School used drugs to lower cholesterol in humans and demonstrated reversal of atherosclerosis in the femoral artery (located in the leg). Other research followed these studies, much of it substantiating the general hypothesis.

By the late 1970s and early 1980s, the reversal of atherosclerosis was considered a fait accompli—most scientists believed that a diet sufficiently low in fat and cholesterol could indeed reverse atherosclerosis in the coronary arteries of humans. For twenty years, heart disease pioneer Nathan Pritikin argued the case to scientists and the American public, but he was criticized by researchers because he hadn't proved the claim in the laboratory.

Compliance Is the Key to the Cure

And then came the most celebrated reversal study yet, the Lifestyle Heart Trial, done by Dean Ornish, M.D., director of the Preventive Medicine Research Institute in Sausalito, California. In that study, a group of middle-aged men and women—all with proven atherosclerosis—were placed on a vegetarian diet, low in fat and cholesterol. They stopped smoking, exercised three hours per week, and were instructed in stress management techniques. They were compared with a group of people of similar age and similar degrees of illness who did not get the vegetarian diet, exercise, smoking cessation, and stress management. These people, who were called the "control group," got the usual care for heart disease patients. Both groups were followed for one year, after which angio-grams—an X-ray test that reveals the extent of the plaques clogging the coronary arteries—were performed on both groups.

The scientists reported that eighteen of the twenty-two people who had adopted the special diet, exercise, and lifestyle program showed sig-nificant reversal of atherosclerosis in the coronary arteries. In fact, the amount of reversal was not only significant, but astounding. Eighty-two percent of the experimental group showed reversal of their lesions. Most of those in the control group—the patients who received the usual care—showed progression of their disease: The plaques got bigger.

Following this study, scientists in Heidelberg, Germany, placed eigh-teen people on a low-fat, low-cholesterol diet, coupled with an exercise program consisting of bicycle riding thirty minutes per session, up to six days per week. These patients were compared to a control group that re-ceived no special advice or follow-up. Compliance to the program was mixed; some people followed the diet and exercise program closely, others did not. The results demonstrated how much compliance paid off. After one year, seven of the people who followed the special diet and exercise program had experienced regression of atherosclerosis in their coronary arteries, as measured by angiograms. In patients who received no special care, regression was found in only one.

This study confirms what I tell my patients all the time: Compliance is the key.

Cholesterol Level: The Best Single Predictor of Health

Diagnostic tests usually have high degrees of specificity, but one test re-veals a great deal about general health. That test is cholesterol level. Re-search has consistently shown that lowering blood cholesterol is directly tied to curing heart disease. But when you consider declines in blood cholesterol, two factors are very important: the total cholesterol level

Cholesterol Changes (11 days)
(for entire group)

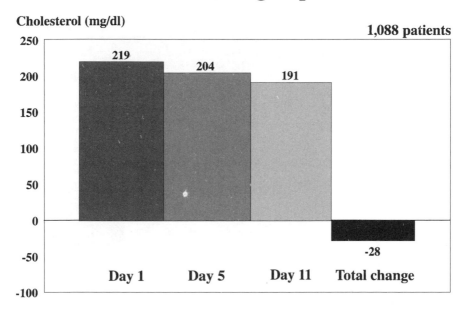

Cholesterol (mg/dl)

1,088 patients

Cholesterol levels decrease on the average 15 mg/dl in five days (approximately 3 mg/day) on a low-fat, no-cholesterol, high-fiber, high-carbohydrate diet. After eleven days the average reduction is 28 mg/dl. This data is from over 1,000 participants studied at the McDougall Program at St. Helena Hospital in the Napa Valley, California.

and the degree of decline in cholesterol after you've adopted the McDougall Program. The amount of your drop in blood cholesterol is sometimes a greater indicator of improved health than the actual number of your total cholesterol, especially those first few cholesterol readings that you get *after* you've adopted my program. Some patients who come to my program in the St. Helena Medical Center with cholesterol levels of 300 mg/dl or more leave my center with cholesterol levels of 200 mg/dl or less. Some of these people are disappointed, however. They tell me that they wanted to get to 150 mg/dl, which is ideal. And they ask me why they didn't see greater declines in cholesterol.

I tell them two things: First, I ask these people to be patient. Many of

Cholesterol Changes (11 days)
(based on initial values)

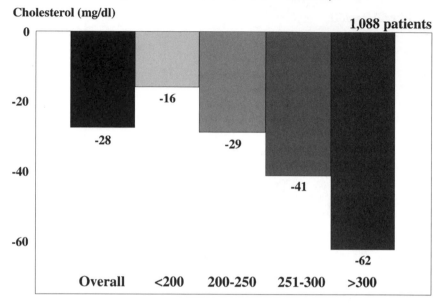

Cholesterol (mg/dl)

1,088 patients

"The sicker you are the better you get." In nicer words, those who begin the program with the highest cholesterol levels realize the greatest changes (because they have the largest margins for improvement and were likely eating the unhealthiest foods before they started the program). This data is from over 1,000 participants studied at the McDougall Program at St. Helena Hospital in the Napa Valley, California.

us have been abusing our health for decades before we adopt the Mc-Dougall Program. Once you begin the diet, blood cholesterol levels drop precipitously, but the fat and cholesterol that have been stored in your tissues for many years will now be dumped into your bloodstream for some time to come. That will keep the cholesterol levels up for a while, even though you are eliminating it from your body. Sometimes, I prescribe cholesterol-lowering over-the-counter and prescription medications to help get those cholesterol levels down even further and faster. Nevertheless, the relatively diminished cholesterol in the blood will bring about tremendous improvement in health. People in this situation still feel better and their chances of suffering a heart attack will be greatly diminished, for all the reasons I described earlier. In other words, they can still enjoy the first stage of healing, despite their relatively high total cholesterol number, as long as their compliance on the program is good.

The second thing I tell people is that the percentage drop in cholesterol is often enough by itself to create reversal of atherosclerosis. Some patients experience reversal after they've dropped their total cholesterol levels sixty points, but still have cholesterol levels well into the 200 mg range.

Another good indicator is the direction of your LDL cholesterol. Is it going down or up or staying the same? Studies have shown that regression of atherosclerosis in the coronary arteries can occur when LDL cholesterol levels fall 40 to 45 percent from their pretreatment levels. That means that if you start out with an LDL level of, say, 230 mg/dl (which is dangerously high), and you drop that LDL level to 130 mg/dl or below, you stand a good chance of reversing your atherosclerosis—if you maintain that level for at least a year, and preferably two. These enormous benefits can occur even though an ideal LDL cholesterol is below 100 mg/dl. The point I try to emphasize to my patients, therefore, is the direction of the cholesterol levels—is your cholesterol level falling?—and how much of a fall the person has experienced.

It should be emphasized, however, that we are talking about a cholesterol level that's declining *as a result of improved dietary practices*. There's no protective effect of a total cholesterol level of, say, 200 mg/dl or more if you are still eating a high-fat, high-cholesterol diet. Such a cholesterol level, coupled with a high-fat diet, is a sign of illness and a need to make changes, fast.

The Magic Number is 150

Still, we should have a goal to shoot for, one that has been shown to have a protective effect against heart disease. And that goal is a cholesterol level of 150 mg/dl. The research has consistently shown that people who have cholesterol levels of 150 or lower have virtually no sign of heart disease.

In an article entitled "Atherosclerotic Risk Factors—Are There Ten or Is There Only One?" William Clifford Roberts, M.D., editor in chief of the *American Journal of Cardiology*, argued that there is only one risk factor for heart attacks and angina due to atherosclerotic coronary artery disease: *a serum cholesterol greater than 150 mg/dl.*

As for the level of "good" cholesterol in your bloodstream, Dr. Roberts states that HDL should only be considered important if the HDL level is low, while at the same time LDL is high and total cholesterol is above 150 mg/dl. These three factors must exist together for HDL to be a factor.

Of the other eight risk factors that are typically associated with heart disease, six of them (male sex, family history of coronary events in a person less than 55, smoking, high blood pressure, diabetes, and severe obesity) only affect people with elevated cholesterol levels (over 150 mg/dl). The other two commonly cited "risk factors"—clinical evidence of heart artery disease and peripheral vascular illness (either of the brain or leg)—are not risk factors at all, but symptoms of already-existing artery disease.

Dr. Roberts points out that international population studies show a virtual absence of atherosclerosis-related diseases when cholesterol levels remain below 150 mg/dl. Even those people with diabetes and/or hypertension show no evidence of increased risk of heart attacks as long as their cholesterol levels are below 150 mg/dl.

The McDougall Diet Is the Traditional Human Diet

For more than a decade, I have maintained that the ideal cholesterol level for my patients is less than 150 mg/dl. Some doctors label my recommendation impractical, yet admit that it is scientifically sound. The reason they believe it's impractical is because they do not believe people will stick to my dietary program long enough to achieve this cholesterol level. Over the years, this criticism has gradually diminished, however, because scientists are recognizing that people not only stick to my program, but they actually enjoy eating this way. Once they learn how to prepare the McDougall foods, they wouldn't go back to their old habits.

In fact, the McDougall diet is close to the one humans have been eating for most of our evolution and close to the diet that is still eaten in traditional cultures the world over. We've already discussed the Chinese in Chapter 1, but the Japanese—a highly advanced and industrialized nation—follow a regimen closer to my own than the American norm. And their rates of heart disease—and, indeed, their life spans—are proof of the effects of this diet.

Japanese women are the longest-living people on earth, with a life expectancy of 82.5 years. Japanese men have a life expectancy of 76.2, according to research conducted by the United Nations. American women rank sixteenth in the world, with a life expectancy of 78.6; American men are twenty-second, with a life expectancy of 71.6. While there are numerous factors involved in the longevity equation, one factor stands out: The Japanese eat relatively small amounts of fat, especially saturated fat. Clerical workers in Osaka, who consume a high-fat diet by Japanese standards, get 22.9 percent of their total calories from fat, and only 5.9 percent from saturated fat. Japanese living in rural Akita, whose diets haven't changed much in centuries, eat only 14.4 percent total calories in fat, and only 3.3 percent in saturated fat. These people are eating mostly grains, vegetables, and fruit, and very little animal food. Overall, the Japanese have one of the lowest heart disease rates in the world.

Therefore, when I recommend a mostly vegetarian diet, I'm not asking people to do something bizarre, or out of the ordinary. All I'm asking is that we go back to doing what people have been doing for a million years or so. From the standpoint of long human experience, the American diet is the anomaly. It is the first time large numbers of humans have consumed so much animal foods, fat, refined foods, and artificial ingredients. The American diet is just a fad, soon to pass.

From my standpoint, the failure of the medical profession to encourage people to adopt the traditional human diet—the low-fat vegetarian diet—as the primary therapy for heart disease contributes to the 1.25 million *preventable* heart attacks that take place in the United States each year, including the 768,000 fatal heart attacks.

Diet Versus Drugs: Which One Provides the Better Results?

I will deal with specific drugs and their side effects in Chapter 12, but for now let me say in general that drugs do not lower the cholesterol level as effectively and as safely as a healthy diet does. Drug therapy can be a good second line of offense, particularly when we have trouble getting the cholesterol level down into the safest ranges for those in great immediate need of treatment. But I would be doing my patients a disservice if, by giving them a prescription for a cholesterol-lowering drug, I lessened their resolve to maintain a healthy diet.

Drugs are not as effective as diet at reversing atherosclerosis. In fact, when scientists compare the studies on people who attempted to reverse atherosclerosis with drugs versus those who used diet and lifestyle alone, diet comes out the winner by far.

In one major study, the Cholesterol-Lowering Atherosclerosis Study (CLAS), 188 nonsmoking middle-aged men who had undergone bypass surgery were divided into two groups: one that got high doses of a cholesterol-lowering drug (colestipol) and a niacin supplement, and one that got a placebo (a pill with no therapeutic value). Both groups were told to eat a low-fat, low-cholesterol diet, but no intensive educational effort was made to change behavior. Both groups had angiograms done at the outset of the study, and at its conclusion two years later. You would think that the high doses of the cholesterol-lowering drug would cause significant reversal, but that was not the case. The researchers discovered that only one in six participants (16 percent) of the drug group experienced discernible reversal of atherosclerosis, even though compliance was considered excellent and, overall, cholesterol levels were reduced by 24 percent. In the placebo group, 2.4 percent experienced reversal. Neither group fared very well when compared to the Lifestyle Heart Trial, in which 82 percent of the people who followed the vegetarian diet, exercise, and stress management program experienced reversal.

After evaluating the results of studies using cholesterol-lowering drugs to reverse the atherosclerosis, Marvin Moser, M.D., professor of medicine at Yale School of Medicine, noted, "Other studies have failed to demonstrate significantly different degrees of progression or regression of coronary lesions with the use of clofibrate or cholestyramine [cholesterol-lowering medications] compared with placebo." In other words, drugs alone do not do that much better than a sugar pill.

The evidence consistently shows, however, that dietary means alone can bring cholesterol levels down 25 percent or more, particularly when that diet is a vegetarian diet similar to the one I advocate. And of the various kinds of vegetarian diets in existence today, the one with the greatest cholesterol-lowering effect is one that avoids all dairy products and eggs. When scientists compared two vegetarian groups, one that followed a strict vegetarian diet (without dairy and eggs) and another that included dairy in their diet, the researchers found that the strict vegetarians had cholesterol levels that were, on average, thirty points lower. The strict vegetarians had cholesterol levels of 133 mg/dl—way below the 150 mg/dl ideal. The lactovegetarians had total cholesterol levels, on average, of 161 mg/dl. Moreover, the lactovegetarians had LDL cholesterol levels that were 24 percent higher than the strict vegetarians'—97 mg/dl for the lactovegetarians versus 78 mg/dl. It's important to point out, too, that the strict vegetarians were people with jobs and families and bills to pay and all the stresses of daily life. They were not in controlled environments; nor were they protected from the influences and temptations of the standard American diet. Yet, they had no trouble sticking to their diets, and keeping their cholesterol levels down to the ideal levels.

And all the benefits of a vegetable-based diet add up to better health for everyone. Just ask George Phelps, a 61-year-old financial adviser living in Visalia, California.

George had a heart attack in 1990, when he was 57. One day in January of that year, he got dizzy and nearly passed out. He was taken to the cardiac care unit at his local hospital where tests showed he had suffered a heart attack. Doctors insisted he have bypass surgery immediately. "I had heard Dr. McDougall on the radio and told my doctor, 'Hey, I'm not doing anything until I talk to this guy.' My doctor responded with, 'You need to have a bypass right away.' I called Dr. McDougall and had my records sent to his office. He looked at them and told me I didn't need the surgery. I asked him how I should deal with my doctor, who was pressuring me to have the bypass. He told me to copy the chapters of his book *McDougall's Medicine: A Challenging Second Opinion* that dealt with heart disease and show them to my doctor, which I did. I showed them to both my general practitioner and my cardiologist. After reading them, the cardiologist said that he wished that he had written them. I adopted the McDougall Program and it changed my life."

When George started the McDougall Program, he weighed 195 pounds (which was about 40 pounds overweight), had a cholesterol level of 230 mg/dl, and—as he likes to put it—was "a human grease pit. I ate a lot of fatty foods. I used to drink a quart of milk at a single sitting." Over the next four months, he lost 40 pounds; his cholesterol level fell to 155 mg/dl, and he regained his youthful fitness. "I walk, do stretching exercises, jump rope about eight minutes a day, and can do seventy-five push-ups at a crack. Today, I feel great and I look ten years younger. When I went back to my doctor, his jaw dropped. Now, both my doctors are practicing the McDougall Program and they're recommending it to their patients."

Triglyceride Changes (11 days)
(based on initial values)

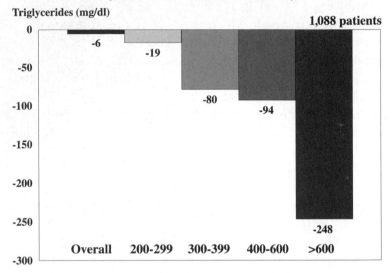

Overall, triglycerides decrease 6 mg/dl in 11 days. People starting with levels above normal (200 mg/dl) show much greater reductions—for example,
248 mg/dl in those starting with levels over 600 mg/dl—by following a high
complex carbohydrate, low-fat diet with regular exercise. Restriction of fruit,
juices, and other simple sugars provides added benefit (see Chapter 5,
page 75). This data is from over 1,000 participants studied at the McDougall
Program at St. Helena Hospital in the Napa Valley, California.

Triglycerides confused with cholesterol

Triglycerides are often confused with cholesterol because people with
elevated cholesterol levels often have high triglyceride levels. Years of
unhealthy eating can cause both to go up in sensitive people. However,
many people have one elevated without the other.

Triglycerides are the fats found in the blood. Cholesterol is a waxy
substance chemically distinct from fatty triglycerides. You might picture
triglycerides as the fat that rises to the top of chicken soup as it cools in
the refrigerator. After a blood drawing, fat rises to the top of the vacuum
tube—like the chicken soup—forming a yellow layer as the red blood
cells settle to the bottom of the tube. The more triglycerides the thicker

the layer of fat at the top. Normal triglyceride levels are below 200 mg/dl. The highest levels I have seen in patients have been in the 5,000 to 6,000 mg/dl range. In these cases the fat rises to the top of the vacuum tube before the needle is removed from the patient's arm. Triglyceride values can change 100 mg/dl in a matter of hours, especially after eating.

A high triglyceride level is recognized as a risk factor for the development of heart disease; however, its importance is of some debate. Blood cholesterol is a much more reliable predicator of a person's risk of heart disease than are his triglycerides. The diet for the McDougall Program for a Healthy Heart can cause a dramatic drop in elevated triglyceride levels in a few days.

CHOLESTEROL VARIATIONS

When measuring cholesterol and triglyceride values, you must take into account your present health, fasting state, and posture. Ideally your time without food should be the same before each test, your eating patterns the previous day should be similar, and tests should be taken after maintaining a similar posture. Ideally no alcohol should be consumed within three days of the test, and you should not be under any unusual stresses, like an illness or pregnancy.

If an unexpected result is obtained, then assume one of the values is not a true representation of your levels—a variation or error occurred. Your response should be to obtain further test results in order to obtain an accurate picture of your cholesterol and triglycerides. An ideal cholesterol is less than 150 mg/dl and triglycerides should be less than 200 mg/dl (ideally about 100 mg/dl). Based on multiple tests, assess your condition and determine your need for further treatment. You may wonder why your blood tests change so much.

Behavioral Sources

Diet: Saturated fats (especially palmitic acid) and dietary cholesterol raise cholesterol. Each increase of 100 mg of dietary cholesterol/1,000 calories raises blood cholesterol by 10 mg/dl (after 500 mg of cholesterol daily the effects are much smaller). Cholesterol absorption through the intestine varies among people from 18% to 75%; greater absorption means higher blood cholesterol. Coffee (especially unfiltered) raises cholesterol slightly. Complex carbohydrates and monounsaturated and polyunsaturated fats lower cholesterol levels; oat bran modestly lowers cholesterol and other dietary fibers lower cholesterol mainly by replacing saturated fats. Fish oil inhibits synthesis of VLDL triglycerides.

Obesity: Weight loss lowers triglycerides about 40% and LDL cholesterol (LDL-C) by 10% and increases HDL cholesterol (HDL-C) by 10%.

Smoking: Increases LDL-C and triglycerides and decreases HDL-C by 11% to 14% and is dose-dependent, meaning the decreases in LDL and HDL depend on the number of cigarettes smoked.

Exercise: Lowers triglycerides and LDL-C, and increases HDL-C.

Alcohol: Greatly increases triglycerides, increases HDL-C, and decreases LDL-C.

Clinical Sources

Cholesterol and triglycerides increase with various stresses on the body, for example, during infection. During pregnancy total cholesterol and LDL-C increase and triglycerides often more than double. In the winter cholesterol is 2.5% higher on average than in the summer.

Sampling Sources

Fasting: Triglyceride levels are lowest about 3 A.M., rise after midafternoon, and then decrease until after midnight. Triglycerides increase after eating, but eating has little effect on cholesterol. Prolonged fasting for six days raised total cholesterol and triglycerides by 18%, and decreased LDL-C by 22% (as fat came out of the body fat to supply energy needs). When juice is added to a ten-day fast (reducing use of body fat), total cholesterol falls 21%.

Posture: Standing concentrates the blood (water pools toward the legs with gravity, as blood components float) and raises cholesterol and triglycerides about 10% compared to a sample taken after thirty minutes of lying down.

Analytic Sources

Instruments: Precision and accuracy of modern instruments is remarkably good. Calibration and standardization with reference laboratories is improving the accuracy—there must be less than a 3% variation.

Biologic: Cholesterol measurements varied 2.5% within the day; 4.8% within the week; and 6.1% within the year. Triglycerides varied greatly, as much as 36% within the day. Triglycerides are greatly affected by eating, physical activity, emotions and other stresses.

Part II

THE PROGRAM: DIET, EXERCISE, AND LIFESTYLE

5. McDougall's Heart-Healing Diet

- *Healthy eating is a lot more delicious and varied than most people realize.*
- *In time you'll learn to love the foods, as your cooking ability improves and tastebuds adjust.*
- *While you're learning, your health will be improving with each passing day.*
- *In order to achieve maximum benefit, you should follow the program faithfully.*

So, let's get right down to basics. The first thing you should realize is that the foods that make up my program are not only delicious and varied, but provide all the nutrients your body needs, and in optimal amounts. You don't have to measure anything; you don't have to worry about getting adequate calcium or iron or protein or carbohydrates. It's all here, and in the most healthful quantities. If you follow this program faithfully, your blood cholesterol level usually falls dramatically in days. If you are overweight, it's almost a certainty that you'll lose weight— effortlessly. You won't have to count calories or starve yourself, either. Eat all you want of the foods recommended below. You'll still shed unwanted pounds. Meanwhile, your energy levels will increase significantly. Your mind will also become clearer and sharper. For the vast majority of those who strictly follow this program, angina pain will dramatically decrease or disappear. Your blood pressure will drop (if it's now too high). Many other cardiovascular symptoms will fade away.

Before you make any significant changes in your diet, lifestyle, and medication, you should consult your physician and remain under his or her guidance. This is very powerful medicine and therefore it may be essential to have medical guidance as your condition improves with the McDougall Program for a Healthy Heart.

I must emphasize that compliance is the key to this program. By fol-

lowing my recommendations faithfully and consistently, you are laying
the foundation for what can be termed a phoenixlike restoration of your
health. Those parts of your psyche that have been telling you for years that
you will never regain your youthful vitality and appearance are wrong.
Stick to this program and you will witness your own transformation.

The diet is broken down into three categories of foods. The first contains
those foods that you can eat without limit, except the limitations imposed
by the size of your stomach (and your good sense). The second group contains foods that can only be eaten in limited amounts, and then only for
those who are free of certain conditions. If you currently suffer from the
conditions named below, you should avoid the foods listed in group II.
The third group contains foods that should be avoided completely.

The McDougall Diet

I. Eat all you want of the following foods:

- **Whole grains,** including amaranth, barley, brown rice, buck-
  wheat, bulgur, corn, millet, oatmeal, quinoa, wheat, and whole wheat
  berries. Also, a wide variety of noodles made from these whole
  grains and lightly sifted grains.
- **Whole grain flour products,** such as whole grain noodles and
  whole grain breads, including wheat, rye, sourdough wheat and
  rye; multigrain breads made of whole, unrefined grains. One caveat,
  however: *Do not eat any flour product that contains oils or fats.
  Oils and fats are often hidden in baked flour goods. Read the labels
  carefully!*
- **Potatoes, sweet potatoes, and yams.**
- **Squashes,** such as acorn, buttercup, butternut, hubbard, and summer.
- **Beans and peas,** including aduki, black, black-eyed peas, chickpeas,
  fava, green peas, kidney, lentils, lima, mung, navy, pinto, soybeans
  (yellow and black), split peas, and string beans.
- **Green and yellow vegetables,** such as broccoli, brussels sprouts,
  cabbage, celery, Chinese cabbage, collard greens, endive, escarole,
  kale, leeks, lettuce (dark), mustard greens, sprouts, and watercress.
- **Round vegetables,** such as cucumber, okra, onions, pepper (red,
  green, and yellow), and tomato, and a wide variety of **mush-**

rooms, including button, cèpe, cremini, oyster, portobello, and shiitake.
* **Root vegetables,** including beets, carrots, daikon radish, parsnips, red radish, rutabaga, turnips.
* **Mild spices and cooking herbs,** including allspice, anise, basil, bay leaf, caraway, cardamom, cayenne, cilantro (coriander leaves), cinnamon, cloves, cumin, dill, fennel, garlic, ginger, mint, mustard, nutmeg, oregano, pepper, rosemary, saffron, sage, tarragon, and thyme.

II. Eat limited amounts of the following foods, but only if you do not currently suffer from one or more of the illnesses described below.

* **Fruit, fruit juice, and dried fruit**—limited to two to three servings per day.

Caution:

Research has shown that fructose, the type of sugar found in the greatest concentrations in most fruit, significantly raises blood triglyceride and cholesterol levels, especially in sensitive people on a high-fat diet.

Fruit contains three types of sugars: fructose, glucose, and sucrose. Of these three, fructose is the most abundant in the vast majority of fruits. Fructose is also present in honey (in very high quantities), table sugar, and many refined foods in which fruit sugar is added. In addition, many juices and drinks are sweetened with fructose. High-fructose corn syrup is one of the most common sweeteners used in packaged foods today. Again, reading labels is a must.

Fructose increases LDL and VLDL particles in the blood, which cause atherosclerosis and heart disease. Meanwhile, fructose does nothing for HDL, the good cholesterol. Since LDLs and VLDLs increase, and HDLs remain constant—which in this case means they become proportionately lower to LDLs and VLDLs—the net effect of fructose can be to increase your risk of heart disease.

This rise in triglycerides and cholesterol is small and nonthreatening in people who have low triglycerides and eat a low-fat, high-fiber diet. But if you eat a high-fat diet and eat lots of fruit, you're placing yourself at risk. Not surprisingly, dietary fat and fructose combine synergistically to drive both triglycerides and cholesterol levels even higher.

What is most disturbing is that fructose seems to have the most deleterious effect on people who are already at risk of heart attacks and strokes, those who already have elevated triglyceride levels, those with diabetes and high blood pressure, and postmenopausal women. (You will recall from Chapter 1 that postmenopausal women are at greater risk of having a heart attack than premenopausal women.) In these people, the rise in triglycerides and cholesterol resulting from fruit intake appears to be higher than in healthy adults.

My Recommendation:

Avoid fruit, fruit juice, and other simple sugars if your blood triglyceride level is above 150 mg/dl or if you have heart disease, high blood pressure, or diabetes.

- **Sugar and sweeteners.** Use the same criteria for sugar as was described for consumption of fruit. White sugar, known as sucrose, is a disaccharide composed of glucose and fructose.

Sugar can be eaten in small amounts, but only if your triglyceride level does not exceed 150 mg/dl, and you do not suffer from high cholesterol, heart disease, high blood pressure, or diabetes. Avoid all foods that contain sugar, along with fats and oils. All sugars drive up triglyceride levels, though sucrose and glucose don't elevate blood triglyceride and cholesterol levels nearly as much as fructose.

Sugar is sugar. There is little difference in nutritional effect among honey, maple syrup, molasses, brown sugar, or white sugar. They are all simple carbohydrates, best described as "empty calories." They contain no fiber, protein, or fat, and contribute little or nothing to vitamin and mineral needs. Artificial sweeteners have their drawbacks, too. Their taste is not as pleasant as that of natural sugars, and they can cause unpleasant reactions, such as headaches, in sensitive people. A few people claim even more severe reactions. Artificial sweeteners can increase your appetite and encourage weight gain.

- **High-fat plant foods.** Limit your intake of high-fat plant foods, including nuts, nut butters (such as peanut and sesame butters), seeds, seed spreads (tahini), avocados, coconut, olives, and soybean products, including tofu (which contains approximately 54 percent fat). These vegetable foods are all high in fat, and may indirectly increase your risk of heart attack and other cardiovascular diseases.

- **Salt.** Salt is permissible in small amounts—½ teaspoon per day—unless you suffer from heart failure, salt-sensitive hypertension, or edema (water retention).

Only a fraction of people with high blood pressure experience an elevation in blood pressure when they consume salt. Nevertheless, whenever possible, use salt-free seasonings and spices and herbs that can serve as healthful alternatives to salt. When using salt, sprinkle it on the surface of food to get the maximum flavor with the minimum amount used.

A few light sprinkles of salt will be enough for most people. Each half teaspoon of salt adds only 1,150 mg of sodium. This generous amount used daily will please most people's palates. Altogether, with the sodium in the basic foods, this amounts to a total of 1,450 mg a day; 550 mg below the 2,000 mg "low-sodium" diet served to patients dying of "heart disease" in your local hospital's intensive care unit. To bring the sodium intake up to the average of more than 5,000 mg used daily by most Americans, you would have to pour more than 2 teaspoons of salt daily on the surface of your starch-based meals. This amount of salt would make the food unpalatable for most people.

Soy sauce provides a flavorful alternative to plain table salt. Don't be fooled into thinking there is no sodium in soy sauce. The regular varieties have 800 mg of sodium per tablespoon, the low-salt varieties have 500 mg per tablespoon. When choosing a brand of soy sauce, avoid the ingredient monosodium glutamate (MSG). Many people have reactions to this substance, and, of course, it represents another source of sodium. Soy sauce is also sold under the name Tamari. There are variations to the taste of soy sauces, depending upon the producer. Probably you will develop a preference for one brand.

Canned tomato products commonly contain large amounts of sodium. If you are salt-sensitive you will need to purchase the low-sodium varieties. For salt-free alternatives, use chopped fresh tomatoes in place of canned tomatoes, and in place of tomato sauce puree fresh tomatoes in a blender.

- **Alcohol.** Moderate alcohol consumption—by that I mean less than 2 ounces per day—is permissible if your triglycerides are below 150 mg/dl. Alcohol raises triglycerides in the blood and, when drunk in excess, can cause a number of cardiovascular diseases, including high blood pressure, heart failure, stroke, and cardiomyopathy (a disease that reduces the ability of the heart muscle to contract). Alcohol is related to many other illnesses as well, including cirrhosis of the liver, breast cancer, hepatitis, and disorders of the nervous, digestive, urinary, and reproductive systems.

Several studies have shown that people who drink 2 ounces of alcohol or less per day tend to live longer than those who abstain entirely, or who drink more than 2 ounces per day. Moderate amounts of alcohol raise blood levels of HDL cholesterol.

Two 12-ounce beers contain approximately 1 ounce of alcohol. Six ounces of wine contain 1 ounce of alcohol. A 3-ounce glass of distilled spirits contains 1 ounce of alcohol.

GUIDELINES FOR USING SUGAR, SALT, AND SPICE

Avoid Salt	Avoid Sugar	Avoid Spice
if you have:	if you have:	if you have:
high blood pressure	high triglycerides	gastritis
heart muscle failure	high cholesterol	colitis
most kidney disease	hypoglycemia	sensitive intestine allergy
swelling (edema)	diabetes	

III. Avoid the following foods.

1. Eat no animal foods. Avoid all foods of animal origin, including the following: red meat, poultry, fish, seafood, eggs, milk, butter, cheese, yogurt, and sour cream. These foods contain extremely high quantities of fat and cholesterol. In fact, animal products are the primary source of saturated fat in the diet. Saturated fat, as we've already seen, dramatically raises blood cholesterol and leads to atherosclerosis and heart disease. All forms of fat increase your chance of contracting diabetes, cancer, obesity, and other degenerative diseases.

Animal foods are also loaded with protein. Protein demineralizes bones and leads to osteoporosis. Excess protein also causes kidney disease and kidney stones. Protein from animal sources has been linked to several kinds of cancer as well.

Animal foods contain no fiber, which is essential for healthy elimination of waste from the body. Fiber also lowers cholesterol levels and regulates blood sugar and insulin levels. The two latter benefits help to control appetite. High-fiber diets increase food satiety and satisfaction, and depress hunger, which allows you to lose weight while you feel full. Finally, foods of animal origin are low in many essential vitamins and minerals.

Avoid low-fat dairy products. Once milk protein enters the bloodstream, it is perceived by the body as a foreign substance. The immune system reacts to the protein as it would to any other antigen: It makes antibodies to neutralize it. These antibodies may mistakenly attack the arteries themselves, initiating the early injury stage of atherosclerosis. They may also attack and destroy enzyme systems that remove cholesterol from the body. High levels of antibodies to milk proteins are often found in severe atherosclerosis.

So it is not just the cholesterol and fat in dairy products that damage the arteries; dairy proteins are also involved. Therefore, people looking to prevent heart attacks should avoid the low-fat dairy products as well.

2. Eliminate all oils. Oil is a liquid fat. Most of us think of various types of vegetable oils as containing only polyunsaturated or monounsaturated fats and therefore safe for the heart. The fact is that all oils damage the arteries and cause progression of atherosclerosis, as we saw in Chapter 3. Vegetable fats cause sludging of the blood and diminish oxygen flow to the heart and other tissues. People with heart disease are in no position to decrease the amount of oxygen that flows to their heart.

All fats increase weight. As I always say, the fat you eat is the body fat you wear, and weight is a risk factor in heart disease. In addition to these illnesses, oils have been linked to gallbladder disease and diabetes, also a risk factor in heart disease.

3. Avoid sulfur dioxide and MSG. Many people have allergic reactions to sulfur dioxide or MSG (monosodium glutamate). Sulfur dioxide, sodium metabisulfate, and potassium metabisulfite—referred to as sulfite agents—are often used as preservatives on light-colored, dehydrated (dried) fruits, such as apples, apricots, bleached raisins, pears, and peaches, and in wines (even nonalcoholic wines and beer).

They are also commonly used in restaurants to preserve the fresh looks of salads, uncooked vegetables, avocado dips, and shrimp. Salad bars can keep greens from wilting and turning brown for days with a few sulfite sprayings. You may get a hint of whether or not the salad ingredients are preserved with these chemicals by the amount of ice used around the salad bowls—the more ice, the less likely sulfites have been used. But just to be on the safe side, ask the waitperson. Some people have severe reactions to these substances, including asthma attacks, weakness, tightness of the chest, and—rarely—shock and coma.

MSG is a sodium salt of one of the most common amino acids found in proteins. It is used as a flavoring agent in cooking and in a wide variety of processed and packaged foods. The most common unpleasant reactions to MSG are headache, nausea, lightheadedness, increased salivation, fullness, and heartburn. Less frequent symptoms include warmth (burning), tightness, weakness, tingling and pain of the chest, arms, neck, and/or face; thirst, sore throat, asthma, and psychiatric reactions. Cooks in some Chinese restaurants use this flavor enhancer liberally; thus, the reaction is commonly known as "Chinese restaurant syndrome."

HEALTHFUL ALTERNATIVES

Don't Eat	*Healthful Substitutes*
Milk (for cereal or cooking)	Nonfat soy milk Rice Milk (recipe on page 294) extra water
Milk (as beverage)	None; drink water, herb tea, or cereal beverages
Butter	None, or Corn Butter (recipe on page 302) as spread
Cheese	None; or Melty Cheese Sauce (recipe on page 323)
Cottage cheese	None
Yogurt	None
Sour cream	None
Eggs (in cooking)	Ener-G Egg replacer (for binding)

Don't Eat	Healthful Substitutes
Eggs (for eating)	None
Meat, poultry, fish	Starchy vegetables, whole grains, pastas, and beans
Mayonnaise	None
Vegetable oils (for pans)	None; use Teflon, SilverStone, or silicone-coated (Baker's Secret) pots and pans
Vegetable oils (in recipes)	None; omit or replace with water, prune puree, or applesauce for moisture
White rice (refined)	Whole grain (brown) rice or other whole grains
White flour (refined)	Whole grain flours
Refined and sugar-coated cereals	Any acceptable hot or cold cereal (see list on pages 267–68)
Coconut	None
Chocolate	Carob powder or nonfat cocoa powder
Coffee; decaffeinated coffee	Noncaffeinated herb tea, black teas, cereal beverages, hot water with lemon
Colas and un-colas	Mineral water or seltzer (flavored or plain)
Table salt	Salt-free or low-sodium seasoning mixes, low-sodium soy sauce
Table sugar	None if you have heart disease or elevated cholesterol or triglycerides; otherwise, use honey, pure maple syrup, or pure fruit spread sparingly

Three Guidelines for Healthy Eating Patterns

1. Eat until you're satisfied. As long as you are eating the prescribed foods, you can eat until you are full without worrying about proportions or calories or your cholesterol level. On this diet, your cholesterol level will fall and your risk of heart disease will fall with it.

As an added bonus, you'll likely lose weight—even while you eat until you are full. (For more information about weight loss and a program to lose weight healthfully and rapidly, see my book, *The McDougall Program for Maximum Weight Loss*.)

For those of you who need to lose large amounts of weight, you will want to limit your intake of flour products, including breads, bagels, and pastas. Instead, make rice, corn, potatoes, and green and yellow vegetables the mainstay of your meal plan. But don't go hungry!

2. Eat frequent meals if it helps your compliance. Some people find it easier to stay on the diet if they eat four or six small meals per day, as opposed to three meals daily. Eating more frequently does not necessarily mean having a higher cholesterol level or even being overweight. In fact, research has shown that those who ate small, but frequent meals (seventeen meals a day in one study) lowered their cholesterol more effectively than those who ate fewer larger meals. The same study also showed that obese people tend to eat fewer, but larger, meals than lean people. Eating only one or two times a day signals your body that you are fasting. This only encourages your body to want more food when you finally do sit down to a full-course meal. Fewer meals, therefore, often translate into more food at each sitting, which can mean a stronger desire for foods outside the McDougall Program for a Healthy Heart. Many people feel that if they remain sated, especially when they've first started the diet, it's easier to adjust to the new foods and stay with the program.

Fill your plate with a reasonable amount of food. After you have finished that portion, wait about twenty minutes for digestion to start. You will find your hunger drive diminishing quickly. If you're still hungry after twenty minutes, then have seconds and again wait. This is a variation on the importance of frequent meals. You move from a gorging pattern to grazing, with greater satisfaction of hunger, and less food intake.

3. For maximum satiety and satisfaction, include beans and legumes in your meals. Legumes, which include all beans, peas, and lentils, contain large amounts of protein. They are rich in carbohydrates and contain soluble fiber, which binds with cholesterol and helps to eliminate it from your body. Fiber also increases the transit time of your food and aids in digestion. Finally, beans are rich and luscious foods, which improve the satisfaction of a meal. There are so many ways that you can prepare beans and so many delicious spices that can be added to them. (See Mary's recipes in Part IV.)

However, you should limit your beans, peas, and lentils to one cup a day, on the average, to protect yourself from any adverse effects of too much protein and the possible loss of calcium from your bones.

Whole Foods Provide Complete Nutrition

As I mentioned earlier, my diet provides all the nutrition your body needs to be strong, healthy, and vital. Studies have shown that a single starch-based food, such as potato, combined with a fruit or a vegetable, provides all the protein, essential fats and amino acids, vitamins, and minerals needed by adults and growing children. Even extreme examples of starch-based diets have been shown to be nutritionally adequate.

Whole grains and vegetables are the principal sources of antioxidants and other immune-boosting nutrients. Squash, yellow and orange vegetables, and leafy greens are the greatest sources of vitamins A and C. Whole grains provide a range of vitamins and minerals, including vitamin E. Grains are abundant sources of fiber and complex carbohydrates, which are the body's primary source of energy.

The only nutrient that may be deficient on a strict vegetable diet is vitamin B_{12}, which is present in animal foods, including fish. If you follow the McDougall Program for a Healthy Heart strictly for more than three years—without eating any animal foods as part of your regular diet— you should take a vitamin B_{12} supplement (5 micrograms daily). This rule also applies to pregnant women and nursing mothers on the Mc-Dougall Program.

PROGRAM MODIFICATIONS

Occasionally, variations in the McDougall Program are made for individuals. Common dietary modifications include:

- *For faster weight loss:* Eliminate all flour products (breads, bagels, pastas, etc.) and increase your consumption of green and yellow vegetables.
- *For weight gain:* Increase flour products, add dried fruits, and occasionally include high-fat plant foods.

- *To relieve indigestion (gastritis):* Try eliminating all raw vegetables (especially onions, green peppers, cucumbers, and radishes), fruit juices, and hot sauces.
- Limit legumes (beans, peas, and lentils) to 1 cup per day because of their higher protein content.
- *For people with kidney and liver disorders and those with gout and osteoporosis:* Severely restrict protein from beans, peas, and lentils.
- Limit fruits to three servings per day because of the simple sugars.
- *For people with elevated blood triglycerides:* Restrict all simple sugars (especially those from fruit and fruit juice).
- *For people with food allergies or sensitivities:* Eliminate troublesome foods from the diet or restrict them according to your own needs. For details on nutrition and medical issues refer to *The McDougall Plan, McDougall's Medicine, The McDougall Program,* and *The McDougall Program for Maximum Weight Loss.*

Meal Planning: How to Substitute and Add Flavor to Your Healthy Foods— Without a Lot of Effort

When planning home-cooked meals for yourself and your family, begin by deciding how much time you are willing to spend in the kitchen. If you have been the kind of cook who burns a slice of animal flesh on two sides and calls that dinner, the healthy (fast) alternative is to microwave a potato or two and boil a bag of frozen vegetables. These foods provide excellent nutrition and their taste can be enhanced by adding bottled no-oil salad dressings, salsas, spaghetti sauces, ketchup, or barbecue sauces (see the list of Canned and Packaged Products on page 266).

On the other hand, if you like to spend time in the kitchen, cooking meals from scratch, then a starch-based diet can be as rich, as varied, and as flavorful as anything prepared in the finest restaurant. The recipes in our books contain detailed instructions for preparation of ingredients, and accurate preparation and cooking times to help you. The instructions are written simply and completely, so that even a novice cook should be successful on the first try.

Planning Ahead Makes Everything Easier

Begin by taking a few minutes to plan your menu for the week. Write down the ingredients you'll need to buy at the supermarket and health food stores. A written list will save you time and money. Plan your meals around a starch food for each meal. Introduce variety by choosing different starches, in order to avoid serving pasta three days in a row.

Hearty Breakfasts

Traditional breakfast foods, such as toast, cereals, pancakes, and waffles—all made of whole grains—are included on the McDougall Program. Only a slight variation in the ingredients of these foods need to be made. Many people can't imagine eating a breakfast cereal without milk or cream. The simple solution for a hot cereal is to make it with a little extra water and top the mix with a sweetener like brown sugar or applesauce, if your health allows. If you need to pour something white on a hot or cold cereal, use rice milk or nonfat soy milk. Rice milk has a lighter, sweeter taste than soy milk and is much lower in fat content. Made from fermented brown rice, it is white in color and has a consistency resembling cow's milk. Rice milk can be found in most natural foods stores or can be made at home.

RICE MILK

Blend 1 cup of cooked whole grain (brown) rice with 4 cups of water in an electric blender. Add 1 teaspoon of vanilla for flavor (optional). Filter through a strainer to remove coarse rice husks.

Hash brown potatoes are a favorite in our home. They can be made from scratch or purchased frozen in boxes and bags. One type of hash brown, called "potatoes O'Brien," is cut into quarter-inch chunks, and can be found mixed with onions and green peppers. Pour the desired amount of potatoes from the bag into a nonstick fry pan or a nonstick wok, and cook for 20 to 25 minutes on medium heat, stirring occasionally. Compressed square patties of shredded potatoes sold in boxes of four to eight are my favorite. These become brown on a nonstick griddle after about 10 minutes per side at medium heat on a gas stove. (Cooking on an electric stove takes a little longer.)

Variety in our breakfast of hash brown potatoes comes at the dining table. Our daughter, younger son, and Mary top their potatoes with three different brands of bottled mild salsa. Our older son uses ketchup. I use a mixture of Lea & Perrins Steak Sauce and Bull's Eye Barbeque Sauce (quite a tangy taste). The possibilities for toppings are endless: Try oil-free salad dressings, horseradish, Tabasco, Worcestershire sauce, packaged (or leftover) soup, or spaghetti sauce.

Bagels, toast, or rice cakes, either plain or topped with no-sugar jams, are fast and simple breakfasts. Recipes for more complicated breakfasts can be found in Part IV of this book. There's nothing sacred about what you eat for breakfast. I'm sure you've had leftover pizza or a burrito for breakfast in the past. You can do the same with healthy foods. The first meal of the day in Asian countries is often the same as the middle and last meals: rice and vegetables.

Hot drinks for breakfast should be noncaffeinated, such as cereal beverages like Postum, Cafix, and Pero. Herb teas are satisfying selections. Some people enjoy hot water with lemon juice. Traditional cold drinks are fruit juices, although some people can't tolerate them well because of indigestion caused by acidity. They also raise triglycerides and cholesterol in sensitive people.

Tasty Lunches

Because it falls in the middle of the day, lunch is usually quickly prepared, eaten almost as fast, and forgotten in no time. Leftovers make lunch easy. Among the leftovers that commonly find their way to our lunch table are bean dishes, grain dishes, and soups left to thicken as they cool. Also, you can make wonderful sandwiches from lettuce, sprouts, sliced tomatoes, onions, and leafy greens. For more flavor, add dashes of Tabasco, barbecue, or steak sauce, or of an oil-free salad dressing, or of one of the many mustards available.

Do you fill your pita bread pocket too full, and then have trouble holding on to it? Here's a way around that dilemma: Cut the pita bread in half around its *edge—rather than cutting it along its equator—*leaving two flat circles. Layer the foods you want over one half and cover with the other; eat the combination like a sandwich or with a fork and knife. You can also spread leftovers on your circles of pita bread and add garnishes and sauces to them; then roll up the filled circle like a burrito.

Some instant dry soups packaged in paper containers make excellent lunches. Just add hot water and wait a couple of minutes for lunch to be ready. Instant soups come in many varieties (see the list of Canned and Packaged Products on page 266).

Potatoes are a great foundation for lunches as well as breakfasts. Bake, boil, or microwave them. Cut them crosswise in half, split them lengthwise down the middle, or mash the whites, or skins and all, before adding the chosen topping. Instant dry soups can be made with half the recommended volume of hot water, and then poured over a cooked potato, providing a substantial covering with spicy flavors. Or top your potato with oil-free salad dressings, salsas, barbecue sauces, ketchup, steak sauces, horseradish, Tabasco, Worcestershire sauce, spaghetti sauce, or any other oil-free, animal product–free favorite sauce.

If you pack a lunch for work or school, use covered plastic containers. Carry cooked potatoes in a sealed plastic bag. Soups and other liquids can be stored hot or cold in a thermos. Fresh tap water, bottled water, bottled mineral water, juices, and bags of herb teas are convenient beverages for packed lunches.

Satisfying Dinners

Your dinners will be planned around starches, with the addition of fresh or frozen vegetables and fruits, mixed with your favorite seasonings. Your first goal is to decide on a few selections that please everyone who will share the meals.

First Rule: Keep It Simple

When we first started eating this way more than fifteen years ago, Mary would make three or four different dishes for each meal in an effort to imitate the American style of serving a main dish, two or three side dishes, and a dessert. She soon learned that too much variety makes for too much work. The modern practice is an anomaly. Your grandparents and mine probably kept meals simple: porridge for breakfast, soups for lunch, and a stew for dinner. You too should plan your meals around a single dish, possibly supplementing it with a salad or vegetable side dish. Think of pasta with a topping, or rice covered with a sauce, or just plain soup and wholesome bread.

Make Quantities

The serving size may cause you some concern if you are cooking for only one or two "small eaters." But we suggest that you still make at least the full quantity called for by a recipe and refrigerate or freeze the leftover portions. This will save you preparation time later—and money, too. It will also provide you with something tasty on short notice. All of these foods freeze well, except the ones made with arrowroot or cornstarch, which become sort of lumpy when frozen. If you plan to freeze foods containing these thickeners, you should separate and freeze the surplus amounts without adding the cornstarch or arrowroot. Add the arrowroot or cornstarch to the separated portions later, when you heat them.

Make an extra effort to have on hand portions of frozen beans and rice. Doing so will cut down on preparation time for recipes that use these slow-cooking foods.

Two Weeks of Sample Menus for
The McDougall Program for a Healthy Heart

These are only sample suggestions—you do not have to follow this menu. In fact, you will probably find the program more enjoyable if you go through the recipes and make up a menu plan of the foods you already like. Repeat selections as often as you like—most people enjoy a limited selection of items they eat over and over again. Bread and bagels should be made without oil or dairy products and may be found in most supermarkets. Assorted green and yellow vegetables may be added to any menu as desired. Baked tortilla chips made without oil may be purchased in most natural food stores.

DAY 1

BREAKFAST

Cooked Cereal
Bagel
Herb Tea

LUNCH	DINNER
Spicy White Bean Spread	Italian Potato Salad
Pita Bread	Tomato Spinach Risotto
Assorted Chopped Fresh Vegetables	Fresh Bread
Water or Soda Water	Herb Tea or Water

DAY 2

BREAKFAST

Pancakes
Herb Tea

LUNCH	DINNER
Mexican Corn Soup	Garbanzo Salad
Fresh Bread	French Bean Casserole
Water or Soda Water	Herb Tea or Water

DAY 3

BREAKFAST

Breakfast Tortillas
Herb Tea

LUNCH	DINNER
Aram Rolls	Portuguese Bean Soup
Spinach Cilantro Dip with	Macaroni and Oaty Cheese
Baked Tortilla Chips	Herb Tea or Water
Water or Soda Water	

DAY 4

BREAKFAST
French Toast
Herb Tea

LUNCH
Corn Chowder
Fresh Bread
Couscous Salad
Water or Soda Water

DINNER
South of the Border Salad
Kelly's Manicotti
Herb Tea or Water

DAY 5

BREAKFAST
Hash Brown Potatoes
Herb Tea

LUNCH
Garbanzo Spread
Fresh Bread
Assorted Chopped Fresh Vegetables
Water

DINNER
Dilled Broccoli Soup
Fried Rice
Herb Tea or Water

DAY 6

BREAKFAST
Cooked Cereal
Herb Tea

LUNCH
Quick Bean and Vegetable Chowder
Fresh Bread
Water or Soda Water

DINNER
Curried Corn Salad
Stuffed Twice-Baked Potatoes
Rich Brown Gravy
Herb Tea or Water

DAY 7

BREAKFAST
Breakfast Tortillas
Herb Tea

LUNCH
Healthy Heart Burgers
Whole Wheat Buns
Water or Soda Water

DINNER
Creamy Vegetable Soup
Garbanzo a la King
Fresh Bread
Herb Tea or Water

DAY 8

BREAKFAST
Pancakes
Herb Tea

LUNCH
Three Potato Chowder
Fresh Bread
Water or Soda Water

DINNER
Burman's Perfect Salad
Southwest Vegetable
Griddle Cakes
Fast Chili Topping
Herb Tea or Water

DAY 9

BREAKFAST
French Toast
Herb Tea

LUNCH
"Cheese" Spread
Pita Bread
Assorted Chopped Fresh Vegetables
Water or Soda Water

DINNER
Italian Broccoli Salad
Basque Paella
Herb Tea or Water

DAY 10

BREAKFAST
Hash Brown Potatoes
Herb Tea

LUNCH	DINNER
Hearty Bean Soup	Hot Cole Slaw
Fresh Bread	Southwest Kasha Bake
Water or Soda Water	Herb Tea or Water

DAY 11

BREAKFAST
Cooked Cereal
Bagel
Herb Tea

LUNCH	DINNER
Black Bean and Orzo Salad	Chard and Squash Soup
Baked French Fries	Potatoes Mexicali
Water or Soda Water	Pita Bread
	Herb Tea or Water

DAY 12

BREAKFAST
Breakfast Tortillas
Herb Tea

LUNCH	DINNER
Craig's Favorite Noodle Soup	Southwest Salad
Fresh Bread	Blanco Mexican Chili
Water or Soda Water	Herb Tea or Water

DAY 13

BREAKFAST

Pancakes
Herb Tea

LUNCH	DINNER
Monica's Burrito Filling	Tortilla Soup
Whole Wheat Tortillas	Southwest Jambalaya
Water or Soda Water	Fresh Bread
	Herb Tea or Water

DAY 14

BREAKFAST

French Toast
Herb Tea

LUNCH	DINNER
Vegetable Soup	Kit's Mock Guacamole with
Fresh Bread	Baked Tortilla Chips
Water or Soda Water	Julie's Black Bean Torta
	Herb Tea or Water

Adjustment Is Only a Matter of Time

This diet, if followed properly, can make you well. All you need is the willingness to eat these foods. At first, giving up all those fatty foods that have made you ill seems difficult, if not downright hard. Yet, if you give my program a few weeks, you'll be wondering how you ate any other way. I can't tell you how many thousands of people have told me that when they first adopted the diet, they thought they'd never be able to change. And then, after a day or two, they began to like the McDougall foods. And after a week or two, they actually found themselves craving the very foods that were making them well. They were enjoy-ing—even delighting in—foods that are the best form of medicine.

If you think that this cannot happen to you, please give yourself the chance to be proven wrong. Give the program a few weeks, two months perhaps, and witness the transformation of your health, your physical vi-tality, your appearance, and your tastebuds. Once you see the results and begin to enjoy the food, you will not want to live any other way.

6. McDougall's Exercise for Healthy Hearts

- *The first rule for exercise: It should fun.*
- *You don't need a lot of exercise to derive a lot of benefit.*
- *Exercise reduces stress and boosts optimism.*
- *Walking is still the best exercise for your heart.*

Exercising after a diagnosis of heart disease can be frightening for the obvious reason that you're afraid of bringing on a heart attack—or, for many of you, a second heart attack. Paradoxically, exercise—coupled with the correct diet—is essential to restoring the strength of your heart. My father was one of the many millions of people who learned this lesson.

After my father had his first heart attack, he suffered all the same doubts about his body and especially his heart that most people who have had heart attacks experience. Would he be able to do any kind of physical exercise ever again? he wondered. Would his life suddenly be restricted? Within three weeks after suffering a heart attack, he was walking five times a week—a mile at a time. And within a month, he had answered all his nagging doubts. He could recover not only his health, but his strength. And, no, he would not become an invalid. Just the opposite: Dad was as active in his sixties as most men are in their forties and fifties.

After he reached his early seventies, he had some setbacks, which brought on another heart attack in 1994. In August of that year, he came to visit me and he was clearly timid about pushing himself physically. We were in the backyard pool together. I asked him why he was only wading, not swimming. My dad was a terrific swimmer; as a youth he had been on the navy springboard diving team and used to love the water. But now he was worried about what the strain of swimming might do to him, and confided as much to me. "I really don't see any problem with it, Dad," I told him. "But you do whatever makes you comfortable." With that, I walked back to the house to make us lunch. When I looked into the backyard, I saw my dad swimming laps in the pool and doing great. From that point onward, he was free of most of his fear. He didn't push himself too hard. He respected the need for gradual improvement, but he didn't let the fear keep him from regaining his health and his strength.

I tell this story because I know how afraid people are after they've been diagnosed with heart disease or had a heart attack. That fear can stop you from exercising, which would be a mistake for most heart patients. At the same time, everyone with heart disease must be cautious. That's why I strongly urge everyone with a history of heart disease or other health problems to have a medical examination by their doctor before they start an exercise program, even the gentle recommendations I suggest in this chapter.

At the same time, I want you to know that exercise can be safe. All you need is a brisk little walk three to five times a week. If your health permits and you want to do more, by all means enjoy a more physical workout. But remember, exercise must be fun if it is to be maintained, and you needn't do any more than walk regularly to improve your cardiovascular and muscular fitness, and maintain it for life.

Aerobic Exercise Boosts Oxygen Intake—
and Oxygen Means Life

For most people, I recommend aerobic exercises, and the one I think is best for people with heart disease is walking. It's safe and it provides an excellent aerobic workout, even if you do nothing more than stroll. Other aerobic exercises include jogging, bicycle riding, cross-country and downhill skiing, tennis, basketball, and racquetball.

Aerobic exercise causes you to inhale greater quantities of oxygen into your lungs, which means that you increase the amount of oxygen flowing to your heart, brain, muscles and tissues throughout your body. This also increases the amount of oxygen your muscles can absorb and utilize.

The amount of oxygen the muscles use declines as we get older, setting off an array of symptoms normally associated with aging, such as a loss of stamina, alertness, and resistance to disease. Conversely, regular aerobic exercise increases the amount of oxygen your muscles utilize, which in turn increases your stamina and mental acuity, and boosts your immune system. It also does wonders for your heart.

Too Many Benefits to Count

There are so many benefits that are derived from exercise that it's difficult to name them all. And as long as you don't overdo it, exercise boosts your immune system. Here again, we see that moderation really is the key: Small amounts of exercise done three to five times a week—for at least thirty minutes per session—is best for your health in every respect. Pushing yourself too hard depresses immune function and consequently lowers your resistance to infection with viruses and possibly other diseases like cancer.

When you exercise, you force your heart to beat faster in order to provide more blood and oxygen to muscles throughout the body. By doing so, you are requiring your heart to pump more blood per beat in order to meet the body's needs for blood and oxygen. In effect, your heart is being trained to work more efficiently. It is capable of pumping much more blood than it could in the past, in the same amount of time.

Once the heart gets in better shape, it starts to slow down. Why not? It can now do the same amount of work with less effort. This means that as your heart rate slows, your heart can rest longer between beats.

Changing Blood Chemistry for the Better

Even small amounts of regular aerobic exercise pump up your high-density lipoprotein. As your HDLs increase, your risk of heart attack decreases. Remarkably, HDLs rise even faster among those who are overweight and haven't been on an exercise program before.

You may be under the impression that you have to do a lot of exercise to improve your HDL level, but that isn't the case. Even regular strolling increases HDL levels. A study published in the *Journal of the American Medical Association* (December 1991) showed that strolling at a leisurely pace of about three miles per hour significantly increased HDLs in fifty-nine women, who walked between twelve and twenty minutes per session, three to four times per week.

Exercise also lowers triglyceride levels, which makes your blood less viscous and less likely to sludge. That, of course, improves the flow of oxygen to muscles throughout your body, including your heart muscle. Finally, exercise lowers blood pressure. For many, exercise alone can normalize blood pressure.

Not surprisingly, these and other benefits have a rather striking effect on longevity.

Boost Your Chances of Living Longer

In November 1989, the *Journal of the American Medical Association* published the landmark study done at the Institute for Aerobics Research and the Cooper Clinic of Dallas that showed that even small amounts of exercise increased longevity and prevented major diseases. The scientists examined the impact of exercise on mortality of some 13,344 people, and found that exercise not only increased longevity, but also significantly reduced the risk of contracting heart disease and cancer. Unlike previous research, which depended on questionnaires to determine fitness, the scientists in this study conducted treadmill stress tests on all the participants and thus determined their fitness and cardiovascular health. Following the examinations, each man and woman in the study was placed in one of five groups, based on his or her degree of fitness. The categories ranged from sedentary people who engaged in no exercise at all to well-conditioned athletes who ran marathons. Not surprisingly, those who exercised the least died the soonest. Remarkably, the scientists found that the greatest health benefit fell to those in the second level of fitness, the people who only walked a half hour a day, three or four times a week. These people had less than half the chance of suffering a heart attack or contracting cancer than those who lived sedentary lifestyles. Remarkably, the mortality rates among the four groups that exercised—which included walkers, well-conditioned athletes, and even men and women who ran marathons—differed only slightly.

The research showed that small amounts of exercise provided the biggest benefit.

Other research has confirmed this finding. A study of 16,936 Harvard alumni, aged 35 to 74, found that those alumni who burned 500 to 3,500 calories per week on exercise showed significantly lower rates of mortality, especially from cardiovascular and respiratory diseases, than those who lived sedentary lives. Mortality rates were one-fourth to one-third lower among those who expended 2,000 calories per week in exercise than among those who did no exercise at all.

Mortality rates are one thing, but the quality of life is quite another. You may live to be 70 no matter what you do, but whether or not you enjoy those years is everything. Health problems can make your 70 years on this planet a living nightmare. On the other hand, you can adopt the McDougall Program for a Healthy Heart and do a great deal to change the quality of those 70 years, including getting out each day and doing a little walking. Whether or not you live a year or two longer is almost beside the point. What you really want is to feel good and enjoy your life.

Reduce Stress, Improve Your Mood, and Lower Anxiety

As a sales manager at a large corporation, with nine people to supervise and the kind of job that requires frequent travel all over the country, Carol Major, 57, has all the ingredients of high stress and burnout. She manages to control the stress and avoid the related problems that are so common in her profession. How does she do it? "Exercise and the McDougall diet," says Carol. "Exercise helps me keep the stress level down and the job in perspective."

Carol, in fact, does a catalog's worth of physical exercise each morning. She begins with some stretching and some calisthenics (to keep her legs, stomach, and hips tight) and then does thirty minutes on her exercise bicycle. She also walks about a mile and a half a day.

Carol had aortic valve replacement surgery done in 1983; before then she could not exercise at all because her heart problems caused her to suffer chronic fatigue. After the surgery, she was permitted to exercise more frequently, but she still lacked the kind of energy she wanted, and felt she could have. A few years later, she discovered the McDougall Program through my books and radio shows. Since then, Carol says, "I've become totally convinced that this way of eating is the best way for me. I've got lots of energy and I feel great. I also see that whenever I go off the diet, I feel sluggish. But with the energy I have, I can do the exercises I like to do and I can keep my job's stress level down."

* * *

The benefits of exercise affect every area of your life. Regular exercise elevates your moods, improves your sense of well-being, raises your self-esteem, boosts your immune system, and increases your energy.

People who previously suffered chronic emotional problems reported feeling less stress, less anxiety, and fewer sieges of depression after they began exercising, according to a study published in the July 1991 issue of *Postgraduate Medicine*. These same people reported experiencing an increased capacity to handle stress without succumbing to negative thinking and emotional depression. The study also found that with consistent exercise, people undergo a kind of emotional transformation. They report feeling emotionally brighter, healthier, and more positive about life in general.

This is not simply talking oneself into a good mood. Exercise changes brain chemistry, which is the basis for many emotional disorders. After just twenty minutes of running, the brain increases its production of beta endorphins, which are morphinelike compounds that create the "natural high" runners frequently report. Even depression has been shown to be relieved with exercise.

A study conducted on police officers examined the psychological effects of aerobic exercise on one group, anaerobic exercise (in this case weight training) on another; and no exercise at all on a third. After ten weeks, the police officers who did the aerobic exercises reported greater improvements in well-being and greater reductions in stress than those who did the weight training, although both of these exercise groups reported significant improvements in mood and stress than the group who did no exercise at all.

Nature's Second-Best Beauty Treatment

Part of the reason people feel so good after they exercise is because they look good. Only a healthy diet has a greater impact on your appearance than exercise, but when the two are put together they are the surest road to physical beauty that I know of. Exercise burns calories, which means it lowers your weight. It will take off those oil and fat rolls on the stomach, thighs, and buttocks. It will make your skin healthier, brighter, and more alive.

As I showed in *McDougall's Program for Maximum Weight Loss*, there is no better approach to weight loss than a low-fat, no-cholesterol diet combined with a moderate exercise program. By following my diet, you can eat all of the recommended foods you want and still lose weight. Exercise makes you lose weight faster.

The Best and Safest Exercise for the Heart

Twenty minutes or more of brisk walking each day will change your life, especially if you are now out of shape and overweight. Walking provides all the benefits of a good aerobic workout, without the dangers that competitive sports present. Fifteen minutes of brisk walking—about four miles an hour—will burn almost as many calories as jogging that same mile. Yet, walking doesn't present the risk of injury or heart attack that jogging does.

Walking is safe if you have had a heart attack because there's little chance of overexerting yourself. If you feel angina pain come on, stop walking and rest until it passes. Then resume your walk at a more leisurely pace.

Tips to Make Your Walking Safe, Rewarding, and Comfortable

1. **"It's the shoes! It's gotta be the shoes!"** Yes, the shoes count. Be sure your walking shoe has a firm heel that will keep your foot tightly secured in the shoe. It should have a thick, resilient sole to cushion the impact of your foot against the ground. The shoe must also provide plenty of arch support. It must also have a wide toe. Don't buy shoes with a pointy toe; they will cause painful feet and possibly bunions later in life. Some experts recommend that a walking shoe should be a half-size larger than the size you're used to in order to accommodate a thicker sock (sometimes even two socks per foot) and to give your foot plenty of breathing room. Obviously, you don't want a shoe that's too big, but you may want to try a walking shoe that's a half-size larger to see if it feels better on your foot.

2. **Warm up and cool down.** Before you start your walk, do ten minutes of gentle stretching exercises. This will prepare your muscles and heart for your workout. To start up immediately, without a little warm-up stretching, may shock your muscles and cause cramping

later on. After you've walked, do another five or ten minutes of light stretching. This will allow your muscles and heart to cool down and resume their normal respiration.

3. Start slow and gain momentum. Don't launch yourself into your walk at top speed. Start out slow and work your way up to a more brisk pace as you feel your circulation improving and your energy rising. Also, you do not want to put too many demands on your heart immediately. If you are beginning an exercise program, you only need to reach 60 percent of your maximum heart rate to condition your heart, muscles, and respiratory system.

To find your maximum heart rate, subtract your age from 220. If you are 40 years old, your maximum heart rate would be 180. That means that a 40-year-old only needs to get his heart rate up to 108 and keep it there for fifteen to twenty minutes to enjoy a fitness-improving workout. For those who are more physically fit, 90 percent of maximum heart rate provides maximum conditioning. For a 40-year-old, that means 162 beats per minute.

4. Do three sessions per week for starters. If you are out of shape, have been diagnosed with heart disease, or have suffered a heart attack or a stroke, begin a walking program that concentrates on the amount of time you walk, rather than on distance or speed. I recommend that you start walking three times per week, and that each session last fifteen to twenty minutes. Avoid hills and walk on relatively flat surfaces. Maintain this practice for two to four weeks, until you feel your strength improving. Then, depending on your physical reaction to these sessions, increase your time to twenty-five to thirty minutes. After a few weeks, maintain at least the same thirty-minute session, but gradually increase your speed and distance walked within that thirty minutes. Eventually, try to increase your speed, distance, and time walked, until you've reached a point that provides you with a good workout that fits your schedule.

5. Can you walk and talk at the same time? One of the best ways to monitor your workout—and one of the simplest—is to see if you can talk effortlessly while you are walking. As long as you can talk easily while you are walking, you're not overexerting yourself. If you have trouble talking, you're walking too briskly and pushing yourself too hard. Slow down or rest.

Periodically, you may want to monitor your heart rate. While resting, place your first two fingers on your carotid artery in your neck, below the ear and jawline. Count the pulse beats as you count down ten seconds on a watch, and then multiply by six.

Heart rate is directly related to your oxygen consumption and the intensity of your exercise. As heart rate increases, so, too, do oxygen consumption and intensity level.

6. Hike in atmosphere. Walk in places that inspire you: forests, parks, meadows, and along rivers. For many, the ideal place to walk is down Main Street or in the local shopping mall. The ideal place lifts your mood; it gets your mind off your problems, and makes you lighter of spirit. In any case, change the locations from time to time. Make new discoveries in your hometown.

7. Become a social walker. Hike with friends and even join one of the many walking clubs. Many of these clubs conduct guided excursions through beautiful forests and natural wonders all over the country, and right in your own backyard.

8. Tune into tunes. Music makes exercise fun and easier. People who listen to music while they exercise, in fact, exercise longer than those who do not listen to music while working out. As we all know, music lifts the spirit, and the spirit lifts the body. It boosts your mood and gives you rhythm, which makes your exercise session more fun, less painful, and longer lasting.

9. Vary your walk with a world of machines. Stationary bicycles, treadmills, StairMasters, and NordicTrack skiers are just a few of the incredible array of exercise machines available today. You can walk, climb stairs, row a boat, cycle, and cross-country ski all in front of your television set or CD player. Put on your Walkman and do several miles in your living room. Many of these machines monitor heart rate and show how many calories you've burned in a given exercise session.

10. Walk *in* water. Water dramatically reduces the gravitational pull on your body, making you lighter and putting less stress on your joints. Chin-deep water, for example, makes you only one-tenth of your normal weight. That means there's a lot less stress on your back, knees, ankles, and feet. Water aerobics are wonderful for anyone with arthritis, back injuries, or weight problems, or for women who are pregnant. Most local YMCAs, YWCAs, and health clubs offer water aerobics classes for children to senior citizens.

11. Use the local resources. Most adult education programs, colleges, and universities offer surprisingly inexpensive health and fitness programs. Many of them have sliding-scale rates to fit most people's budgets. Many adult education programs offer very inexpensive yoga classes that incorporate light stretching and breathing exercises— a great way to improve your fitness and reacquaint yourself with your body, especially if you haven't exercised in years.

12. Trip the light fantastic and rekindle the heart. Walk to the music. Just about every town in America has dancing clubs. Square, contra, modern, jazz, and ballroom dancing are great forms of aerobic exercise. Take your spouse or find a partner and give your heart a workout, in more ways than one.

Warning #1: Change Your Diet Before Exercise

As I have stressed throughout this book, animal fats and oils lead to sludging of the blood, atherosclerosis, and thrombosis. And all three lead to heart attacks and strokes. If you continue to eat a high-fat and high-cholesterol diet, and then begin an exercise program, you're placing your life in jeopardy. Don't do it. Adopt the McDougall Program for a Healthy Heart. My diet will thin your blood, and take the pressure off your plaques and make them less likely to rupture. As I've said, you'll start to enjoy the cardioprotective benefits of my program within hours of eating McDougall foods. Once you've begun the diet, start the walking program described above. Begin gently and gradually build your fitness and endurance. But do *not* start exercising without adopting the diet.

Warning #2: See Your Doctor Before You Begin

Your doctor will provide you with the best guidance as to how soon you can begin your program. He or she may want to give you a complete physical, basic blood tests, including a cholesterol, triglycerides, and blood sugar, an EKG, and/or a stress treadmill test. Once your doctor gives you the green light, start the walking program, and start to enjoy the many benefits of exercise.

7. The McDougall Way to Calm the Mind

- *There are many roads to Rome, but only two that I am certain of.*
- *Practice the McDougall Program for a Healthy Heart with loved ones and friends.*
- *The McDougall Program for a Healthy Heart is the basis for peace of mind.*

Diet and Exercise Reduce Stress

Chronic stress, as we all know, leads to illness—in a few direct and many indirect ways. Stress increases muscle tension, raises blood pressure, adversely changes respiration, kidney function, and hormones. Psychological stress has been shown to concentrate the blood, which results in a slight rise in total, HDL, and LDL cholesterol. Indeed, stress is a contributor to many of the illnesses we face today. But the biggest way stress induces harm is by causing you to practice more self-destructive behavior. When under stress you drink more coffee and alcohol, smoke more cigarettes, eat more rich food, and abandon exercise routines. When a stressful project ends you may find yourself wanting to celebrate with a steak dinner with all the trimmings followed by cheesecake.

If you can separate the stress from the injurious responses then you will likely suffer very little real damage. The body is designed to take a considerable amount of stress without becoming diseased, but its tolerances for destructive eating and living are small. Throughout human history and in all of the world today stress is a part of people's daily lives—bills must be paid, marital discord abounds, family members become ill and die—yet heart disease is only common where people eat the rich Western diet. You will never have full control of the stresses in your life, but beginning today you can permanently change your diet and lifestyle.

Everyone handles stress in his or her own way. For some, meditation or prayer provides a heightened sense of harmony and well-being in the face of life's trials. For others, long walks in the woods or along the ocean are sources of inner peace. Whatever works for you, I urge you to do it. As a medical doctor, I feel my expertise lies in a scientific approach to your physical health.

I can also demonstrate the many positive effects good health practices will have on your mind and well-being. As I showed in the previous chapter, exercise alone will reduce stress. In addition, researchers have demonstrated that a diet made up of whole grains and fresh vegetables and fruits changes brain chemistry. According to research at the Massachusetts Institute of Technology, a single meal of brown rice, vegetables, and fruit increases brain levels of serotonin, a neurotransmitter that boosts your sense of well-being, helps you relax, improves your concentration, and enhances your sleep. If you eat well and exercise, your stress levels will decrease: You'll think clearer, you'll have a greater sense of well-being, and you'll have abundant energy to address your problems head on. With all of this going for you, I believe your chances of finding a solution for your problems are excellent.

Love Is Still Among the Best Medicines Known

In addition to diet and exercise, I encourage people to get their relatives and friends to practice the McDougall Program with them. I suggest this for two very important reasons. The first is that most of us need support when we make a major life change, and adopting the McDougall Program for a Healthy Heart qualifies as a major change in anybody's book.

The second reason I encourage people to adopt this program with loved ones is because we need someone to share our experience with, to talk to about the new diet and food preparation, and to discuss our progress on the program. In short, we need intimacy.

This has been demonstrated repeatedly in large- and small-scale studies. One of the earliest was the study of 7,000 people in Alameda County, California, in which researchers found that those who had strong community ties—that is, those who were married, had close personal friends, and affiliations to church or civic groups—had lower rates of disease and mortality than those who were unmarried and were socially isolated.

Later research shows an even more direct link between intimacy and heart disease. At Duke University Medical School, researchers found that those who suffer a heart attack and have no spouse or close personal friend are three times more likely to have a fatal heart attack within five years of the original event than those whose hearts are equally damaged, but have an intimate relationship.

The Duke University research is based on a nine-year follow-up study of 1,368 patients who were initially admitted to Duke for cardiac catheterization to diagnose heart disease. For people with both minor and severe heart muscle damage due to a heart attack, the results were consistent. People with this degree of heart damage generally face about a 40 percent chance of dying within five years. The Duke University researchers found that those who were married or had a close intimate relationship reduced their risk of suffering a fatal heart attack to 20 percent, while those who lacked intimacy raised their chances of dying to 60 percent. That's a threefold difference, strictly on the basis of close, personal relationships.

When you adopt the McDougall Program for a Healthy Heart, you have to acknowledge that you're doing something out of the norm. You're to be congratulated about that. You're courageous and wise to stand up and refuse to follow the herd, because in the case of the American diet, the herd is heading right for the cliff and it's a long fall. Nevertheless, you also need support in what you are doing. For that reason, I recommend that you gently, gradually, and gracefully teach your friends and loved ones how to eat better and prepare delicious foods that will support their health. Wherever possible, join others who are eating in similar ways.

People all over the country have formed little potluck gatherings that feature McDougall foods and offer the opportunity to share experiences on the program with others. They swap recipes and provide lots of very useful information. I also offer a bimonthly newsletter that offers support to people following my program and reports the latest McDougall events (Call [800] 570-1654 to order the newsletter or write to The McDougalls, P.O. Box 14039, Santa Rosa, CA 95402).

Finding Peace of Mind

Once you change your diet and begin a healthy exercise program, your ability to put things in perspective will be greatly enhanced. So many people have reported that after they adopted the diet and exercise program, they saw life differently. They weren't overwhelmed by their issues. They were able to discern their priorities more clearly.

No one put it better than Carol Major, the sales manager profiled in the previous chapter: "After I started eating this way and exercising, I made up my mind that my work is only a job. The company I work for is a business. It's not my family. If I'm going to be stressed, I'm going to be stressed about my family and that's all. I also decided that I was going to do the best job I can at work every day, but once I leave the job, the work day is over. I'm not there anymore. The more I take care of myself, the better I am at doing this."

I have met many people in their forties, fifties, and sixties ready to retire from an active business life for medical reasons, because they felt so poorly. If not overtly ill, they had lost the spark of life that kept them on the leading edge of their field. After a change in diet and a little exercise they were back enjoying a productive, exciting day—full of energy and enthusiasms that they had lost only a few years before.

In the end, health is achieved by effectively balancing many factors in our lives—family, work, finances, friendships, spiritual life, and play, just to name a few. The question that I always confront is this: How can any of us give attention to all of the factors in our lives if we are less than healthy ourselves? The truth is, it can't be done. No matter what approach you take to your own well-being, your first and most fundamental concern must be your own physical health. If you attempt to establish peace of mind but eat poorly and do not care for your physical body, you are only fooling yourself. As your health deteriorates, your life will seem increasingly overwhelming. And guess what? Your stress levels will increase in direct proportion to your decline in health. Not only will you fail to achieve peace of mind, but you will suffer physically as well. On the other hand, if you take care of your body and conduct yourself along the lines of your philosophical, ethical, and spiritual beliefs, your health will be as good as it can be—which for most people means radiant good health.

The McDougall Program for a Healthy Heart is the basis for such an approach to life.

Part III

THE BEST
MEDICAL CARE
YOU CAN GET

8. Dangerous Habits and How to Change Them

- *The first step to changing behavior: Focus on what you are doing.*
- *Cigarettes, arteries, and the blood: a deadly combination.*
- *Surprising truths about coffee, tea, and alcohol.*

Before You Fight Your Habits, Focus on Them

Having habits is part of being human. So is having to break them. Most of us maintain our habits by shielding ourselves from information that reveals why a particular food or drink is harmful to us. We'd rather remain unconscious of both the habit and its consequences. That's a mistake, I believe, because it actually makes it much more difficult than you realize to change your habits. Information alone, if allowed simply to gestate in our consciousness, causes a slow change in behavior. Of course, all change requires willpower. But your will is easier to engage when you realize the consequences of your habit. Something in the psyche—perhaps it is the will to live—starts to marshal your psychic resources in the direction of new, life-supportive behaviors.

Therefore, I offer you two very effective ways to help make changing your habits a little easier. First, embrace the information that reveals why this food, or that drink, or the cigarette is hurting you. Don't block it from your mind. Just let it in. Read about the substance in question. Listen to informed people who talk about the substance. Talk to your doctor about the eating, drinking, or smoking. You don't have to do anything about the habit at first. All you have to do is learn as much as you can about the effects of the food you are habitually eating, or the drink you're addicted to, or the cigarettes you may be smoking. Let the information seep into your consciousness. Give it a little time to take effect.

Second, reflect on how this particular food, drink, or cigarette makes you feel. If you're addicted to coffee, reflect on the coffee when you experience that nervous tension late in the afternoon or start to worry excessively (some people can get a little paranoid), especially about little things. Notice how the substance, whatever it may be, affects your body or changes your personality, your outlook on life, and your relationships. Note all the symptoms that may be related to the harmful substance: Does it cause palpitations, irregular heartbeat, fatigue, mood changes, muscular tension, worry? Are there lingering effects?

The more conscious you become of the health effects of the substances you ingest, the easier it is to change your life. Information changes behavior. Just look at all the people who have given up red meat or dairy products or cigarettes during the past twenty years. They had no more willpower than the rest of us. The world is changing because information about the relationship between diet and health is increasing. That information has a power all its own. All we have to do is allow the right information into our lives, embrace it, and let it redirect our desires. Pretty soon, you're living in an entirely new way. You're healthier, happier, and more alive. Everything you do is a little easier because you took a huge burden off your body, mind, and spirit.

Therefore, allow me to inform you briefly of some of the effects of certain substances that many of us consume habitually.

Cigarettes

In addition to the chemical additives, tars, and nicotine that fill the lungs and bloodstream—substances that give rise to disease by themselves—cigarettes are among the most powerful free radical producers we can be exposed to. Cigarette smoke is rife with these highly reactive molecules that, once inside your cells and bloodstream, break down DNA, sometimes causing cancer, and oxidize LDL particles, thus creating atherosclerosis. As I described in Chapter 2, once they are oxidized, LDL cholesterol particles are consumed by white blood cells, called macrophages, which become engorged with the decaying cholesterol. Together, the diseased macrophages and the LDL combine to form a fatty streak in your arteries that will eventually grow into a full-blown atherosclerotic plaque if you continue to consume cholesterol in excess. The road to heart disease is a simple little formula: The more oxidized LDL you have in your bloodstream, the more plaque clogs your arteries. This is one important reason cigarette smokers have such high rates of heart attacks and strokes. More of the LDL cholesterol in their bloodstreams is being oxidized and turned into atherosclerosis than in the nonsmoker's bloodstream.

Antioxidants (especially vitamins C, E, and beta carotene) inhibit the oxidation of LDL particles, and thus offer some protection against heart disease. A study in the *American Journal of Clinical Nutrition* showed that cigarette smokers have lower levels of antioxidants, especially vitamin E, in their bloodstreams. This occurs because their antioxidant reserves are depleted in the face of such high levels of free radicals in their bloodstreams and tissues. The lung tissues of smokers have lower levels of vitamin E than that of nonsmokers, as well.

At the same time, the tiny sacs within the lungs, called alveoli, show higher inflammation and higher concentrations of white blood cells, reflecting the increased immune response that occurs in smokers. The immune systems of smokers must continually deal with the onslaught of so many foreign and poisonous substances that they are in a constant state of red alert.

In addition to oxidizing LDL particles, smoking increases the rate at which platelets coagulate and form clots. These clots, as I discussed in Chapters 2 and 3, create the vast majority of heart attacks. Finally, smoking also oxidizes polyunsaturated fats, making them a greater threat to health.

Smoking not only makes the LDL particles more dangerous, but increases LDL and triglyceride levels. It also decreases HDL cholesterol by 11 percent to 14 percent and is dose-dependent (meaning that the more you smoke, the more damage done).

Coffee

There is considerable controversy raging over whether or not coffee contributes to heart disease. A 1990 report published in the *New England Journal of Medicine* found no relationship between coffee intake and heart attacks. Other research has shown exactly the opposite results, including a study also published in the *New England Journal of Medicine* showing a 2.5-fold increase in the risk of heart attacks among those who drank five or more cups of caffeinated coffee per day.

Why can't we get a straight answer? One reason may lie in the inherent problem of studying coffee drinkers. As a group, they are more likely to be cigarette smokers. They also tend to consume more animal foods, which, of course, are rich in fat and cholesterol. These factors are going to drive up their cholesterol levels and confound the study results. Also, the differing amounts of coffee consumed by each person in the study may confuse the results. Two cups of coffee per day, or even four cups for that matter, may not cause apparent health problems. However, one study has shown that six cups per day increases the risk of heart disease. Other research demonstrated that nine cups of coffee per day increases that risk 2.2 times over that for people who drink less than one cup per day.

Nevertheless, some of the confusion may be cleared away by a study published in the May 1990 *Lancet*, which showed that the type of brewing method used determines the cholesterol-elevating effect of the coffee. Filtering coffee through a paper filter removes a substance that causes total cholesterol and LDL cholesterol to increase in the blood. The caffeine in coffee does not raise cholesterol levels; therefore it is not surprising that decaffeinated coffee raises cholesterol as much as regular coffee.

Nevertheless, beyond the questions of cholesterol level are the troubling effects of caffeine—or perhaps I should say *after*effects. Many people drink coffee for its buzz—the heightened state of alertness and mental acuity it provides. There's no question that under certain situations, such a state of mental clarity and keenness is desirable. Yet, we all know that there's a downside. In addition to the pleasant and positive effects there are side effects, which include anxiety, nervous tension, tremor, and, for many, confusion. Drinking coffee results in excessive insomnia, muscle tension, and headaches. The caffeine raises blood pressure, heart rate, and frequency of irregular heart rhythms (arrhythmias).

Indigestion is almost a universal side effect with both caffeinated and decaffeinated coffee. Loose stools and sometimes diarrhea, along with an urgency to urinate, make serious coffee drinkers aware of the location of all the public rest rooms in town. And all of it adds up to more discomfort than the drink is worth.

Tea

A cup of tea contains about one-fourth of the caffeine that most cups of coffee contain, which makes it less stimulating and nerve-racking. Interestingly, tea also contains antioxidants and thus may offer some protection against heart disease, cancer, and other degenerative diseases. Research has demonstrated that regular consumption of Japanese green tea is associated with lower rates of cancer. One of the reasons for this protective effect is the high level of antioxidants found in green tea. In a study reported in *The Lancet* scientists reported that black tea contains as many antioxidants as green tea, and thus may offer the same protection.

Alcohol

One of the most popular episodes shown on *60 Minutes* was entitled "The French Paradox" (November 17, 1991), which reported that the consumption of wine by the French protected them against the heart disease–producing effects of their high-fat diet. The popularity of this message is of no surprise. People love to hear good news about their bad habits.

The French have three times less heart disease in each age category than Americans. The reasons given for this difference were: The French do not eat between meals; they take more time to eat their meals, as opposed to our habit of rapid gorging of fast foods; and they do not eat the amount of processed foods that Americans consume. Also, the French eat more of their dairy products as cheese than as milk.

One researcher, who based his ideas on rat experiments, speculated that cheese did not cause as much artery damage as milk does. Nevertheless, there is no scientific basis for such a suggestion, and the literature—such as a 1992 study in *The Lancet* has refuted it. Other investigators have suggested that the French love for garlic may be a lifesaver.

The question is this: Is there really a paradox?

The apparent difference between French and, say, American heart disease rates may be an artifact of the traditional French diet, which currently is changing, unfortunately. During the past twenty-five years, the French diet has become much higher in fat and lower in alcohol than in the past. Data from the United Nations Food and Agriculture Organization (FAO) has found a 40 percent increase in fat consumption by the French during the past twenty-five years. The proportion of fat consumed in France increased 29 percent from 1961–63 to 39 percent in 1986–88. Heart disease takes decades to develop; thus, the heart disease rates may not have had time to catch up.

Fat consumption for Americans reached 39 percent of their total calories in the 1950s, and has remained at or above that level ever since. Since the French intake in fat and alcohol is now approaching that of the Americans, there is every reason to believe that with sufficient time they will suffer the same death rate from heart disease as we do. As of now, they have only had four to six years of high-fat eating compared to more than fifty-plus years for Americans.

Pros and Cons of Alcohol Consumption

The research on alcohol may, on the surface, present a contradictory picture. There are some benefits to moderate alcohol consumption, but on the whole they are small in comparison to the dangers of excessive intake of alcohol. Since stories of the "French paradox" began to surface, the scientific literature has reported a number of articles on the relationship between heart disease and alcohol, particularly red wine. This benefit is not new news. During my days in medical school, I saw firsthand in autopsies that skid-row alcoholics often had the cleanest arteries. Their diet was, of course, mostly "liquid vegetarian" in the form of alcoholic beverages, often wine. They were, however, not known for their longevity—just their clean arteries.

The research clearly shows that moderate consumption of alcohol—defined as about an ounce (20 to 30g) of alcohol a day, or two to four drinks a day—is associated with a 40 percent reduction in the incidence of heart disease. Beer, wine, and spirits seem to be equally protective. One of the reasons moderate alcohol consumption is associated with a reduction in the incidence of heart disease is that it raises HDL cholesterol levels. HDL, you will recall, helps reduce the likelihood of heart disease by removing cholesterol from arteries and tissues, and out of the body through the feces. However, the HDL-raising effects of alcohol are not a straightforward equation, meaning that higher amounts of alcohol do not give you more HDL in your blood.

HDL cholesterol can be divided into smaller parts, or subfractions. Subfraction HDL_2 changes very little with alcohol intake, whereas HDL_3 rises substantially when alcohol is consumed. The early research suggested that only HDL_2 levels were associated with changes in a person's risk of heart disease. However, more recent research has shown that both subfractions are associated with lower heart disease rates. Also, the more recent studies report that both types of HDL rise with alcohol consumption. However, elevation of HDL cholesterol appears to account for only half of the protective effect of alcohol. There's more to it than just HDL.

Alcoholic beverages, especially red wine, contain powerful antioxidants. These substances prevent LDL particles from being oxidized and thus forming atherosclerotic plaque in the arteries. Antioxidants, including quercetin, epicatechin, and resveratrol, are found in the nonalcoholic components of wine. Red wine diluted a thousandfold with water has been shown to inhibit LDL oxidation significantly more than vitamin E (a-tocopherol).

In addition, wine seems to thin the blood, thus preventing clots from forming. A heart attack occurs as a consequence of two unhealthy conditions: the rupture of volatile atherosclerotic plaques and the creation of large artery-blocking clots that form on top of the ruptured plaque (a process called thrombosis). While animal fats promote the rupture of plaques and the formation of large clots, alcohol decreases the clotting activity of the blood, and thus reduces the chance of a heart attack. This occurs because alcohol inhibits the tendency of platelets to aggregate to form blood clots. A study of 1,600 people showed small amounts of alcohol reduced the tendency of their platelets to aggregate. This effect of thinning of the blood can also increase bleeding tendencies and may account for the increased risk of hemorrhages in heavy alcohol users.

Adverse Effects on the Heart

Heavy alcohol consumption over time can damage the liver so severely that it can no longer synthesize HDL cholesterol, dramatically increasing the risk of atherosclerosis. Excessive alcohol consumption is the second most common cause of elevated triglycerides (diabetes is the first). Moderate alcohol intake shows no consistent effects on triglyceride increases, however. Elevated triglycerides are associated with an increased risk of heart attacks, diabetes, and high blood pressure. They can become sufficiently elevated to cause inflammation of the pancreas.

Another cardiovascular disease associated with alcohol consumption is heart failure. Heart decomposition typically occurs in men between the age of 30 and 55 years who have ingested at least 3 ounces (80 g) of alcohol daily for a minimum of ten years. Chronic excessive alcohol consumption is a major cause of cardiomyopathy—a severe form of heart muscle failure. There is also an increased incidence of sudden death that peaks at about the age of 50 in alcoholics. Bouts of heavy drinking have caused the onset of irregular heart rhythms. The most common arrhythmia associated with alcohol is atrial fibrillation.

Heavy drinking was twice as common in men and seven times as common in women who suffered brain hemorrhages. Acute heavy alcohol consumption is also characteristic of young adult stroke victims. People who decrease their alcohol intake soon lower their risk of strokes.

Social drinking is associated with a small rise in systolic blood pressure (the top number). In heavy drinkers the rise may be substantial. This increase in blood pressure may be caused by the effects of alcohol on blood pressure–elevating hormones (aldosterone, renin, and catecholamines) and by an increase in the activity of nerves that cause blood vessels to constrict, thus increasing the resistance to blood flow within the arteries.

The benefits for the reduction of heart disease with the moderate use of alcohol revealed by scientific research have caused some doctors to advocate temperate drinking. But, the overall effects on health are negative, especially for people who fall within the 10 percent of the population who are problem drinkers. Obviously, we are all responsible for our own behavior and ultimately each of us must decide if he or she is abusing alcohol or not. When it comes to matters of public health policy, however, physicians must take a responsible and sober approach. Our position cannot be one of advocacy of alcohol, nor should we blur the issues that surround the use of alcohol, especially since alcohol is often linked to many serious social problems, such as drunk driving, violence, and family abuse. Although moderate use of alcohol reduces risks of heart disease, it dramatically increases the risks of dying from other causes, such as cirrhosis of the liver, cancer, violence, and accidents. For example, people over the age of 35 with a previous arrest for driving while impaired (DUI) have nearly twelve times the risk of dying in an auto accident compared to controls with no history of a DUI offense. Obviously, the first indication a person has problems with alcohol deserves serious attention. Regardless of how mixed the messages may seem, efforts by everyone in our health care system should be to decrease the use of alcohol.

Having habits are part of our birthright, but a part we can change with the right information and a little effort. This chapter is a step in that direction, I hope. Now, ask yourself, "How do these substances make me feel?" Then ask yourself, "Wouldn't I be a lot better off without them?"

9. How to Deal with Your Doctor

- *Don't forget that you are the one buying the services.*
- *Take responsibility for your health.*
- *Your time is valuable, too.*
- *Listening is an art your doctor can learn (if he or she hasn't learned it already).*
- *A good doctor-patient relationship improves health outcome.*

In a perfect world, you would automatically get the best possible medical care simply by showing up at your doctor's office. And, in fact, the most fundamental truth in the doctor-patient relationship is that both parties want the same thing: for you to get well. Your doctor has worked long and hard to be able to provide services that help to create that happy state of health for patients. Unfortunately, this is not a perfect world and the doctor-patient relationship is no different from any other type of human relationship. It's full of obstacles, barriers, and assorted potholes that can get in the way of good communication and essential care. Not surprisingly, these obstacles can cause problems.

According to a Gallup poll conducted for the American Medical Association, 75 percent of patients complain that doctors keep them waiting far too long in waiting rooms. Seventy-one percent believe that doctors do not spend enough time with their patients. More than half of patients (57 percent) believe that their doctors do not explain things well enough, and an equal percentage believe that doctors do not care as much about patients as they used to. Perhaps for all of these reasons, a significant majority of people—67 percent—believe that doctors are in the profession for the money. These are just a few of the problems that get in the way of the doctor's and the patient's central objective: to dispense and receive the best care possible.

Most patients do not know doctors well enough to understand why barriers between doctor and patient exist, and consequently are surprised and even shocked when they don't get the kind of care they want. It is not my intention to criticize either side, but to help patients get the most out of their time with doctors, so that they can have the best chance of regaining their health. Therefore, I'm providing you with this summary as a guide to getting along with your doctor, especially when you face a serious health issue and want to do everything in your power to encourage your own speedy recovery.

You'd be surprised how much influence you have over your doctor's behavior toward you, and indeed over the entire medical community. Patient demands for nutrition information and preventive health measures have triggered a revolution in health care. The doctors aren't leading the way in this revolution—laypeople are. In the same way, real improvements in your relationship with your doctor are not only possible, but very likely *if* you are clear about what you want and demand the best treatment possible. Since you are the one paying for the services, you shouldn't hesitate to make such demands.

Take Responsibility for Your Health

Some of the most powerful tools for improving your health are entirely at your command. You can eat well. You can exercise daily. And you can change the habits that are causing your health problems. None of these steps requires anything from your doctor. In fact, they are entirely your responsibility.

Taking responsibility for your health will do two things immediately. First, it will encourage you to adopt the McDougall Plan for a Healthy Heart fully and faithfully, which will dramatically improve your health. Second, it will help you to create a healthy relationship with your doctor. Your doctor is not your mother or father taking care of you. This is a business relationship, not a parent-child relationship, and you must treat it as such. A great many failed relationships between doctor and patient have occurred because patients have had inappropriate expectations of their doctors. There's a lot your doctor *cannot* do for you that is essential to your recovery.

Nutritional Ignorance in Medicine

As a rule, doctors do not dispense good nutrition information. Part of the reason may be that only a minority of physicians receive any training in nutrition while they are in medical school. Currently, only 29 of the 129 medical schools in the United States have required nutrition education courses. A 1993 survey of 30,000 physician-members of the American Medical Association (with 3,400 responding) found that less than one-quarter of doctors actually ask their patients about their diets, and only one-third of them incorporate recent nutritional information in their practice.

It's not that doctors disagree with such information. In fact, the doctors, who were surveyed by the Nutrition Information Center at New York Hospital–Cornell Medical Center, agreed with such statements as "diet has an important role in disease prevention," and "doctors should spend more time exploring dietary habits during patient evaluation." They even agreed that "in many cases, medication could be reduced or eliminated if patients followed a recommended diet." Nevertheless, the great majority of these doctors didn't incorporate these beliefs in their medical practice.

As recently as 1987, the *Journal of the American Medical Association* reported that fewer doctors believed that lowering blood cholesterol levels could prevent heart disease than people in the general public. They reported that only 64 percent of doctors believed that heart disease could be prevented by eating foods lower in fat and cholesterol, but 72 percent of the general public believed such dietary changes could prevent heart disease. Once again, the general public was ahead of medical doctors.

Become the Expert

No one cares more about you than you do. You need to be intimately involved in every step of your care. You should ask for specific information and research that support the advice your doctor is giving you. You should also ask him or her for the information packet that comes with any prescription so that you can be aware of a drug's side effects, and whether it will interact with other drugs, or foods, or should be taken if you have other illnesses.

By being responsible for your health, you have empowered yourself and your immune system to rally against all forms of adversity. A growing body of research has demonstrated that people who actively participate in their own recoveries experience higher rates of recovery, even from very serious illnesses. Those who persist in emotions that make them feel like victims actually weaken their immune systems and their efforts to recover. People who take responsibility for their health are less likely to surrender to any obstacle that stands in the way of recovery, and that includes any problem that arises in your relationship with your doctor. If a doctor brusquely brushes you off, or refuses to give you information that you need, you are more likely to correct the situation if you are being responsible for your own recovery. You'll either encourage the doctor to change, or you'll change doctors.

Be a Wise Medical Consumer

How is it that we can be so discerning when we purchase a piece of electronic equipment, and be so passive when buying medical care? Perhaps we feel that the CD player is more understandable than the workings of our bodies. In any case, we often surrender the whole effort at making wise choices about how we are treated, and by whom. The many consequences of this passive patient population are costly, both in terms of unwise medical decisions and unnecessary tests and surgery.

When deciding on a doctor, choose someone who has the specific skills you need. This seems like common sense, but you'd be surprised—especially in this age of specialization—how many people simply show up at a doctor's office thinking that he or she knows everything there is to know about all aspects of medicine. If you are pregnant, you want a doctor who is a good catcher and has a kind and friendly disposition to welcome your baby properly into the world. If you're in need of a surgeon, you want someone with a steady hand, a clear eye, and a reputation for cutting straight and true. You do not want someone with a reputation for taking out more than is absolutely necessary. In both of these hypothetical cases, you'll have to do a little digging—no more than you would do to find out if you're buying the right piece of stereo equipment.

The Kind of Doctor You Need While on the McDougall Program

If you have heart disease, are currently on medication, and have begun the McDougall Plan for a Healthy Heart, you want to find a doctor who has experience and knowledge in reducing the medication people take, and even taking people off drugs entirely. This is not as common as it sounds. Many doctors know how to write prescriptions and put people on drugs. Many know how to alter medications, shifting from one drug to another. *Only a minority of physicians have experience and know-how in taking people off medication.* Most doctors prescribe drugs with the intention that the patient will take them for life—that's what the drug companies taught them to do. Also, people expect to take drugs, which means they do not expect to get well!

When I practiced medicine in Hawaii and made rounds in my local hospital, I used to overhear doctors and nurses say to one another with trepidation: "There goes the doctor who takes people off medication." It was as if I was doing something wrong. What I threatened was their belief that medication is good for patients! I had to reeducate my health care professionals to believe that *healthy people don't take medication; sick people do.*

In most cases, drugs do not cure you of illness. They merely treat the symptoms that arise from the underlying disease. Only by correcting an unhealthy diet and lifestyle—the cause of our underlying problems—can we cure the illness. The McDougall Program for a Healthy Heart will treat the underlying disease and thereby free you of the symptoms.

You'll also need a doctor who keeps you informed of certain important tests, most notably your total cholesterol, triglyceride, blood sugar, uric acid, and blood pressure. Do not be satisfied with the words, "It's in the normal range," or "It's okay," or, "You're a little high," or worse yet, "Don't worry about it, I'm the doctor here." These words are in fact symptomatic of a parent-child relationship with your doctor. Be clear about the numbers and know the goals you are shooting for. By knowing your numbers, you will be more likely to stick with the program and appreciate your results.

Your Time Is Valuable—Even in the Doctor's Office

Doctors are notorious for keeping people cooling their heels for unreasonable periods of time in waiting rooms. Such behavior is not only poor business practice, but simply rude. Sure, there are medical emergencies on occasion, and no one—whether you are a homemaker, a salesperson, or a doctor—can stay perfectly on schedule. There are going to be delays in all of our lives; we all get behind on occasion. But it shouldn't be the rule, and if it is, something's wrong. With too many physicians, the problem is chronic and offensive, especially since such delays can easily be corrected by improving the doctor's scheduling and by eliminating the practice of double bookings for the same appointment hour—a practice far more common than many people think.

A former office nurse explained to me that her boss would look in the waiting room when he first arrived in the morning. If fewer than fifteen people were waiting for him, his ego was hurt. Apparently, his fragile image depended on having a crowd of people eager to see him. He would sulk if he didn't have a large audience.

Typically, patients tolerate such offenses. They imagine that doctors get behind on their appointments because they are selflessly serving, and therefore are not aware of the clock. Ironically, people do not expect the doctor's altruism to extend to their patients' schedules. Waiting patients get tense and blood pressures rise because they have other appointments to keep, too, and their lives are being disrupted by such delays.

The most dramatic reaction to a two-hour wait I ever heard about was from a quiet 80-year-old grandmother who had patiently sat for over two hours in her doctor's waiting room. When she was finally called, she walked into the doctor's office, picked up his overstuffed wastebasket, and poured the contents onto his desk. She then walked out without explaining. The doctor later called to discover the reason for her reaction and wisely apologized. Perhaps this experience improved his scheduling skills.

One way to relieve an overcrowded waiting room filled with unhappy patients is to relocate some of them to examination rooms. You are lulled into thinking your wait is almost over. No such luck. You soon realize that this is another way station that requires another thirty to sixty minutes of waiting—only this time you're half-naked and freezing to death!

Some conscientious people try to make the most of the waiting by bringing paperwork or a good book to the doctor's office. This may keep the blood pressure down for a while, but the annoyance still gets to people and it doesn't solve the problem.

Nevertheless, there are ways of cutting through the kafkaesque world of the doctor's waiting room. Here are some suggestions:

1. Make the first appointment in the morning or the first after the lunch hour.
2. Call ahead to see if the doctor is running on time.
3. Have the nurse call you half an hour before he will be ready to see you.
4. Explain that your time is valuable too, and you don't want to be kept waiting longer than fifteen minutes in the future.
5. Choose your doctor or medical clinic based on their business practices. Shop around for medical businesses that respect your time.

Make the Doctor Take Time and Listen

You just spent fifty-two minutes sitting in the waiting room and you're now face to face with your doctor. Before saying hello she reaches for her prescription pad—a gesture of impatience that pressures you to hurry up and get the problem out, so the doctor can see the next person. She is abrupt and begins examining you while you are still trying to explain why you are here. You feel additional pressure because you know there are fourteen other people who have waited just as long as you have to see the doctor and you don't want to keep them waiting any longer either.

Studies of doctor-patient interviews reveal that many doctors are rude and abrupt, interrupt patients before they actually report their true concerns, and often fail to discover the true medical problem that caused the patient to seek treatment in the first place. Researchers at the University of Rochester Medical School have found that physicians all too often seize the first complaint offered by a patient, assuming it to be the most important one. However, research has shown that there is little or no relationship between the order in which patients bring up a particular concern, and the importance of that concern. Experts in the doctor-patient relationship point out that patients typically have three problems that they wish to report in the average doctor visit. Many people leave the most important and sensitive issue for last. One study showed that a majority of patients were interrupted by their doctors within eighteen seconds of beginning to explain their problem. *Eighteen seconds!* There's no way these people were going to get to their deeper and more sensitive concerns.

These behaviors are both transparent and avoidable. Here are some of the things you can do to protect yourself.

1. When making an appointment, tell the receptionist that you need extra time. Doctors do not like having a reputation for rushing patients through visits. When a doctor gets word that you requested a longer appointment, he is placed on notice. He'll want to avoid any appearance that he's like one of those other doctors who put people on conveyor belts.

2. Once in his office, state your problems and explain that you don't want to feel—or be—rushed. If you feel hurried, ask him to call you later to discuss the issues that you didn't have time to cover or ask him if you could make another, longer appointment at some time when you could converse unhurried.

3. Have a written agenda. Refer to your list of questions when you sit down with your doctor. The list provides formal parameters for your meeting and prevents you from forgetting important questions that you might otherwise neglect to ask, especially if you are being pressured to move along quickly. If you're shy about asking questions, simply hand the list to your doctor and let her answer the questions one at a time. If you don't cover all your points in the time allotted, give the doctor your list and ask her to call you later with her answers.

Making the Most of Your Appointments

There are several steps you should take to ensure that you make the most of your time with your doctor, and thus get the best possible treatment. Here are a few suggestions.

1. Ask about the doctor's fees prior to services, and whether or not insurance is accepted, particularly with special services or tests that you may need.

2. Make your needs known prior to the visit, including tests you may already know are necessary. For example, many people choose a specialist to do one or more series of tests: cholesterol level, EKG, treadmill stress test, or PAP smear. State any unusual treatment that you are coming for, and specify any paperwork that the doctor must fill out (such as insurance forms or employer health records).

3. Take a spouse or a friend into the doctor's office to act as an advocate for you. A third party is usually more objective. He or she may also help you remember important questions. In any case, there is strength in numbers. You take some of the pressure off yourself, and don't feel compelled to agree to any test or treatment that makes you feel uncomfortable. Ask any car salesman if this approach works. They love to see a man alone in their showroom.

4. Discuss your condition thoroughly. Be sure to ask about the actual benefits and risks of any test or treatment. Also, ask what would happen if you refused a test or a treatment. You'd be surprised how often "no treatment" is the best option. Finally, ask about alternative approaches to your problem.

5. Ask for written material that explains your condition, the treatment involved, and your options. Ask for references for additional information on your condition. This way, you'll be able to study the problem at a more relaxed and clearer moment.

6. Unless there is a real emergency concerning your condition, never make a decision while in the doctor's office. Go home and think about the recommendations, talk to friends, nurses, other doctors. Read articles. Seek second opinions from other health professionals.

7. Revisit your doctor after you have done extensive research and ask more questions. If you are not absolutely certain that you have explored the issue thoroughly, make another appointment with your doctor and talk it over further. Don't be a hasty or foolish consumer.

8. Second opinions should come from doctors who truly have a fresh viewpoint on your problem. Don't ask the first doctor for a referral; he'll send you to someone who agrees with him. Ask for a referral from friends, or—best of all—from someone in the medical business, such as a hospital nurse who works side by side with these doctors and sees their successes and failures. Call the experts whose names appear on the research papers that examine your type of problem. The authors usually have a passionate interest in your disease. You can contact these people by letter or phone. A visit may be well worth the time and expense.

9. Seek out the medical research in libraries. Scientific papers are easily understood with a little effort. Library computers make research almost effortless. For a small fee your librarian will research your problem and provide you with a list of references and article summaries. The articles that interest you can be requested for further study. The research papers your doctor gives you will likely reflect her beliefs. Remember, in most cases there are many highly acceptable ways to approach medical problems. Only by informing yourself thoroughly can you know which method is best for you.

10. Ask your doctor what questions he would ask if he had your condition. Ask how he would go about making sure his treatment was the best available. What would he read? Who would he consult? Where would he be treated?

There's an Ordinary Man or Woman Inside the White Coat

It's useful to keep in mind that doctors are often under enormous and sometimes dispiriting pressures. As I explained earlier, I went through my own professional crisis as a plantation doctor practicing in Hawaii. I had gone into medicine with the intention of making people well, but when I got out of medical school and started practicing, I found that my patients were not recovering as I had hoped they would. At first I was dismayed, then discouraged, and then depressed. I confided to one colleague that I wasn't a good doctor because people in my practice weren't getting well. But when I checked with my colleagues, I found that their experiences were no better than my own. It wasn't until I began to research the underlying causes of diseases that I realized why my methods were not working. A lot of the standard practices simply don't work. That's when I changed my approach to health care, and started to help people actually recover their health.

As I became more experienced in medicine, I learned that my crisis was typical for young doctors. The vast majority of people who go into medicine are highly idealistic. In the early stages of one's career, the belief in the infallibility of medicine causes a great deal of ego inflation. The doctor not only feels virtually invincible against disease, but also makes the mistake of taking full responsibility for the successes and failures of patients. With time, however, the doctor begins to see the limits of his or her methods, and the painful side effects of various treatments. Should the doctor admit such limitations and accept the fact that she is not omnipotent? Or should she persist in this lofty social role, even if that role is unsupported by the evidence emerging from her practice? This question naturally precipitates an internal conflict.

How the doctor answers that question will decide how his practice and career proceed, and how he relates to patients from that moment onward. Many of the offensive behaviors displayed by some doctors are actually the methods used to prevent patients from discovering their limitations, and from seeing any doubts the doctors harbor. They discourage questions by treating the patient as if she were incapable of understanding the technical issues involved. The use of medical terms is one of the more common defensive techniques used by physicians to subtly undermine the curiosity and probing of laypeople. It should be remembered that the need for the doctor to be all-knowing arose in part because patients didn't know how to be responsible for their own health, or didn't want to be. We've all participated in the creation of many false expectations.

Today, the attitudes of both patients and doctors are changing. Suddenly, many patients want to be involved in their treatment and to be responsible. In effect, patients have turned the tables on doctors. Naturally, a certain amount of time is needed to change the patterns in our culture.

In the meantime, patients who insist upon being enlightened will often see the defensive side to their doctor, especially if the doctor has emerged from her medical crisis by trying to keep the image of omniscience intact. If a patient's probing continues, a doctor's response may become hostile. Impatience and anger toward a patient almost always work. Such statements as, "Who's the doctor here and who's the patient?" or "When did you get your medical degree?" will keep even the strongest patients in line.

Your doctor has not been trained in ways of improving basic human relationships, communications, and business skills. Many doctors simply neglect these essential areas, thinking perhaps that their only job is to evaluate patients objectively, write prescriptions, give orders to hospital staff, and check on the patient's progress or lack of it. Many doctors believe, incorrectly, that when it comes to dispensing health care, it's still a seller's market. It isn't. And the doctor who persists in that belief is in jeopardy of going out of business. The combination of a wide variety of issues facing doctors, and their general resistance to improving their communication skills, can add up to a less than satisfactory relationship with patients.

Don't Act Like You're Better Than Me

I was raised in a family where doctors were considered right up there next to God. When I suffered my stroke, I realized how human doctors really are. This experience was an awakening on many levels for me. It demystified doctors. I realized that their powers were extremely limited. I say all of this to encourage your participation in your own recovery. Obviously, there are many doctors who are gifted healers and exceptional men and women. I hope that yours is exactly this type of human being. But no matter how good your medical care may be, I want you to honor your own intelligence and to understand that your participation in the healing process is essential to your recovery.

Eventually, doctors will become more like teachers, giving people the information they need to be well, rather than parents, dispensing pills and potions that the patient knows little about, but consumes like a compliant child. The future of the doctor-patient relationship is one of greater communication and increased cooperation. It is a return to an older way of dispensing health care. Or, as Hippocrates, the Father of Medicine, said: "It is not enough for the physician to do his duty; he must also receive cooperation from the patient."

When the Patient and Doctor Work Together

People who take an active participation in their own recovery fare much better than those who are passive and accepting. This attitude also applies to the way people relate to their doctors. A study in the October 1991 issue of *Diabetes Care* reported that patients who maintain more control during their doctor appointments experienced a 15 percent drop in their blood sugar levels just two months after seeing their physicians. One possible explanation for this phenomenon is that with better communication between doctor and patient, the patient better understands what to do and therefore can carry out the doctor's instructions. Other research has supported the conclusion that patients report better health and fewer symptoms after they've seen their doctors.

Now is the time for you to take control.

10. Beware of the Hospital Diet

- *Hospitals can be dangerous places.*
- *Hospital diets promote disease.*
- *You can protect yourself from a second heart attack.*

Each year, more than 300,000 people die in hospitals after suffering heart attacks. They do not die in emergency rooms, but as inpatients in coronary care units or regular hospital wards. Another 90,000 people die as inpatients after suffering strokes that also occur in hospitals, bringing the total number of dead from these two cardiovascular diseases—*in hospitals*—to approximately 400,000 per year. Many of those deaths were preventable.

You should be aware that on the doctor's order sheet in the coronary care unit an order for a laxative and a stool softener is already typed in for all patients to help counteract one of the most notorious effects of the low-fiber hospital diet. This same diet contains enough salt, fat, and cholesterol to keep people's blood pressures, blood sugars, cholesterols, and triglycerides dangerously high. Of course, all of this continued disease requires more medication from the pharmacy, and possibly more surgeries. An argument could be made that these highly profitable departments owe the food service a kickback for all the business it creates.

I want you to know the dangers you will face when you enter a hospital and begin eating the standard hospital diet. That diet, by itself, is enough to keep you from leaving the hospital alive, and you had better understand that danger right from the start.

Change Your Diet Right There in the Hospital

If you are lying in a hospital bed right now after being diagnosed with heart disease, or having had a heart attack, you do not need to be frightened any more than you already are. That fear, however, can be put to good use by letting it motivate you to make changes in your way of life. I'm sure you've already acknowledged the need to change, and now that you're reading this book, you know what to do to protect yourself. The question you're probably asking yourself is *when*—as in, When should I begin to change my diet and lifestyle? The answer to that question is your next meal.

The most powerful tool that you have control over right now is your diet. A healthful diet can protect you against any further heart trauma. An unhealthful diet can push you headlong into greater danger. If you already have had a heart attack, and now find yourself in a hospital bed being served the hospital diet, I urge you to make some essential changes today. Many foods can be avoided and new ones can be added to your diet simply by asking the hospital staff to provide you with a healthy diet. Here's what you can do.

Your first move should be to call the hospital dietitian and clearly explain that you will be changing your diet, as of this moment. Explain to the dietitian what you want to eat based on the following recommendations. If necessary, remind the dietitian that it is unconscionable to feed a patient dying of heart disease a high-fat, high-cholesterol diet.

Avoid the following:

- All animal foods, especially red meat, dairy products, and eggs. As you will see shortly, the hospital diet is based upon these foods and all of them contribute to heart disease and increase the chances of another heart attack. Chicken and fish are very poor second choices—loaded with cholesterol and fat.
- All margarine and refined foods that contain fat.
- All oils and oily foods, including salad dressings.

Eat the following:

- All grains, especially oatmeal (always available in hospitals), rice (brown rice if possible), whole wheat or rye toast (without the butter), Wheatena, Cream of Wheat, and any other grains that are available. Often, hospital staff can make brown rice or some other grain upon request.

- All the vegetables that are available, especially leafy greens (collards, kale, mustard greens, and others), all types of lettuce, broccoli, cauliflower, salad, carrots, and squash. All of these vegetables are rich sources of antioxidants, which prevent the oxidation of LDL cholesterol in the bloodstream and therefore help heal the atherosclerotic plaques. (See Chapter 12 for more on antioxidants and other natural remedies to lower cholesterol and prevent atherosclerosis.)
- Eat moderate amounts of fruit. One or two pieces of fruit per day is a good source of fiber and many antioxidants, but an excess of fruit provides the body with too much fructose, which may contribute to heart disease. (I discuss fruit in great detail in Chapter 5.)

If possible, ask family members and friends to bring you healthful cooked meals to eat while you are in the hospital. They can also bring a wide variety of ready-to-eat foods that are rich in fiber, such as rice cakes, whole grain crackers, and a loaf of whole wheat bread. See pages 266–85 for the list of McDougall OK'd Canned and Packaged Products.

If altering your diet is impossible in the hospital, change it immediately upon being discharged from the hospital. But before you decide that changing your diet now is too much trouble, please read on.

The Vulnerability of Heart Patients

Most of the people who have just had a heart attack do not realize how vulnerable they are to suffering a second heart attack. I tell you this not to scare you, but to protect you. To delay the essential preventive changes any longer is to put yourself in greater jeopardy.

In an editorial for the September 1989 issue of *The American Journal of Cardiology*, William C. Roberts, M.D., the journal's editor, outlined both the important risk factors and the vulnerability of patients who have recently had a heart attack. Here is a summary of Dr. Roberts's key points:

1. No matter what the patient's blood cholesterol level was at the time of the heart attack, it was too high.

As any cardiologist will tell you, many people who suffer heart attacks and strokes often have total cholesterol levels well within the so-called "normal" ranges. In fact, the normal ranges are dangerous, especially for people with preexisting heart disease.

The average cholesterol level in the United States today is 210 mg/dl. For decades, doctors considered that level to be normal and even healthy, but today we have learned otherwise. In fact, the rates of heart disease increase sharply with cholesterol levels over 180 mg/dl. *The Seven Countries Study,* conducted by Ancel Keyes, the founding father of cardiovascular epidemiology from the University of Minnesota School of Public Health, showed that the lowest death rates due to heart disease occur among those with cholesterol levels below 180 mg/dl. When your cholesterol level reaches between 180 and 200 mg/dl, your death rate doubles—that is, you're twice as likely to die as someone with a cholesterol level below 180 mg/dl. Once your level reaches 200 mg/dl, the death rates climb sharply and steadily, especially after you reach or surpass 240 mg/dl.

Hence, you can have a cholesterol level that is quite "normal," even "average," and still have a heart attack.

2. The greatest threat to having a *second* heart attack is the fact that you've had a *first* heart attack.

Having a heart attack dramatically increases your chances of having another one, simply because this is a very reliable sign that your heart arteries have very severe disease. Meanwhile, the factors that give rise to the original heart attack—atherosclerosis and the likelihood of thrombosis—are still present, and probably being promoted by the foods you choose every day, including those you eat in the hospital.

This point is graphically demonstrated by the experiences of people who have survived an initial heart attack. More than nine out of ten of them will have another one. And the chances of such a person dying of a heart attack are greater than 90 percent.

3. The first six months after a heart attack is the time when you face the greatest danger of suffering a second attack, one that could be fatal. Overall, between 15 and 20 percent of patients die within six months of having a heart attack, even after they've survived the initial event and hospitalization. This points to the necessity of immediate diet and lifestyle changes.

4. The higher the blood cholesterol level—including the LDL level—the greater the chance of suffering a heart attack. As I've already shown, total cholesterol and LDL contribute directly to cardiovascular disease and heart attacks.

5. The greater the percentage drop in blood cholesterol, the greater the reversibility of atherosclerosis and the opening of the patient's arteries. As I discussed in Chapter 4, reversibility depends in large measure on how far your cholesterol level falls. That drop in cholesterol also reflects a diminished likelihood of forming clots in the arteries that bring on a heart attack. These factors reduce your chances of having another heart attack.

Despite the vulnerability of a patient who has suffered an initial heart attack, having a second heart attack is not a fait accompli, no matter how bad the odds sound. People can overcome these bad odds by adopting my program. As Dr. Roberts points out, the single best "deterrent" to having that second heart attack is the lowering of total blood cholesterol level.

Unfortunately, the hospital diet will not lower your cholesterol level. On the contrary, the hospital diet will likely encourage the progression of the disease, and contribute to the chances of a second heart attack.

AHA Diet: Disguised and Dangerous

The hospital diet is supposed to approximate the American Heart Association's Step 1 regimen—the diet prescribed to lower blood cholesterol levels—which derives less than 30 percent of its calories from fat and contains less than 300 mg of cholesterol per day. Of that 30 percent, less than 10 percent is supposed to come from saturated fat, or animal foods. This is considered a "low-fat" regimen, according to the American Heart Association (AHA).

You should understand that this AHA diet looks pretty much like the one that causes most people to wind up in the hospital in the first place. It includes lean meats, chicken with the skin removed, fish, milk and milk products, and no more than three eggs per week. It contains lots of refined foods, such as white bread, white rolls, crackers, and margarine. It includes coffee, decaffeinated coffee, and sugar, as well. It's hardly a therapeutic regimen, at least by McDougall standards.

In fact, the AHA's 30 percent fat regimen is regarded as a "prevention" diet, not a therapeutic program. As we will see shortly, the regimen's preventive effects—even for healthy people who have not suffered a heart attack—are dubious at best.

In any case, the diet offered at most hospitals is not prepared by hospital personnel; it is contracted out to one of the big hotel chains, such as the Marriott Corporation, whose business executives and dietitians administer the food service and control the bottom line. Food services in hospitals are less a therapeutic program than a corporate concern. Hence, the Marriott Corporation's standard "Fat/Cholesterol Controlled Diet" reads like an open buffet at the local American Association of Retired Persons' convention that would take place at, say, your local hotel. Included in the "Main Fare" for lunch is "Philadelphia Steak Sub," or "LS [low-salt] Chicken Tetrazzini," served with a "savory cream sauce." The Dinner menu includes "LS Pork Cabbage Soup," "Baked Meatloaf *with LF Brown Gravy* [their italics] and "Turkey Broccoli Divan," described on the menu as *"Sliced Turkey with broccoli spears drizzled with a light cream sauce."* The meal is accompanied by a variety of desserts, including "Angel Food Cake," white bread, dinner rolls, wheat bread, and margarine.

And this is pretty much the standard fare for people in the hospital. When Rob Bryant of northern California had his bypass before he began the McDougall Program in 1990, he ate lean steaks, pork chops, ham, and scrambled eggs and bacon in the hospital. I can only guess that his physicians didn't feel it necessary to educate Rob as to how he could avoid having a second bypass by adopting a low-fat diet.

Most of the people who adopt my program come to me after they've exhausted other conventional medical choices. Many of them have had lots of experiences with doctors, medical tests, and hospitals. Virtually all of my patients describe the diets they ate in hospitals in the same terms: tasteless foods with plenty of fat and cholesterol. It's little better than the standard American diet, and unconscionably low in whole grains, vegetables, fruits, fiber, and antioxidants.

"It's tragic," said William Castelli, M.D., the director of the Framingham Heart Study. "And sometimes it's enough to kill people."

Not only can mistakes be made in the menu, but it's difficult to monitor the fat and cholesterol content of a diet that includes meat, chicken, eggs, and dairy products. Let us assume for the moment that by some mathematical and culinary miracle these meals derive less than 30 percent of their calories from fat and contain less than 300 mg of cholesterol. (We'll suspend our skepticism.) The AHA's 30 percent fat diet is still not a safe regimen for most people, especially those who suffer from heart disease. Indeed, every person who enters a hospital because of some form of heart disease should be asking himself whether the "Fat/Cholesterol Controlled Diet" is a *safe* way to be eating. I think not.

The Disease Gets Worse on the AHA Diet

Numerous studies have examined the effectiveness of a low-fat, low-cholesterol diet alone, or combined with drugs designed to lower blood cholesterol and even reverse atherosclerosis. In many of these studies, the AHA's 30 percent fat diet was eaten by the control group, the group that receives no special treatment and is considered the "baseline" group, to be compared against the "experimental" group. The experimental group in studies is the one that receives the "special" treatment, that is, the diet or drug that scientists want to test to see what effect, if any, it has on people.

Many of the studies examining the effects of diet and/or drugs on blood cholesterol and atherosclerosis were done by David Blankenhorn, M.D., a scientist at the University of Southern California who, before his death, was considered the preeminent authority on reversal of atherosclerosis. In one study done by Dr. Blankenhorn, a 30 percent fat regimen was used by the control group. The results showed that many of the people in the control group experienced *progression* of their coronary atherosclerosis. In other words, the cholesterol plaques in the arteries leading to the heart got worse! In one study, progression of atherosclerosis occurred even when people took cholesterol-lowering drugs. That, of course, meant that the diet had pumped enough fat and cholesterol into the bloodstream to overcome the cholesterol-lowering effects of the drug, and thus increased the likelihood of heart attack or stroke.

Other studies have confirmed these findings. In a study done at the University of Minnesota, 85 percent of patients on a diet similar to the Step 1 diet showed a definite worsening of their coronary blockages after ten years. This, in fact, has been the consistent finding in studies in which the AHA diet was used.

The AHA diet does not greatly affect cholesterol levels. Research published in *The New England Journal of Medicine* compared the effects of a cholesterol-lowering drug alone and in combination with a low-fat, low-cholesterol diet similar to the AHA's regimen. The regimen used in the study contained less then 30 percent fat, with less than 7 percent of that fat coming from saturated fatty sources. It also contained less than 200 mg of cholesterol. Like the Step 1 regimen, this diet—called the National Cholesterol Lowering Education Program Step 2 diet—allowed a wide variety of animal foods, including lean meats, eggs, and dairy products. And, not surprisingly, the regimen achieved essentially insignificant drops in total cholesterol levels among the participants. The average reduction in total cholesterol was a paltry 15 mg/dl—a reduction that amounted to only 5 percent! A 5 percent reduction in cholesterol is not going to affect the course of the disease very dramatically, if at all.

By comparison, people with similar initial levels of cholesterol (251–300 mg/dl) on the McDougall Program at St. Helena Hospital were studied. In eleven days, there was a 41 mg/dl drop in cholesterol, which represents a 16 percent reduction. Of course, our diet contains no cholesterol and is only 7 percent total fat.

Without improving blood cholesterol levels, the diets that are routinely dispensed in hospitals—even the "low-fat, low-cholesterol" varieties—only serve to support the disease and thus increase the risk of suffering another heart attack.

It's Time to Update the AHA Diet

Given the vulnerability of people who have had a heart attack, and the recognition that lowering cholesterol is the best treatment, the AHA's diet and the National Cholesterol Lowering Education Program's diets appears downright irresponsible. The AHA's diet is an old instrument that has yet to catch up with the enormous body of evidence and expansion in understanding of how heart attacks and strokes occur, and what we must do to prevent them. Unfortunately, even though the scientific evidence is overwhelming on this subject, there is little sign that the AHA and thousands of hospitals will make long-overdue adjustments to protect people.

Many factors influence the kind of treatment you receive from your doctor and hospital, and among the most important of these are the financial costs involved. Hospitals are businesses and as such are run by businesspeople concerned about the bottom line—not by nutritionists or physicians.

Walter Willet, M.D., Ph.D, Professor of Nutrition and Epidemiology at the Harvard Medical School, and one of the top cardiovascular researchers in the country, thinks people should seriously consider alternatives to the AHA diet. In an interview, Dr. Willet said, "In addition to the concern over the diet's saturated fat and cholesterol is the fact that it reduces HDL cholesterol. You've also got partially hydrogenated vegetable oils in the diet [found in margarines]," which also contribute to heart attacks.

Dr. Willet pointed out that the AHA's recommendations make no mention of the need for antioxidants. Antioxidants stop the oxidation, or the decay, of lipids, which triggers the atherosclerotic process. Research has shown that by increasing consumption of vegetables rich in antioxidants, you can significantly reduce the risk of heart disease and heart attacks. The AHA's recommendations place no importance on the need to boost your antioxidant intake.

The reason for this delay in implementing the current scientific data is that most hospital administrators do not believe that people will make the appropriate diet changes to save their own lives. Furthermore, most of the hospital staff still eat the rich American diet that is causing all of this death and disability. They can't see beyond their own dinner plates.

Mortality Falls When Heart Victims
Adopt a Vegetarian Regimen

In 1992, the *British Medical Journal* reported a study in which 406 patients who had recently had heart attacks were studied to see what effects, if any, immediate changes in diet would have on mortality rates after one year of treatment. The patients were divided into two groups. "Group A" was given a "semi-vegetarian" diet that consisted of vegetables, fruit, dried legumes, nuts, and small amounts of fish; these people were asked to eat at least 400 grams per day of fruits and vegetables, along with their standard rations of beans, split peas, lentils, nuts, and fish. "Group B" was instructed to follow the AHA diet, but received no additional advice.

Both groups were fed their respective diets while they were still in the hospital recovering from their heart attacks, and were asked to follow their programs for one year after discharge.

After one year, the researchers found that the people following the near-vegetarian program had better compliance, and had dramatically lower total cholesterol levels, lower LDL cholesterol, and higher HDL cholesterol. The vegetarians also had lost more weight and had far fewer fatal and nonfatal heart attacks than those following the AHA's diet.

The researchers concluded that "comprehensive diet changes initiated within 48 hours of myocardial infarction" were associated with greater weight loss, lower cholesterol levels, and fewer fatal and nonfatal heart attacks in "Group A" than in those following the AHA diet.

Hospitals are missing a tremendous opportunity to help people change their lives for the better. After a heart attack or bypass surgery, the patient's full attention is focused on never repeating this experience. The introduction of a highly effective, easy-to-understand program to prevent further heart disease would be obviously welcome.

The McDougall Program for a Healthy Heart Brings Immediate Protection

The Key Is to Stop Plaque Rupture— Especially After a Heart Attack

You can save your own life while you are in the hospital by making proper food choices. One of the great benefits of the McDougall Program for a Healthy Heart comes during the first few days after you adopt the program, during which time you experience an immediate lowering of blood cholesterol. That lowering of cholesterol causes the lipid pool inside the plaque to drain, thus stabilizing the plaque and reducing the risk of rupture. It is the rupturing of these unstable plaques and the subsequent thrombosis that gives rise to most heart attacks and strokes. And these ruptures occur in people with "normal" cholesterol levels being fed the hospital diet.

For all of these reasons, I maintain that, if possible, the person who has recently suffered a heart attack should adopt my program while he or she is still in the hospital! Obviously, the patient depends on the hospital dietitian, family, and friends to make McDougall foods available, but it's important.

It's equally essential that you maintain the diet once you are out of the hospital. This is the best way I know to bring down your cholesterol level into the safe ranges. On the McDougall Program for a Healthy Heart, it is not uncommon for people with high cholesterol levels (over 300 mg/dl) to see declines of 100 mg within the first ten days on the diet.

If you are unable to change your diet in the hospital, then you should change it immediately after you have been discharged. One of the biggest problems with the hospital diet is that it deludes people into thinking that this is a safe way of eating—it is, after all, what the hospital is giving you. But the hospital is teaching people the wrong lesson. This regimen is not only unhealthy, but will cause you to wind up right back in the hospital (if you are lucky enough to survive another heart attack or stroke). Greater changes are needed to protect yourself.

Ray Mattos can tell you that there is no greater protection against such a fate than the McDougall Program for a Healthy Heart.

In July 1977, when he was just 48 years old, Ray had a massive heart attack. Four months later, he underwent a quadruple bypass operation, in which four coronary arteries were replaced. Ray had had a history of heart disease leading up to the first heart attack, and he limped along at a greatly reduced pace for the next eleven years.

In 1988 he came to my program at St. Helena Hospital. He arrived with a cholesterol level of 325 mg/dl, and was headed for a second heart attack. After two weeks of eating McDougall foods, his cholesterol level fell to 158 mg/dl, and he hasn't had a problem with his heart since. He's also lost a few pounds on the diet, too, going from 180 when he arrived at St. Helena's, to 155, which he has easily maintained for the past seven years.

11. How to Interpret Heart Tests

- *A good history provides most of the diagnosis.*
- *Patients, not test results, should be treated.*
- *Don't let one test cascade into another.*
- *Know the purpose of each test.*
- *Know the long-term consequences of each test.*

As soon as you see your doctor for possible symptoms of heart disease, you wade into a stream of events whose powerful current seems enough by itself to carry you on to further tests and procedures, including surgery. You may feel swept along in this process. You need to be cautious every step of the way. This is not to say that you should avoid visiting your doctor and listening to his advice. On the contrary, seeing your doctor is an essential part of getting well, especially since her diagnosis will help you make the appropriate changes in your life.

Tests, by themselves, are frightening. Our very lives seem to depend on the little numbers and graph lines that are derived from blood analysis or highly complex machinery. You are expected not only to deal with all the frightening symptoms of your illness, but also to be some kind of math wizard, suddenly adding up the numbers and making appropriate decisions. Patients easily become overwhelmed and intimidated. Throw into the equation the fact that not all tests are necessary, and some are even dangerous, and you've got the basis for mounting anxiety.

In order to help you gain a greater sense of personal control in the situation, I have described all the standard diagnostic tests performed in coronary care. I've also provided the kind of information your doctor will derive from these tests, and what the possible results of each test might mean. So let's examine the individual tests, beginning where every physician begins, with a personal medical history.

1. PERSONAL MEDICAL HISTORY AND PHYSICAL EXAMINATION

How a personal history and physical examination are done:
Your doctor will ask you a series of questions and then check your heart, eyes, lungs, reflexes, and other parts of your body, especially those related to any risk factors for heart disease that you may exhibit. The entire history and exam will take less than an hour.

Why they are done:
A personal history and physical exam are your doctor's first attempts at putting together the clues that reveal the underlying cause of your symptoms. The doctor will ask you about the symptoms or illnesses you suffer from now, or may have suffered in the past; he or she will ask about medications taken, whether or not any specific illnesses run in your family, and whether you are allergic to certain drugs, such as penicillin. Many physicians feel that if the diagnosis is not made after taking the patient's history, it's unlikely to be made by the addition of a physical examination and any other tests. While this wisdom is a basic part of medical training, it's also one of the first lessons forgotten by most doctors when they start seeing patients.

The doctor will conduct a physical examination. If you present symptoms of heart disease, your doctor will pay close attention to the condition of your heart, and check for any major risk factors for coronary heart disease. He or she will also order a series of diagnostic tests, beginning with a blood cholesterol test. Test results provide doctors with objective evidence of disease, or what is typically referred to as a *sign*. A symptom is evidence of a disorder that the patient is aware of, such as pain. A sign is objective evidence of disease that is detected by the physician, usually through the use of tests.

Risk Factors for Heart Disease

When a physician examines you, he or she will be looking for clues to the cause of your problems. Major risk factors for heart disease, which your doctor will look for, include the following:

Heredity. Genes play a role in determining your vulnerability to heart disease. However, only a tiny percentage of people are unable to offset this genetic vulnerability by improving their diets and life-styles. Virtually everyone—no matter what his or her family history has been—can prevent heart disease through proper diet and activity.

Male sex. Men have a greater risk and a higher incidence of heart disease than women, especially premenopausal women.

Increasing age. This is more of a risk factor for people who grow old on the typical American diet, rich in fat and cholesterol, than for those who eat diets made up primarily of whole grains and vegetables.

Cigarette smoking. A major cause of atherosclerosis and heart disease.

High blood pressure. Hypertension directly contributes to heart disease, heart attacks, strokes, and kidney disease.

Blood cholesterol level. Elevated cholesterol is a major risk factor.

Diabetes. Diabetics often have high cholesterol levels and much higher rates of heart attacks, peripheral vascular disease, kidney disease, and disorders of blood vessels.

Obesity. People who are more than 30 percent over their ideal weight are far more likely to suffer from cardiovascular diseases than those who are at normal weight.

Physical inactivity. Sedentary lifestyles increase the stress upon the heart, making the heart muscle work harder to pump the same amount of blood than hearts that are physically fit.

Stress. This least definable and tangible risk factor, like other risk factors, is dramatically improved by healthful diet and lifestyle.

In addition to these major risk factors are several physical symptoms that suggest the presence of heart disease. Among them are:

Angina pectoris. Pain in the chest, often brought on by physical exertion or changes in temperature; pressure or dull ache in the center of the chest.

Abnormal heartbeats. Irregular beating (arrhythmia), rapid beating (tachycardia), or fluttering.

If you present one or more of the major risk factors, your doctor will likely order a series of tests.

My advice:

Seeing your doctor and undergoing a medical history is essential. If you present one or more risk factors, signs, or symptoms, a cholesterol test and an EKG are the next steps in the process. If you have no symptoms, signs, or risk factors, you may still choose to have a cholesterol level test. No other test provides more insight into your current health status, and your chances of contracting heart disease in the future.

Ophthalmoscopy

In evaluating the extent of atherosclerosis and heart disease, a useful test often performed as part of the physical examination is a *funduscopic exam*, otherwise known as ophthalmoscopy. A funduscopic exam of the eye allows the physician to look at the blood vessels, nerves, retina, and other tissue, all located behind the eye.

Why the test is done:

Ophthalmoscopy is an important part of a routine physical examination and a complete eye exam. The exam can reveal possible causes of eye disorders (such as cataracts and glaucoma) and headaches. It can also be used to view the tiny blood vessels behind the eye, and thus tell the physician if there is significant atherosclerosis, signs of high blood pressure, or diabetes.

How the test is done:

The physician uses an instrument called an ophthalmoscope, a small, handheld device that has a light attached to it and a lens through which the doctor can look into the patient's eye. The lens magnifies the image the doctor sees by as much as fifteen times. The physician gets very close to the patient's eye and peers through the scope to view the back of the eye. (Occasionally, eye drops are inserted into the patient's eye in order to dilate the pupil.)

The patient is asked to move her eye left, right, up, and down, while the physician examines the inner eye.

Risks:

There are no risks to the patient associated with the test itself, though the drops used in the test may cause nausea, dizziness, and dry mouth. Patients undergoing funduscopy should have someone else drive them home after the exam is performed, if eye drops are used.

2.   BLOOD CHOLESTEROL TEST

Why the test is done and what it will tell your doctor:

Checking your blood cholesterol level is essential in determining your risk of coronary heart disease. I cannot overstate the value of this test. An initial test can serve as a baseline, to be compared against future readings to determine the direction of your health. The test will tell you much about your cardiovascular health, but will also provide information about your diet—the amount of fat and cholesterol you currently are eating—and your risk of other illnesses, including diabetes, high blood pressure, several forms of cancer, and liver disease. The most important type of cholesterol test is the one that reveals your total cholesterol number.

How the test is done:

A blood cholesterol test is taken by drawing a quantity of blood— usually 7 milliliters—from a vein at the elbow (called the antecubial vein) with a needle syringe. There is no risk associated with the test and only the minor discomfort of having blood drawn.

How you should prepare for the test:

Most doctors prefer their patients to fast at least twelve hours before taking a cholesterol test, because it can provide a clearer and more accurate reading. Cholesterol tests are taken without fasting, but I recommend that a fasting test be taken whenever possible.

You should avoid alcohol for twenty-four hours prior to taking the test. Alcohol will raise your cholesterol level, and may provide an artificial reading, especially for those who drink only occasionally.

Factors that may affect your cholesterol readings:

Among the most common are a wide variety of medications, such as cholesterol-lowering drugs, which will likely provide a lower cholesterol reading. Oral contraceptives, alcohol, and many other drugs tend to increase cholesterol levels. Be sure to tell your doctor if you are taking any medication.

Types of blood cholesterol to be tested for:

Total Cholesterol

This test measures the total amount of cholesterol in your bloodstream without discriminating between the three forms of cholesterol: VLDL, LDL, and HDL. These other fractions of cholesterol can contradict one another and give you an inaccurate and confusing picture of your health. Total cholesterol provides you with the clearest, surest, and most accurate picture of your cardiovascular health.

Blood cholesterol is measured as milligrams (mg) of cholesterol per deciliter (dl) of blood. Below is the meaning of the individual cholesterol levels and the action I usually take when a patient presents such a cholesterol level.

Total Cholesterol Ranges	*Associated Risk of Heart Attack or Stroke*
Below 150 mg/dl	Little or no risk. This is what I consider a safe cholesterol level, and it's what I am shooting for in all my patients.
151 to 179 mg/dl	Low risk, but should be monitored. The research demonstrates that heart attack and stroke are unlikely with a cholesterol level below 180. Still, it's not ideal, and I like the cholesterol level to fall to 150 or below. The person with a cholesterol level of 180 usually needs to make only a few changes to get it into the safe ranges.

Total Cholesterol Ranges	_Associated Risk of Heart Attack or Stroke_
180 to 199 mg/dl	Increased risk, double the heart attack rate of cholesterol levels below 180. Anything between 180 and 200 is a concern to me. I encourage people to be stricter with their diets. If the person has already had a heart attack and has a cholesterol level around 190, I often put them on a cholesterol-lowering medication until the cholesterol falls to a safe level.
200 to 219 mg/dl	Significant risk, with sharply increasing rates of heart attacks and strokes. I regard cholesterol levels in this range as a kind of wolf in sheep's clothing: This is around the national average, but since thousands of people with cholesterol levels in this range have heart attacks each year, I send up the red flag and encourage people to immediately adopt the McDougall Program for a Healthy Heart. A short period on a cholesterol-lowering medication may also be in order until the cholesterol level comes down into the safe ranges.
220 to 239 mg/dl	"Borderline high," says the National Cholesterol Education Program (NCEP). This is dangerously high in my book, and it requires immediate treatment. If diet alone does not bring down this cholesterol level quickly, I usually prescribe cholesterol-lowering medication.
240 to 299 mg/dl	Very high risk of suffering a heart attack or stroke. People with cholesterol levels in these ranges have four times the rate of heart attacks than those who have cholesterol levels below 200. Requires immediate and aggressive treatment.

Total Cholesterol Ranges	*Associated Risk of Heart Attack or Stroke*
Over 300 mg/dl	Extremely high risk of an early death from a heart attack or stroke

My advice:

Everyone over the age of 30—and sometimes younger if there is a family history of heart disease—should know their total cholesterol level, because it shows where your health is heading. Knowing your cholesterol level will help you improve your diet.

Low-Density Lipoprotein or LDL

What your LDL level will tell your doctor:

LDL, the "bad" cholesterol, is the culprit in the creation of atherosclerosis, which in turn gives rise to heart attack and stroke. This test is not as important as total cholesterol. Indeed, if the LDLs are high, the total cholesterol level will also be high.

How the test is done:

LDL level is derived as part of an overall blood cholesterol test. The blood is drawn from a vein by a needle syringe. A level of 130 mg/dl and below is healthy, according to NCEP, but way too high by my standards. Healthy, according to McDougall's standards, is 100 mg/dl and below.

High-Density Lipoprotein or HDL

What your HDL level will tell your doctor:

HDL, the "good" cholesterol, offers a certain amount of protection against atherosclerosis and heart disease. This test measures the amount of HDL in your bloodstream.

HDL cholesterol levels lower than 35 mg/dl—especially when coupled with a high total cholesterol and/or high triglycerides (see below)—are considered a major risk factor in the cause of coronary heart disease. NCEP states that men should have an HDL level of 50 mg/dl or more; women should have an HDL level of 65 mg/dl or more.

How the test is done:

An HDL test is part of an overall cholesterol profile and is derived from blood drawn by a syringe from a vein.

Value of an HDL test:

In my judgment, HDL is an overrated test. Invariably, people will admit to me that they have a high cholesterol level, but they follow that admission with, "but my HDLs are high." This can give a person a false sense of reassurance that his cardiovascular system is healthy, and he fails to change his diet. HDLs go up as your total cholesterol level goes up, and total cholesterol level is the most significant number when it comes to protecting you against heart disease.

People with low total cholesterol levels typically have low HDL levels. For example, a man with a cholesterol level below 150—ideal in my book—may have an HDL level of 25 mg/dl. If you looked at the HDL alone, you might conclude that this man is at risk of developing heart disease, but you'd be wrong. His chances of having a heart attack are tiny in comparison to those of a person with a cholesterol level of 230 mg/dl, and an HDL of 50.

Despite the fact that HDL's importance tends to be overrated, I regard it as a useful secondary diagnostic tool.

How the test is done:

An HDL test is part of an overall cholesterol profile and is derived from blood drawn by a syringe from a vein.

Ratio of HDL to Total Cholesterol

You may hear your cardiologist refer to an "HDL" ratio. I do not place much stock in this number for the simple reason that total cholesterol is much more diagnostic and HDL is not a clear predictor of health. In any case, I want you to know what your doctor may be talking about if he or she makes reference to the HDL ratio.

What this ratio means:

The HDL ratio actually means the amount of HDL in comparison to your total cholesterol level.

How do you figure out your HDL to total cholesterol ratio:

The ratio between HDL and total cholesterol is arrived at by dividing the number for your HDL level into your total cholesterol. For example, if your total cholesterol is 200 mg/dl, and your HDL level is 50 mg/dl, you would divide 200 by 50 and get 4, or an HDL ratio of 4:1. If your total cholesterol level is 250 and your HDL is 50, you would divide 250 by 50 and arrive at 5, or an HDL ratio of 5:1. Cardiologists want a low total cholesterol and a healthy HDL level, which drives the overall ratio downward.

Healthy and unhealthy ratios:

Any ratio of 4:1 or above is unhealthy according to most doctors, indicating an increased risk of heart attack and stroke. Ratios below 4:1 are in the healthy ranges.

3. TRIGLYCERIDES

Why the test is done and what it will tell your doctor:

Triglycerides are fat that circulate in the blood. Triglycerides, which are composed of three fatty acids, cause blood platelets and clotting proteins to adhere to one another, which increases the likelihood of thrombosis and heart attack. Triglycerides also cause red blood cells to clump, thus reducing circulation and blood and oxygen flow to cells and tissues throughout your body. Triglycerides also can paralyze insulin and raise blood sugar levels.

I have seen triglyceride numbers well above 5,000 mg/dl. In this case, the blood is so viscous that it looks like coagulated cooking fat. However, people with levels in this range can drop their triglyceride levels to below 1,000 within twelve days on my program.

Triglycerides by themselves are not a direct indicator of your risk of heart disease. However, when coupled with a cholesterol profile, your triglyceride test reveals a great deal about the fat, cholesterol, and sugar content of your diet and your risk of heart attack and stroke. It is an important test.

How the test is done:

Triglyceride analysis is usually done along with a blood cholesterol test. It is derived from a 7-milliliter quantity of blood drawn from a vein.

There is no risk involved and only the minimal discomfort associated with a puncture of the skin and blood vessel.

How you should prepare:
It's essential to fast from food and alcohol for twelve to fourteen hours before taking a triglyceride test, since eating will dramatically raise triglycerides. You can drink water, however.

How to interpret the results:
Blood levels between 40 and 150 mg/dl are healthy for men; blood levels between 35 and 135 mg/dl are healthy for women.

My advice:
Have the test done as part of your cholesterol profile. It's an important part of the picture. Men and women with high triglyceride levels should adopt the McDougall Program for a Healthy Heart immediately, and especially focus on eliminating fruit, fruit juice, and sugars from their diet. The benefits of lowering triglycerides are highly debated, and elevated triglycerides, in most cases, are much less important than elevated cholesterol when it comes to predicting your chances of getting a heart attack.

4.   SERUM URIC ACID TEST

Why the test is done and what it will tell your doctor:
Uric acid is produced as a by-product of the body's metabolism of purines (metabolites of DNA and RNA) found in protein-rich foods. Uric acid is cleared from the body by the kidneys; therefore, its relative quantity within the blood, determined by the test, can tell you and your doctor much about your diet, and whether your kidneys are functioning optimally. Kidney function is often impaired by high blood pressure, atherosclerosis, diabetes, or some other cardiovascular disorder. High uric acid levels are also associated with a variety of diseases, including gouty arthritis, kidney stones, the possible presence of congestive heart failure, infection, hemolytic or sickle cell anemia, tumors, and psoriasis. Low levels of uric acid may suggest the presence of liver disease. I use this very valuable test as yet another clue to the overall condition of the circulatory system, kidneys, and the person's diet. Uric acid levels often

reflect the richness of a person's diet along with his or her inability to handle such rich foods.

How to prepare for the test:
You'll need to fast for at least eight hours before taking this test.

How the test is done:
A 7-milliliter sample of blood is drawn from the vein at the elbow and analyzed for uric acid levels.

How to interpret the results:
Normal uric acid levels in men range from 4.3 to 8.0 mg/dl; normal uric acid levels in women range from 2.3 to 6.0 mg/dl.

5.   HEART ENZYME TEST *(also known as Cardiac Enzymes or Heart Attack Enzymes)*

Why the test is done and what it will tell your doctor:
Enzymes are proteins that serve as catalysts and controllers of chemical reactions inside cells.

Different types of tissues and cells produce their own characteristic enzymes. Muscle cells, for example, produce their own unique enzymes. Whenever cells and tissues are damaged or destroyed, their enzymes are released into the bloodstream. Since the enzymes have some degree of specificity, they can be used to trace the source of damage. I say "some degree of specificity," because muscle cells throughout the body can release the same enzymes. Also, in the case of the heart, similar enzymes are released by the brain and skeletal tissue.

Nevertheless, when the heart muscle has been damaged, as in the case of a heart attack, it releases three enzymes: *creatine phosphokinase* (also called creatine kinase or CK), *aspartate aminotransferase* (AST, but formerly known as SGOT), and *lactate dehydrogenase* (LDH). Higher than normal blood levels of these three enzymes can therefore suggest a heart attack, which is why doctors test for their presence in the blood.

Since other tissues can release similar enzymes to those of the heart, this test is not definitive by itself. However, these cardiac enzymes are an important diagnostic tool, if a heart attack is suspected. They are especially revealing when your doctors compare the results of this test with other information, including your personal history, cholesterol, and EKG.

How the test is done:

A heart enzyme test is done by taking a routine blood sample, drawn from a vein by a needle syringe. The test is usually repeated for two or three days after the actual or suspected heart attack to monitor the changes in blood levels. There is no risk involved in the test and only a small amount of discomfort associated with drawing blood.

How you should prepare:

Fasting is not necessary for the test.

How to interpret the results:

Here are the general parameters for each of the cardiac enzymes that will be elevated after a heart attack.

• Creatine phosphokinase becomes elevated within the bloodstream four to eight hours after a heart attack, and reaches its peak between twelve and twenty-four hours after a heart attack. It remains high for approximately seventy-two hours, and then begins to fall off gradually. Normal CK levels range from 25 to 130 international units (IU) per liter (L) of blood in men and from 10 to 150 IU/L in women.

Some CK exists in the blood simply because muscle is continually being broken down and replenished. A heart attack will boost blood levels of CK as much as five times the normal rates within the first twenty-four hours.

CK enzymes are found in the heart, brain, liver, and skeletal muscles. Elevations in CK can suggest damaged tissues in any of these locations. The CK can be divided into components that are more specific for heart muscle damage.

• Aspartate aminotransferase (AST) rises quickly during the first twenty-four hours after a heart attack. It usually peaks within forty-eight hours of the event and can remain elevated for up to five days. A heart attack can cause AST levels to rise four to twenty times their normal blood levels. Normal levels in both sexes fall anywhere from 8 to 20 IU/L. AST is found in the heart, liver, skeletal muscles, pancreas, and kidneys.

- Lactate dehydrogenase (LDH) rises during the first day after a heart attack and remains elevated from seventy-two to ninety-six hours after the event. Normal levels in both sexes range from 45 to 90 IU/L. LDH appears in various forms in the heart, kidneys, red blood cells, lungs, and liver. LDH is often elevated and seldom offers a clear insight into the person's condition.

6. ELECTROCARDIOGRAM *(also known as EKG or ECG)*

What it is and what it will tell your doctor:

An electrocardiogram (often referred to as an ECG or EKG, for the German word *electrokardiogramma*) measures the electrical impulses that transfuse the heart and help it pump blood. The heart's electrical impulses emanate throughout the entire body and can be detected at the surface of your skin. Sensitive electrodes that are attached to the EKG machine can pick up these electrical impulses and translate them into waves that are drawn on graph paper. These waves are then interpreted by a physician to reveal the condition of the heart.

Remarkable as it sounds, an EKG can reveal a wide range of abnormalities of the heart. Among them are the consistency and health of the heart's rhythm, and any injury (such as from a heart attack) or scar tissue that interrupts the electrical conduction of the heart. The test reveals the size and position of the heart's chambers, any inflammation in the heart muscle, whether or not there is ischemia (oxygen deprivation) caused by atherosclerosis, and any imbalances in the minerals (called electrolytes) that make electrical flow possible. An EKG also can determine the workings of a pacemaker that might be installed in the heart. For this reason, it is an essential test whenever heart disease is suspected.

How the test is done:

The patient lies down on a table. A technician will clean areas of the chest, arms, and legs and place a conductive jelly on specific locations where the EKG's electrodes will be attached. (For men who have particularly hairy chests, a small amount of hair may be shaved to assure conductivity.) A total of five electrodes (known as leads) are placed on the skin of the chest, wrists, and ankles. During the test, the chest lead is placed in a

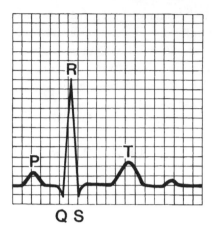

An electrocardiogram (EKG) is an important tool for the diagnosis of heart disease. The waves drawn across the paper represent the movement of electricity through the heart muscle. The P wave occurs with the contraction of the upper chambers, called the atrium. The QRS wave occurs with the contraction of the large ventricles. The T wave occurs at the time of heart muscle relaxation. Changes in this normal pattern can mean heart disease.

series of six positions around to measure the different aspects of the heart's function. The test causes no discomfort and there are no risks involved.

How the results are read and interpreted:

The wave created on the EKG's graph paper can be read by a physician to determine how well the heart is functioning. Each complete wave pattern represents an entire round of expansion and contraction of the heart. A healthy heart creates a standard wave pattern, characterized by four miniwave points, in the middle of which is the characteristic "spike" that rises from the baseline. These five points in an entire wave sequence are labeled P, QRS, and T.

The small rise at the P miniwave reveals the moment just before the atria (or upper chambers of the heart) begin to contract. The QRS segments indicate the contraction of the ventricles, or lower chambers of the heart. The R portion of that segment is the spike, or extreme high point, that jumps out at you whenever you see an EKG tracing. This represents the extreme contraction made by the ventricles, which push blood out to either the lungs or the aorta, depending on which side of the heart we are talking about. (See

Chapter 2 for a discussion of the anatomy of the heart.) The T segment of the wave represents the point at which the electrical potential returns to zero, the moment just before the heart begins another round of beating.

As I said, a normal, healthy heart reveals a steady and consistent pattern on the EKG tracing. However, each form of coronary heart disease—including heart block, or atrial or ventricular fibrillation—is characterized by its own distinct and obviously uncoordinated wave pattern.

My advice:

An EKG provides important clues to the overall cardiovascular picture.

If you came to your doctor with symptoms that suggested possible heart disease, your doctor probably took your personal history and performed cholesterol and triglyceride tests, an EKG, and perhaps a heart enzyme test (if he or she suspected a heart attack). If there are no signs of illness from these tests, you should stop taking tests and begin the McDougall Program for a Healthy Heart, unless your doctor has a convincing argument for your doing otherwise. These tests should have given your physician a very clear picture of what the illness is, and how advanced it is. You have the basis for a confident diagnosis, and you should be able to make some clear decisions.

For a small minority of people, further tests may be necessary, however. The EKG looks at only about fifty heartbeats, a tiny fraction of the workload for a muscle that beats 100,000 times each day. This limited examination of the heart may not reveal why a patient has periodic chest pain. If the EKG revealed no abnormalities, yet mysterious symptoms persist, your physician may request that you undergo an exercise stress test to take a closer look at the heart's activities.

7. AMBULATORY ELECTROCARDIOGRAM
(also known as Holter Monitoring)

What it is and what it will tell your doctor:

Ambulatory electrocardiography, nicknamed Holter monitoring for the scientist who invented the technology, is a portable EKG monitoring device that is worn for twenty-four hours, during which time the patient's heart is monitored continuously. All 100,000 beats of the heart that occur during an average day are recorded, thereby documenting any changes in heart activity or arrhythmias that may be associated with chest pain or discomfort. The test is also used to monitor the hearts of those who have already had a heart attack, are on drug therapy, or have a pacemaker installed in their hearts. The test can be helpful to people who have arrhythmias of mysterious origin. It is not used routinely for people with typical symptoms or signs of coronary heart disease, nor will it provide you with much useful information.

How the test is done:

Electrodes are attached to the chest and side of the body, using adhesive suction cups. The other end of these electrodes are attached to a cassette recording device that is worn on a belt around the waist. The patient is asked to go through a routine day while wearing the device and to record his or her routine activities—as well as any heart symptoms or abnormal physical events—in a diary. The patient should wear loose-fitting clothing and avoid getting wet while wearing the equipment. The recording device weighs approximately 2 pounds and doesn't inconvenience people very much. There are no risks associated with the device and no chance of getting shocked by the electrodes.

How the results are read:

The cassette tape, which records every heartbeat, is scanned by a special high-speed monitoring device and translated into an EKG wave recording, which can be read just as a standard EKG test by a specially trained physician.

My advice:

Take this test only if you fit into one of the above-mentioned categories. Otherwise, stick with the standard battery of tests that include a patient history and a resting EKG.

8.   ECHOCARDIOGRAM (also known as
Cardiac Echo)

What it is and what it will tell your doctor:

Echocardiogram works very much like sonar. The test bounces sound waves off the heart and then receives the impact of the returning vibration, or echo, which is translated into a picture of the heart on a special monitor. It is a noninvasive procedure that examines the size, shape, and motion of the heart, the function of its valves, and its chambers.

There are two types of echocardiograms performed: The M-mode echocardiogram provides a vertical—or up and down—view of the heart. This perspective reveals the workings of the heart's valves and ventricle chambers. The two-dimensional or B-mode echocardiogram offers a cross-sectional or lateral view of the heart, its structures, and its motion. Usually, both types of tests are done on the same patient.

An echocardiogram requires a technician to conduct the test and a specially trained cardiologist to interpret its results. Therefore, before you undergo such a test, be sure of the qualifications of the person evaluating it.

Echocardiogram is used primarily to diagnose the condition of the heart's valves; to evaluate the workings of the heart's chambers and to measure their size; and to determine whether the heart is swollen, and the extent to which the heart's muscles have been damaged after a heart attack. Echocardiogram will tell if the heart's chambers are leaking, whether the heart is degenerating, whether there is fluid leaking from the sac that surrounds the heart (pericardium), and whether or not there are tumors present in the heart.

How the test is done:

The patient lies down on a table and conductive jelly is applied to his chest, over the area of the heart. A transducer, a dime-size device that picks up the returning sound waves, is placed over the jelly. The room lights are dimmed so that the cardiologist can better see the oscilloscope screen, a television-like monitor, used to view the impressions made by the echoes coming back from the heart. The transducer is moved about on the chest to check the heart's function from various angles. An EKG machine monitors the condition of the heart throughout the test.

The patient is asked to breathe slowly and to hold his breath at various points. The entire test takes approximately thirty minutes. It is safe and painless. No X rays are used in the test; no electrical currents are passed through the heart.

My advice:

If an EKG does not provide adequate information, the echocardiogram may well clarify the diagnosis in appropriate cases.

9. STRESS TREADMILL TEST *(also known as Stress Test, Exercise Test, or Exercise Tolerance Test)*

Why the test is done and what it will tell your doctor:

Exercise causes muscles to burn energy and use more oxygen. In order to deliver oxygen to muscles in greater quantities, the body signals the heart to beat faster and pump more blood and oxygen to cells and tissues. For millions of people with angina pectoris, exercise triggers chest pain caused by cholesterol plaques that block the coronary arteries and thus prevent the heart muscle from getting all the oxygen it needs.

An exercise treadmill stress test is performed to determine the severity of atherosclerotic blockage of the coronary arteries. (The diagnosis of heart disease is made by history and a resting EKG.) Since the stress test subjects the patient's heart to varying degrees of exercise, the test is also done to determine how much exercise and physical work the heart can perform before abnormalities appear on the EKG or angina pain manifests. Once this information is obtained, a doctor can advise the patient on how much exercise he or she should do to improve cardiovascular health. A stress test is also used to screen for asymptomatic artery disease and to determine the cause of irregularities of the heartbeat during exercise.

How the test is done:

An exercise stress test is done by having a patient walk at varying speeds on a motorized treadmill while he or she is attached to an EKG machine, as well as heart rate– and blood pressure–monitoring devices. The treadmill is set at a slow speed at first and then incrementally increased to determine the heart's reaction at different degrees of physical exercise, or stress.

Sometimes a stationary bicycle is used instead of a treadmill. The same monitoring devices are used, and the patient pedals the stationary bicycle at varying degrees of intensity while the technician or doctor monitors the patient's heart.

Once the exercise phase of the test is completed—it requires about fifteen minutes—the patient is asked to lie down and undergo a resting EKG, which requires another fifteen minutes. The entire test takes about a half hour.

Think twice before you take this test:

You should not be taking this test if you have any of the following conditions: an aneurysm (a ballooning out of the wall of a vein, artery, or part of the heart), swelling of the heart or the sac that surrounds the heart, uncontrolled hypertension, congestive heart failure, or unstable angina. All too often, a stress test is the conveyor belt to the bypass table.

If you do not have any of the above-mentioned disorders, your risk of suffering a heart attack is small to minimal, especially since the test can be stopped when the patient experiences even the slightest pain. Moreover, it is performed under a doctor's supervision and medication can be given to correct any abnormalities that may arise.

How the results are interpreted:

There are a lot of false readings with this test, especially for women. Between 20 and 30 percent of people with proven heart disease have "normal" stress tests, meaning the test says they are healthy. On the other hand, between 20 and 50 percent of healthy people have "false positives," meaning the test says that they have heart disease when they don't, which of course needlessly upsets people. Therefore, you should not have a stress test if you are otherwise healthy because it could lead you down the road to unnecessary tests and possible surgery.

How you should prepare:

You should be asked by a nurse or doctor not to eat, smoke, or drink any alcoholic or caffeinated beverages at least three hours before taking the test. If the test is negative, you should not pursue any further testing or treatment. If the test is positive, the next step is a thallium scan for patients with suspected coronary artery disease.

My advice:

Ask your physician what information he or she expects to glean from this test that cannot be obtained from a resting EKG or other diagnostic exams. If you fall into any of the above-mentioned categories that suggest possible danger to your health, or if you have a very low risk of having heart disease, seek a second opinion before you take this test.

10.   THALLIUM SCAN *(also known as Thallium Myocardial Imaging, "Cold Spot" Imaging, Myocardial Perfusion Imaging, Thallium Scintigraphy, or Exercise Nuclide Scan)*

Why the test is done and what it will tell your doctor:

A thallium scan is usually done after a person fails a stress treadmill exam: It is performed to determine the extent to which arteries leading to the heart are blocked by atherosclerosis. The test will show the extent to which the patient's heart has been damaged by a heart attack, how much scar tissue is present, and the location of the damaged tissues within the heart. It is also used to determine the condition of bypass grafts, the vessels that have replaced the clogged arteries.

How the test is done:

The patient walks on a stress treadmill while attached to an EKG machine and blood pressure– and heart rate–monitoring devices. The speed of the treadmill is increased until the patient reaches his exercise peak, at which point a small amount of radioactive material, called thallium, is injected into the vein at the elbow. The patient exercises for another minute to keep the blood moving rapidly through the circulation and then lies on his back on a table beneath a special camera (scintillation camera) that can detect radioactive dye in the body. The radioactive emissions from the thallium dye create an impression on the camera's film. The resulting image reveals the extent of the profusion of radioactive dye within coronary arteries and the heart itself.

Ideally, the dye should be uniformly spread throughout the arteries and heart; however, it will not collect in the places where the arteries are blocked with significant amounts of plaque or where scar tissue exists within the heart muscle. These places appear as dark areas on the film and are referred to as "cold spots."

Pictures are taken from various angles, as the patient assumes different postures. The entire test takes about forty minutes.

The only real risk involved in the test is the exercise treadmill portion, which does stress the heart. The dye poses little or no risk. The amounts of radiation are small—about the same exposure to radiation that you would get from a chest X ray.

Tell your doctor if you are taking any medications. Pregnant women and anyone with a history of significant neuromuscular damage, acute heart attack, and acute infections should avoid this test. People with diabetes should discuss the effects of the test with their doctor before agreeing to it.

How the results are interpreted:

The test is highly accurate. Old scars from previous heart attacks will turn up and therefore may confuse the picture somewhat with any tissue damage done by a recent heart attack. Nevertheless, the resulting picture offered by a thallium scan will provide you and your physician with a clear image of the extent of coronary atherosclerosis or heart damage.

My advice:

The test itself is safe and preferable to an angiogram. I am not concerned about the test so much as where the test leads. A thallium scan is usually part of the formula of tests that leads to an angiogram and then to bypass surgery or an angioplasty. *If you pass the thallium scan, it is unnecessary to have an angiogram.* If a significant amount of disease is present, however, the angiogram is the next test to take.

Review the criteria for the angiogram provided below. If you fall into one of those categories, the thallium scan—and even the angiogram— may well be necessary to determine the extent of your disease. In this case, bypass surgery may be the right option for you. However, before you choose bypass surgery or angioplasty, read Chapter 13 carefully. Ask your doctor the questions outlined in that chapter, and determine in advance whether you are a likely candidate for a bypass, based on all the existing evidence of your condition.

If you are not a likely candidate for a bypass, I would forgo the thallium scan and the angiogram, and adopt the McDougall Program for a Healthy Heart to the letter. Continue to have your cholesterol, triglycerides, heart rate, blood pressure, and EKG monitored periodically to keep track of your health.

11. CORONARY ANGIOGRAPHY *(also known as Coronary Arteriography or Heart Catheterization)*

What it is:

Coronary angiography provides X ray pictures of the insides of the coronary arteries and the tissues of the heart. The test is used for several purposes: to determine the extent of atherosclerosis in the coronary arteries; to evaluate the heart's valves (they can be damaged by injury, disease, congenital defect, or heart attack); to assess the internal workings of the heart, its chambers, the heart muscle, and the septum (the thick wall that separates the two sides of the heart); and to evaluate the results of valve replacement and bypass surgery. In the vast majority of cases, the test is done to evaluate the extent of the atherosclerotic plaques clogging the coronary arteries. However, in all too many cases, angiography is a trapdoor that leads directly to bypass surgery. This occurs all too often when the scientific research fails to support a survival benefit for the operations. If the angiogram reveals any significant degree of atherosclerosis in the coronary arteries, the patient is ushered into a bypass operation or a balloon angioplasty, a procedure in which an inflatable device is inserted into one or more of the coronary arteries and expanded to open the vessel passageway. Therefore, if you have this test, plan on confronting the question of whether or not to have surgery.

What the test will tell your doctor:

Among the most important findings the test will provide are the following:

• The interior of the coronary arteries and the degree to which they are occluded by plaque. In general, physicians regard vessels that are occluded by 70 percent or more to be candidates for bypass surgery. Those vessels will be replaced by vein or artery segments taken from the leg or some other part of the body, or balloon angioplasty will be performed. Significant narrowing of the left main coronary artery or the left anterior descending artery virtually guarantees that bypass surgery will be recommended. (However, this may not be your best option—see Chapter 13.)

• Myocardial incompetency, or a weakened muscle. An impaired heart muscle may be caused by atherosclerosis of the coronary arteries, by an aneurysm, cardiomyopathy (a disease affecting the heart muscle), or a congenital defect. The test will show the size and shape of the chambers, the degree to which they are able to expand and contract, and whether or not the beating of the atria and ventricles is coordinated.

• The condition of the heart's valves, and whether they are congenitally deformed or damaged by infection or heart attack.

• The strength of the septums separating both the upper and lower chambers of the heart, and whether any openings exist that allow blood and oxygen to pass into neighboring chambers.

How the test is done:

The patient lies down on a table. An EKG is attached to the body to monitor the heart while the procedure is conducted. A catheter (long thin tube) is inserted into a large artery, usually the femoral artery at the groin or the brachial artery at the elbow, and then gently threaded upward through the body and into a coronary artery. If the test is being done on one or more of the coronary arteries, the catheter will be manipulated successively into the selected arteries. If it's being done on the heart chambers and valves, the catheter may be sent into either the left or right side of the heart.

While the catheter is being maneuvered into place, a physician monitors its progress by viewing it through an X ray machine called a fluoroscope. During the test, the doctor may ask you to breathe deeply or to adjust your position to allow the catheter to move more freely through the artery.

Once the catheter is in place—in either the coronary artery or the heart itself—a dye, or *contrast medium*, is injected. The dye outlines the atherosclerotic plaque and scar tissue that may result from a heart attack. This dye cannot be penetrated by the X rays, and thus contrasts dramatically with the soft tissue, through which the X rays pass easily. On the X ray pictures, the dye appears as opaque or whitish, and reveals the places where atherosclerosis or some other form of heart disease is located. In this way, the physician can determine the extent of the atherosclerosis or a disorder affecting the heart.

In addition to X ray stills, movie pictures are taken of the heart through the X ray device. Patients are often able to see the pictures themselves on monitors.

The test usually takes between one and two hours, but it can take longer if extensive measurements and evaluations are needed.

How does the test feel:

Many patients complain of nausea or light-headedness during angiography, but those feelings tend to pass quickly. The physician may ask you to cough briefly, which usually eliminates the problem. Coughing also clears the dye from the heart. Medication, such as nitroglycerin, may be administered during the test to counteract spasms caused by the catheter.

The dye causes a warm sensation in the chest, which passes a few minutes after it is injected. Many patients experience episodes of chest pain and skipped heartbeats, but these symptoms tend to pass quickly.

If you experience intense pain, dizziness, shortness of breath, or paralysis, or have difficulty speaking, inform the doctor immediately. The test may be stopped.

Is the test necessary?

This test is one of the most overused diagnostic tools in medicine, which is alarming because it is an invasive procedure that presents significant dangers to the patient. In a landmark study published in the *Journal of the American Medical Association*, physicians studied a group of 168 patients who had been scheduled for angiograms, or were strongly recommended to have the procedure by their doctors. After being encouraged to have the test, these same patients were then examined by an independent team of physicians for a second opinion. Of these 168 patients who were told they needed angiograms, 134 (or 80 percent) were found not to need the test. To confirm the second opinion, the scientists then followed the entire study group for nearly four years and found that, indeed, the procedure wasn't necessary for 80 percent of those for whom it was recommended or even scheduled.

The researchers concluded, "In a large fraction of medically stable patients with coronary disease who are urged to undergo coronary angiography, the procedure can be safely deferred. . . . We reasonably conclude that an estimated 50 percent of coronary angiography currently being undertaken in the United States is unnecessary, or at least could be postponed."

The scientists used the following criteria to determine whether or not a person needed an angiogram. If the patient had one or more of these conditions, the physicians recommended the test; if the patient didn't have any of these symptoms, the test was postponed.

• A substantial drop in blood pressure during exercise stress testing, with either chest pain or evidence from an EKG reading that ischemia (or lack of blood flow to the heart) is present. This means that the heart is slowing down and may even be approaching a heart attack during exercise because of insufficient blood flow to the heart muscle when its workload is increasing. If the patient undergoing a stress test did not experience a significant drop in blood pressure approaching peak exercise, he or she did not meet this criterion.

 • A resumption of angina pain and ischemia while the patient is at rest. A further criterion for this point was that the resumption of ischemia must take place after medication for angina and ischemia had previously proved effective. When pain or ischemia resumes, it is a symptom of worsening coronary atherosclerosis.

 • The presence of angina pectoris with pulmonary edema—a very dangerous combination, since fluid is backing up into the lungs.

 • Intolerance of angina or anti-ischemic medication.

 • The presence of primary ventricular fibrillation.

As this study demonstrated, most of the patients who are recommended for angiograms do not have one or more of these conditions. Moreover, the accuracy of these criteria was proved in the follow-ups of patients who deferred the angiograms. Of those who did not undergo the test—and therefore did not undergo bypass or angioplasty—slightly more than 1 percent died of a heart attack.

My advice:

If your doctor recommends an angiogram, do four things:

1. Share the criteria I just described for deciding on an angiogram with your doctor, and ask him if your condition meets any of these criteria. It would be a good idea to go to your local library and get a copy of the November 11, 1992, *Journal of the American Medical Association* and ask your physician to read the article, and then to reconsider your case.

2. Get a second opinion. As the *JAMA* study demonstrates, second opinions are essential, especially before you undergo a procedure that is invasive and potentially dangerous. When getting that second opinion, do not get a referral from the doctor who originally prescribed the angiogram. Get a fresh perspective. (See Chapter 9 for ideas on how to get a second opinion from someone who can give you a fresh perspective.)

3. Read about bypass surgery in Chapter 13 of this book. You and your doctor may decide together that you can forgo the angiogram because you do not meet the criteria described above and would not benefit from a bypass operation, which makes the angiogram unnecessary. The vast majority of angiograms, as I said, lead inevitably to bypass or angioplasty, neither of which is necessary for a great many people who undergo them every year.

4. Begin the McDougall Program for a Healthy Heart immediately. My program treats the disease itself. It significantly reduces chest pain, the risk of clot formation, and eventually the underlying athero-sclerotic plaque.

12. INFARCT IMAGING *(also known as "Hot Spot" Myocardial Imaging or Scintigraphy or Infarct-Avid Imaging)*

Why the test is done:

This test is performed to confirm whether or not a patient has had a heart attack and to determine the prognosis for recovery. When all the previous tests, including heart enzyme, EKG, and thallium scan, have provided equivocal results.

How the test is done:

A small amount of radioactive material (technetium-99m pyrophos-phate) is injected into the antecubital vein at the elbow. The patient waits between two and three hours for the radioactive material to travel to the heart, where it binds with scar tissue or damaged heart muscle that has resulted from a heart attack.

As with a thallium scan, a scintillation camera is suspended over the area of the heart, thus exposing the camera's film to the radioactive particles being emitted from the heart. The particles create an image on the film. In this case, the radioactive dye concentrates in the areas where the heart has been damaged, and thus the "hot spots" reveal the scar tissue and the locations of a previous heart attack.

The entire test takes about an hour, and uses slightly more radioactive material (about 110 millirads, or the equivalent of five chest X rays) than the thallium scan. Pregnant women should not undergo this test.

My advice:

The test is essentially noninvasive and does not present the same kind of risk as an angiogram. Still, all forms of nuclear medicine pose some risk to the patient and therefore should be undertaken only when essential to the healing process. Only a tiny fraction of people with heart disease actually need this test. Before you become part of that tiny fraction, get a second opinion from a cardiologist who is not involved in your case but can read all your other tests. Multiple opinions, in this case, are a good idea.

13. CARDIAC BLOOD POOL IMAGING
(also known as First-Pass or Gated Cardiac Blood Pool Imaging)

Why the test is done:

The test is done to evaluate the strength of the left ventricle, the chamber that pumps blood to the general circulation. The test will tell the doctor whether the left ventricle is effectively pushing out the blood on its systolic or contractive phase (often referred to as ejection fraction). As you will see in Chapter 13, the ejection fraction is important in determining the overall strength of the heart, and whether a patient should undergo bypass surgery. The test also reveals whether there are any tiny openings in the septum where blood might leak from one chamber to another.

How the test is done:

The patient lies on a table and a small amount of radioactive material is injected into a vein in the arm. An EKG machine is attached to the patient, along with blood pressure– and heart rate–monitoring devices. A scintillation camera is poised above the chest area and picks up the radioactive particles as they pass through the heart. In this case, the camera records the initial pass of blood containing the radioactive marker through the left ventricle. Before the radioactive material enters the left ventricle, there is no trace of radiation being emitted from that chamber of the heart. When the material enters the chamber, the radiation levels increase dramatically. At that point, the ventricle contracts and pushes out the radioactively marked blood from the chamber, at which point the radiation levels fall. The relative amounts of radiation being forced out of the ventricle—as compared to what is left behind—will tell the cardiologist the efficiency of the left ventricle. Ideally, the ventricle should push out almost all the blood from the chamber with each contraction. However, weak or diseased hearts expel only a fraction of the blood that has entered the chamber, and are thus said to have low ejection fractions.

An ejection fraction of 65 percent is considered the lower levels of normal: 65 percent of the blood within the left ventricle is pushed out of the chamber, leaving behind 35 percent within the chamber. Ejection fractions below 50 percent are considered definitely abnormal and evidence of a weakened heart.

Because the blood can be traced as it moves through the heart, the cardiologist can also determine whether radioactive trace material is moving through the septum via tiny holes in the septum. Such holes are often referred to as "shunts."

My advice:

The test exposes the patient to relatively small amounts of radiation—about the equivalent of a chest X ray—but like other nuclear medicine tests should be used only when mysterious symptoms persist and all other tests revealed no abnormality. Seek second and third opinions before agreeing to undergo the test.

Tests are not the problem in medicine today. Each of the tests I've described plays an important role in the diagnosis of disease, and each can be significant in the struggle to save lives. The problem is choosing when to undergo certain tests and when to avoid them. Like any tool, diagnostic tests are often used simply because they are there. Don't be a guinea pig or a source of revenue for a hospital that must use diagnostic equipment in order to pay its overhead. Get all the information you need to make the appropriate decisions. That means taking responsibility for yourself: Ask questions, go to the library and do a little digging, and get second and even third opinions. Meanwhile, adopt the McDougall Program for a Healthy Heart. It's the safest and surest path to a healthy heart. It's also the easiest and the cheapest way to avoid a lot of unnecessary tests.

12. "Natural" and Prescription Heart Medications

- *Diet and lifestyle are the foundation for your healing.*
- *There are many safe and relatively nontoxic ways to help you lower your cholesterol level.*
- *Herbs, supplements, and special foods work best in conjunction with the McDougall Program for a Healthy Heart.*
- *Use prescription drugs when the nontoxic methods aren't strong enough.*

Lex Overzet, a retired businessman living in the San Francisco area, suffered a heart attack in 1969, and for most of the next twenty-four years, he served as a kind of guinea pig for medical therapies. He took a lot of drugs and underwent a wide range of procedures and still suffered from serious heart disease. When he arrived at my clinic at St. Helena's Hospital in 1993, he was taking medications for both high cholesterol and hypertension. Nevertheless, his cholesterol level was still dangerously high at 220 mg/dl, and his blood pressure hovered around 160/90 mm Hg. His weight was 190 pounds, way too high for a man who stood five feet seven inches. He also suffered palpitations and periodic bouts of fatigue.

Over the next twelve days, we got his cholesterol level down to 140 mg/dl. His blood pressure normalized (today it is 134/68), and he lost weight. Eventually, he would lose 20 pounds. He also went off all medication; he no longer suffers palpitations, and he's got lots of vitality.

Leonard Ingle of San Mateo, California, had had two balloon angioplasties for coronary artery disease and high blood pressure for fifteen years prior to coming to St. Helena's. He was taking medication for both high cholesterol and blood pressure, and neither of the drugs was doing him much good. However, after having him on the program for about eight days, I was able to take him off all medication. His cholesterol level fell to 134 mg/dl, and his blood pressure normalized, reaching 130/70. It's been normal ever since. "The McDougall Program was very effective," Leonard said recently. "I made a remarkable improvement in my health."

Like so many people who come to the McDougall Program for a Healthy Heart, Lex Overzet and Leonard Ingle discovered that the first and best line of treatment for heart disease is a starch-based diet, rich in complex carbohydrates, low in fat, and absent of cholesterol. However, there are times when I combine my diet with cholesterol-lowering supplements, herbs, or medication. I do this because one of my initial goals for patients is to get their cholesterol levels down quickly. As I have said in previous chapters, lowering the blood cholesterol is a good indication that the healing process has started. The target I set for my patients is 150 mg/dl, or lower. Sometimes, diet alone does not get the blood cholesterol level down far enough or fast enough. Usually, a slow response to the diet is due primarily to poor compliance; that is, those who adopt the diet simply don't follow it closely enough to lower their cholesterol levels significantly. In these and other cases, I prescribe some form of cholesterol-lowering medication.

Drugs and natural cholesterol-lowering herbs and supplements are a second line of defense. They do not substitute for a healthful diet and lifestyle. But sometimes medication is necessary, and when it is, I try to offer the most appropriate form available.

Depending on the patient and his or her specific condition, I often start out with nontoxic herbs and supplements to lower the blood cholesterol. Many times people prefer these so-called natural methods because they don't cause the severe side effects that prescription drugs often do; they can be bought over the counter and they can be self-administered. If the natural therapies are ineffective, however, I prescribe another prescription drug.

Below is a guide to cholesterol-lowering foods, herbs, supplements, and drugs. Keep in mind that all forms of cholesterol-lowering medication work best in conjunction with the McDougall Program for a Healthy Heart. Don't forget: No food, supplement, or drug will replace diet, exercise, and a healthy lifestyle as the first line of defense against heart disease.

Antioxidants: Stopping the Decay of LDL Particles

As you've no doubt figured out by now, I do not like to deal with symptoms as much as I like to deal with causes. Even when I use special foods, herbs, supplements, and medications, I want these substances to address the underlying causes of disease. That way, I know my methods are not just masking the problems, but actually restoring health.

As I showed in Chapter 2, the changes that occur in LDL cholesterol are one of the initial steps in the creation of atherosclerosis. Inside the bloodstream, these LDL particles *oxidize*, or decay, forming highly reactive molecules called *free radicals*.

The antidote to free radicals are foods that are rich in *anti*oxidants, nutrients that slow the oxidation of LDL. In the case of heart disease, antioxidants significantly slow and even prevent atherosclerosis. They also slow the overall aging of the body. Antioxidants are found in whole grains, vegetables, and fruits. You can also use supplements that contain antioxidants.

Free Radicals and Antioxidants

Free radicals are the hot topic in the cause of disease these days, and antioxidants are increasingly viewed as a powerful form of treatment. In an unpublished paper designed to give direction to future research priorities at the National Institutes of Health, longtime antioxidant researcher William A. Pryor, Ph.D., director of the Biodynamics Institute at the Louisiana State University, summarized the potentially protective effects of antioxidants this way: "In the USA, heart and blood vessel diseases account for almost half of all deaths, and cancer for about another one-quarter. The opportunities to control diseases like these through micronutrients is, perhaps, the most exciting prospect for preventive medicine in the coming decade."

As all antioxidant researchers are quick to point out, however, the way to ensure good health and enjoy the benefits of these important nutrients is to get them from food, as part of your diet. A recent study published in *The New England Journal of Medicine* demonstrated that supplementation alone—especially of large doses of antioxidants—may not have a protective effect, and may even be harmful. In *The New England Journal of Medicine* study, the researchers pointed out that "the [beta carotene] dose [used in the study] exceeded by many times the dietary intake of beta carotene in epidemiologic studies that found a strong inverse association between the consumption of carotene-rich foods and the incidence" of disease. In other words, where beta carotene has been shown to be protective, it is usually taken in smaller doses, and as part of food.

In fact, a vast body of research has demonstrated that when these nutrients are consumed as part of a healthful diet—or in conjunction with a diet rich in vegetables and low in fat—they have a powerful protective effect against many forms of degenerative disease, including heart disease and cancer. The point that I want to stress is that you should not be fooled into thinking that you can protect yourself against the poisonous effects of a diet rich in fat, cholesterol, and refined foods by taking supplements. It isn't true, and it can even be dangerous.

Nevertheless, understanding oxidation and antioxidants will help you make healthful diet and lifestyle choices. It will also help to guide you in your decision on whether or not to take supplemental vitamins.

Free Radicals: The Common Denominator in Diseases of Aging

Free radicals occur when atoms inside your cells decay and lose electrons. Like planets revolving around the sun, electrons spin around the nucleus of an atom. The outermost orbit usually contains two electrons spinning in opposite directions. The electrons balance each other, making the atom stable, which means that they are not interested in becoming involved in chemical reactions with other atoms. In effect, they mind their own business. That's good because it means that cells and tissues maintain their integrity. They do not decay.

Oxidation occurs when an atom loses an electron. At that point, it becomes unstable and begins to break down. That means that the building blocks that make up your cells, or an apple, or a steel girder, are breaking up and decaying. Oxidation is a process by which matter decays. You've seen this decay a million times in the browning of an apple. Ordinary rust is a form of oxidation; the atoms at the surface of the iron or steel are rapidly losing electrons and breaking down. In the process, the steel is losing its ordinary properties of strength and durability. When this process occurs in an apple, we say the apple has "gone bad," meaning that it has changed and is no longer edible.

Once an electron from this outer orbit is lost due to oxidation, the imbalanced atom attempts to regain its stability by stealing an electron from a neighboring atom. However, by stealing the electron, its neighbor becomes unbalanced and must do the same to its neighbor. This sets off a chain reaction of thefts, involving many molecules, cells, and tissues. The result is chemical chaos within whole sections of the body. Chains of carbohydrates are broken, proteins are fragmented, and rearrangements are made in the DNA of our cells, the molecule that tells the cell what to do, how to reproduce itself, and when to stop. Oxidized cholesterol, altered by free radical reactions, is incorporated into cell walls and becomes atherosclerotic plaque. The more fat you eat, the more oxidized cholesterol you have in your bloodstream.

Fats are not the only substances to give rise to free radicals, and heart disease is not the only illness caused by such reactive molecules. Alcohol produces oxygen free radicals that can cause alcohol-induced fatty liver damage. Radiation will knock an electron out of orbit, producing a free radical that can then attach to our DNA. The resulting damage to the DNA can lead to cancer. Oxidants found in cigarette smoke damage lung tissues, leading to emphysema. Environmental pollutants, such as formaldehyde, act as free radicals, causing material damage to many tissues and organs. Free radicals participate in most, if not all, human disease. Studies have shown that free radicals are involved in the cause of more than sixty diseases, including atherosclerosis, rheumatoid arthritis, and chronic lung disease. Free radicals also affect the lens of the eye, causing cataracts.

Free radicals occur through normal metabolism. Bruce Ames, Ph.D., one of the preeminent cancer researchers in the world, along with his colleagues at the University of California at Berkeley, has established that a human cell undergoes about 10,000 hits to its DNA per day by free radicals. We don't all develop cancer because enzymes inside the cell repair the DNA. When free radicals form at a rate that exceeds the cell's ability to repair itself, the likelihood of cancer increases dramatically.

Deadly as they are, oxidants are also very useful to the body. Our own immune cells produce free radicals to destroy bacteria and viruses that enter the body and have the potential to cause disease. In this case, free radicals help to save lives.

Although we cannot prevent free radicals from forming entirely, we can limit their numbers, and thereby limit their destructive effects on the body. The best way to do this is to avoid harmful chemicals, cigarette smoke, and foods rich in fat and cholesterol, all of which cause free radicals. Meanwhile, we should eat foods rich in antioxidants, which stop the formation of free radicals. These antioxidant-rich foods are vegetables.

Free Radical Defenses

While free radicals cause the loss of an electron, antioxidants donate electrons to stabilize atoms, molecules, cells, and tissues. They give the very thing atoms and molecules need to reestablish balance and stability and, thus, prevent the theft of electrons from neighboring atoms and molecules, restoring harmony to those parts of our body that were previously in chaos.

Not all antioxidants are derived exclusively from your diet. In fact, your body produces some antioxidants, such as superoxide dismutase, that prevent the formation of free radicals and clean up their effects when, for example, they harm DNA. In addition, two waste products of the body, uric acid and bilirubin, act as free radical scavengers, cleaning up these rascals.

Antioxidant Vitamins

Numerous vitamins act as antioxidants. Among the most common are vitamins C, E, and beta carotene (the vegetable source of vitamin A). Other vitamins that serve as antioxidants are vitamin B6 and glutathione (found in whole grains and many other vegetable foods).

Vitamin Supplements That May Reduce
Heart Attacks and Death

While it is true that a megadose of vitamins may well have a negative effect, smaller doses of antioxidants are associated with lower incidences of all major forms of disease, even among smokers. In men who smoke, carotene (vitamin A) intake was associated with a lower risk of heart disease in the Health Professionals Follow-up Study. Higher intake of vitamin E supplements has been associated with less heart disease in both men and women. In a study involving more than 11,000 men, the incidence of death due to heart disease and other degenerative illnesses declined as vitamin C intake increased.

Some researchers believe that vitamin C is the strongest antioxidant available in the food supply. In a study published in the *Proceedings of the National Academy of Sciences*, researchers reported that vitamin C "is the most effective . . . antioxidant in human blood plasma." These scientists found that vitamin C is "of major importance for the protection against diseases and degenerative processes caused by oxidant stress [free radical formation]," including heart disease.

Research has confirmed that vitamin C is particularly protective against heart disease because it significantly slows—and in some cases halts—oxidation of lipids. Scientists at the University of California at Berkeley have stated that the research on vitamin C "strongly suggests, yet did not prove, that in plasma ascorbate is capable of completely protecting the lipids against detectable peroxidative damage [the oxidation of LDL cholesterol]."

A growing body of evidence shows the protective effects of vitamin E on the heart and blood vessels. Two recent studies on men and women found supplemental vitamin E tablets reduced the risk of dying from heart disease. Doses of 100 to 200 IU (international units) provided maximum benefits. Men who used vitamin E for at least two years showed a 37 percent reduction in fatal and nonfatal heart attacks, while women who used vitamin E for at least two years showed a 41 percent reduction in fatal and nonfatal heart attacks.

In a sixteen-nation, cross-cultural analysis of blood levels comparing vitamin E and cholesterol in middle-aged men, researchers found that the level of vitamin E in the bloodstream provided the clearest predictor of death due to heart disease. A recent study in the *Journal of the American Medical Association* found supplemental vitamin E reduced the progression of atherosclerosis in the coronary arteries of heart patients. It's important to note that research has shown that vegetarians tend to have higher levels of vitamin E in their bloodstreams than nonvegetarians.

Vitamins and Their Cholesterol-Lowering Effects

Vitamin C will also lower cholesterol, and the side effects of its use are few. In studies using 1 g daily there is little or no change in cholesterol.

However, doubling the dose to 2 g per day drops cholesterol by 12 percent. This dose also decreases platelet adhesiveness by 27 percent. Vitamin C deficiency is a common condition in people whose diet consists primarily of foods with almost no vitamin C—meat, poultry, eggs, dairy products, and vegetable oils.

Two hundred milligrams of vitamin E taken daily was shown to lower total cholesterol by 15 percent and LDL cholesterol by 8 percent in four weeks. In patients with cholesterol levels initially over 300 mg/dl, the drop in cholesterol was 31 percent in four weeks. Vitamin E comes in a dry form (without oil), which is preferable to the oil capsules.

Large doses of vitamin B3 (niacin) have been used for years as a very effective treatment for elevated cholesterol and triglycerides. Reductions of 20 to 25 percent in cholesterol can be expected with 2,000 to 3,000 mg of niacin daily. Unfortunately, flushing, gastrointestinal upset, and worsening of diabetes are common side effects. Hepatitis (with elevation of liver enzymes) is also common with the use of time-release capsules. One study reported eight out of fifteen people on time-release capsules developed hepatitis. None of those on regular niacin developed hepatitis. People taking niacin should be under a doctor's care and blood tests for liver enzymes and sugar should be monitored, along with the checks on cholesterol and triglycerides.

I recommend taking niacin only as a last resort, and only under a doctor's supervision. Before turning to niacin, I usually prescribe a bile-acid sequestering resin (see page 186) (cholestyramine) and/or an HMG-CoA reductase inhibitor (see page 186) because the side effects are less severe.

Should You Take Vitamins?

Unfortunately not enough information is available to give a definitive answer, especially one for recommendations to the general public. Long-term benefits and side effects are not known, even though therapy with carotenoids, vitamin C, and vitamin E is unlikely to result in any significant adverse effects.

My greatest concern is that people will think that good health depends on popping a few pills into their mouths each day, and therefore avoid the surest road to good health: diet and lifestyle. I would be very concerned if people decided that 200 IU of vitamin E each day protected them against the effects of bacon and eggs, or cigarette smoking. Those who thought this way would be wrong and would needlessly suffer the consequences.

Nevertheless, I do believe that if you adopt the McDougall Program for a Healthy Heart, you may still want to take supplements for their possible extra benefit. This choice may be especially attractive for those who already have heart disease and have little time to wait. Others in better health may wish to wait for long-term studies for guidance. *Which supplements should you take—if you want to at all—and how much?*

Available research suggests dosages that may be most beneficial with least cost and possibility of side effects. The following supplements and their amounts are provided below as a guideline.

Nutrient	Amount Recommended (Per Day)
Vitamin C	2 g
Vitamin E (dry form)	400 IU
Beta carotene	25,000 IU

People currently taking these doses show no negative side effects. To avoid consuming oil you should purchase a "dry form" of vitamin E. Many different dosages are available from different manufacturers. Fortunately, these three vitamins have very few side effects, and are nontoxic even in large dosages. Some vitamins are toxic in high doses, however.

Beware of Taking Mineral Supplements

Magnesium has been associated with an increase in the incidence of heart attacks and sudden death, especially among people with heart disease, and those who have recently undergone coronary bypass surgery. Physicians and scientists were initially fooled into thinking that magnesium might be good for heart disease patients because previous studies using intravenous magnesium after a heart attack showed a reduction in serious arrhythmias and death. This finding may have been due to a correction of a magnesium deficiency commonly seen in patients taking diuretics and some heart drugs (like digoxin), however. The discovery led investigators to expect similar benefits when this mineral was given orally over a long period of time, but just the opposite result was found. The risk of heart attack, sudden death, and bypass surgery at the end of the year was nearly double in those on magnesium. Therefore, use of magnesium supplements after a heart attack is not advised.

Other mineral supplements can have a negative impact on your heart health. Zinc supplements decrease HDL cholesterol and may increase your risk for heart disease. Seventy-five milligrams of zinc taken daily significantly lowered HDL cholesterol in a twelve-week double blind study (a study in which neither the patients nor the scientists knew who was receiving the zinc and who was receiving a placebo). Dietary iron intake is also associated with an increased risk of dying of heart disease. Iron acts to promote oxidation of cholesterol and thus causes the creation of free radicals. This promotes the production of atherosclerosis and raises the risk of heart attack.

Vitamin and mineral supplements sometimes have a profound effect on the body. This supports my general argument that nutrients are best obtained from food. Like all "drugs," supplements produce some desirable effects and some undesirable ones. Scientists must look for adverse consequences of therapies even when they may initially seem to be harmless, as in the case of magnesium supplementation.

Fiber and Charcoal: Cholesterol Sponges

Dietary Fiber

Water-soluble fibers found in oats, barley, brown rice, dried beans, legumes, and fruit all lower cholesterol and provide many additional benefits, not the least of which is improved digestion. An evaluation of the research on oat bran published in the *Journal of the American Medical Association* showed 3 g of oat bran eaten each day reduces cholesterol by as much as 5.1 to 5.9 mg per liter of blood. Water-soluble fibers found in all of these grains, beans, and fruits tend to work better on people with higher cholesterols (over 200 mg/dl). In one experiment, 2 ounces of oat bran or 3 ounces of dry oatmeal lowered LDL cholesterol levels in people with initially elevated levels by 10 to 15 percent. Total cholesterol was lowered by 3 to 6 percent.

Barley fiber was found to significantly lower blood cholesterol—both total and LDL cholesterol—and was far better at lowering cholesterol than wheat fiber, which is predominantly nonsoluble.

Charcoal

Highly absorbent and safe, charcoal is formed by the controlled burning of an organic material such as wood. To increase the absorbing activity it is then exposed to air or steam at elevated temperatures. This process develops an extensive network of tiny pores. The charcoal is then referred to as "activated," and is twice as potent as charcoal that does not undergo this process. Activated charcoal is an odorless, tasteless black powder with the capacity to absorb a broad spectrum of substances. For this reason, it is often used to absorb various types of poisons taken into the stomach. It also effectively lowers cholesterol.

Charcoal appears to work by absorbing cholesterol-rich bile acids in the intestine. Once absorbed, the bile acids are eliminated along with the charcoal from the intestinal tract as part of the feces. Charcoal is essentially nontoxic. Its principle drawback is that it absorbs and inactivates a wide array of substances. Some of these substances—such as medications—may be necessary for your health.

Preparations:

It is least expensive to buy the charcoal powder in bulk from your local pharmacy, which they will order for you. No prescription is required and the cost is around $10 for anywhere from 120 to 240 g (4 to 8 ounces). Take 1½ to 2 heaping tablespoons (8 g) in a small amount of water, three times a day. More commonly, charcoal preparations are found in expensive capsules intended for relief of intestinal gas.

When 8 g of activated charcoal were ingested by patients three times a day for four weeks, a 27 percent reduction in cholesterol was observed. Seven patients treated with 8 g of activated charcoal, three times a day, showed a 25 percent decrease in total cholesterol, and a 41 percent drop in LDL cholesterol. The charcoal was also found to increase the "good" HDL cholesterol by 8 percent. These results were accomplished with only negligible side effects.

A study of four kidney patients found a drop in cholesterol from 200 mg/dl to 140 mg/dl after taking 35 g of charcoal daily, for four weeks. Triglycerides dropped to less than 150 mg/dl in three patients.

Charcoal proved almost as effective at lowering blood cholesterol as the widely used prescription drug Questran (cholestyramine), without increasing triglycerides, as the drug had. Sixteen grams of Questran were found to lower the blood cholesterol level by 31 percent; 16 g of charcoal lowered cholesterol by 23 percent—a significant reduction in both cases. However, serum triglycerides were increased by cholestryamine but not by charcoal. It should be noted that cholestyramine can cause much more severe side effects than charcoal (see the section on cholesterol-lowering medications for details).

Another study comparing 16 g of cholestyramine with 40 g of charcoal showed reductions of cholesterol of 21.8 percent by charcoal, and 16.2 percent by cholestyramine.

Herbs for the Heart and Blood

Why would a medical doctor show an interest in herbs? Is Dr. McDougall becoming even more unorthodox? Is this final proof that he's really out there on the fringe? Well, don't consign me to any group—even among the revolutionaries—just yet.

What little I learned of herbs in medical school made me suspicious of herbal medications: I believed they were ineffective and/or had serious toxic side effects. In fact, herbal medicine is so far removed from standard orthodox medicine that the twenty-fifth edition of *Stedman's Medical Dictionary* doesn't even include the words *herb, herbal,* or *herbalist* in its lexicon.

These attitudes, though well entrenched among many doctors today, do not reflect the current scientific knowledge of herbs and herbal medicine, however. Research conducted by the National Cancer Institute and many preeminent university research centers has now established that herbs not only are potent forms of medicine, but also can be used safely and beneficially by virtually everyone today.

Webster's dictionary defines an herb as any plant used as a medicine, seasoning, or flavoring. The word drug is derived from the Dutch word *drogge*, which means "to dry." Some of the most beneficial drugs used in modern-day medicine are pharmaceutically altered extracts from plants. For example, the active ingredient in aspirin was originally derived from the bark of a willow tree. The powerful heart medication digoxin (Lanoxin) originally came from the foxglove plant. (In medical school I prescribed an actual herb, digitalis leaf, to patients.) A highly effective drug for impotence, yohimbine (Yocon), is derived from the bark of an East African tree. Vincristine, a powerful medication used to treat children with leukemia, comes from the periwinkle plant. I seriously regret, for the good of my patients, that my medical education lacked the study of herbal medicine. With the help of the many herbalists I have encountered as guests on my radio show I am slowly remedying this shortcoming.

Herbal Preparations

Garlic

Since 1985, nearly 1,000 studies have been published on the medical benefits of garlic and related plants, such as onions and scallions. An extensive review of the studies on garlic in the *Annals of Internal Medicine* found one-half of one clove of garlic daily lowers cholesterol by about 9 percent. The primary active ingredient of garlic is *allicin*, a sulfur-containing compound that, among other things, causes the distinctive garlic odor. However, odorless garlic, depleted of allicin, has also been found beneficial and lowers cholesterol.

The benefits of garlic on the heart are both numerous and impressive. For starters, garlic lowers both total cholesterol, and LDL cholesterol. It also lowers triglycerides. Next, it raises HDL cholesterol, which means that more LDL cholesterol will be taken out of the body. Garlic decreases platelet adhesiveness, and thus inhibits blood clotting, which diminishes the chances of forming thrombi, the clots that form the basis for heart attacks. Garlic also encourages the breakup of incipient blood clots (fibrinolysis) that form in the arteries and cause most heart attacks. Garlic also lowers blood pressure and improves blood flow by reducing the blood's viscosity.

Various naturally occurring chemicals in onions and scallions have similar though less powerful effects as those in garlic.

How Garlic Works

Garlic lowers cholesterol by inhibiting the activity of an important enzyme in the liver that helps transform dietary fats and cholesterol into blood cholesterol. (The name of that enzyme is hepatic hydroxymethylglutaryl coenzyme A, abbreviated HMG-CoA.) The cholesterol-lowering activity of garlic is similar to that of the drug Mevacor (lovastatin), the most popular and effective cholesterol-lowering medication on the market. Garlic is less potent than Mevacor, but after several months of use the effectiveness may become similar.

Garlic's Side Effects

The most notorious of garlic's side effects is, of course, the odor. Other uncommon side effects from garlic include stomach and intestinal upset, asthma, and a skin rash from contact.

The effects of 800 mg a day of garlic powder lowered total cholesterol, on average, by approximately 30 points—from an average of 265.7 mg/dl to 234.1 mg/dl. It also lowered triglycerides from an average of 225.6 mg/dl to 187.8 mg/dl. A garlic smell was reported in 21 percent of patients who actually took the garlic—mostly by spouses— while 9 percent of controls reported smelling garlic, even when it wasn't administered by the researchers. The scientists found that the higher the initial cholesterol the better the results from using garlic. Another study using a similar dose of garlic powder found a significant fall in blood pressure, from an average of 171/102 to 152/89 mm Hg.

Garlic preparations

As little as one-half to one clove of garlic per day has been found to lower cholesterol. Garlic is found in many forms and preparations: Fresh garlic bulbs, dried whole garlic cloves, garlic powder, and Kyolic. Fresh onions also lower cholesterol.

Gugulipid

This plant extract found in health food stores has been shown to lower cholesterol by 21 percent and triglycerides by 25 percent in three to eight weeks. At the same time, HDL cholesterol rose in 60 percent of patients taking gugulipid. Effects are seen within two to four weeks. The dosage used was 500 mg of a standardized preparation three times a day. Gugulipid inhibits the biosynthesis of cholesterol by the liver. No adverse effects on the liver, blood sugar, or other blood parameters were found. The preparation was extremely well tolerated with only mild gastrointestinal (stomach) upset seen in one patient. In another study using 4.5 g per day in two divided doses (three 750 mg capsules morning and evening), cholesterol decreased by 7.8, 15.8, and 21.8 percent at the end of the fourth, eighth, and sixteenth weeks, respectively. Triglycerides also decreased by 6.7, 17.1, and 27.1 percent in the same time periods. HDL cholesterol rose by 36 percent. Gugulipid has also been shown to decrease platelet aggregation and increase fibrinolytic activity in patients, thus decreasing the tendency for the blood to clot and cause coronary thrombosis.

Ginkgo Biloba

Used for millennia by Chinese healers and widely prescribed today by physicians in Germany and France, ginkgo extract is most commonly prescribed for peripheral vascular disease with intermittent claudication (pain in the legs during walking due to a decrease in blood flow to the tissues) and cerebral insufficiency (low blood supply to the brain). Ginkgo results in an increase in blood flow and a decrease in the stickiness of the blood (viscosity). There have been no adverse effects and no known drug interactions. Dosage in most trials is 40 mg three times a day (of a standardized preparation). Treatment must continue for four to six weeks before benefits can be expected.

Capsaicin

Red pepper is a commonly consumed spice worldwide. It has been found to lower cholesterol levels, possibly by inhibiting liver synthesis and increasing excretion of cholesterol. Capsaicin inhibits aggregation of platelets, thereby deceasing the tendency for the blood to clot. This reduced tendency to clot lowers the chance of a blood clot forming in a heart artery and causing a heart attack. Side effects are usually limited to heartburn, rectal burning, and sweating. Capsaicin is best tolerated when taken before meals. Adaptation occurs with time, so increase the amount and potency to tolerance. Begin with low dosages (labeled mild or light) taken before meals; capsaicin is usually found in 500 mg capsules. Adjust the dosage to avoid unpleasant symptoms.

You can find an expert in herbs that can offer you personal help by contacting the American Herbalist Guild, P.O. Box 1683, Soquel, CA 95073, (408) 464-2441; or the American Association of Naturopathic Physicians, (206) 323-7610.

Doctor-Prescribed Cholesterol-Lowering Medications

Below is a list of cholesterol-lowering drugs that are commonly prescribed. I have summarized how each drug works, and provided some of the side effects that may be of concern to patients.

Bile-Acid Sequestering Resins

Cholestyramine (Questran) combines with bile acids and cholesterol in the intestine to form an insoluble complex that is excreted with the feces. Total and LDL cholesterol are lowered. Side effects include constipation (one-third of patients), abdominal discomfort, gas, and nausea. A bleeding tendency from low vitamin K deficiency is rare. **Colestipol** (Colestid) works like cholestyramine, and has similar side effects.

Fibric Acid Derivatives

Gemfibrozil (Lopid) lowers serum lipids (fats) primarily by lowering triglycerides with variable reduction in cholesterol. HDL cholesterol may be increased. Its action may decrease the breakdown of fats and slightly increase cholesterol excretion. Side effects include mostly intestinal disturbances such as abdominal pain, diarrhea, and nausea, as well as fatigue, joint pains, and abnormal liver tests.

HMG-CoA Reductase Inhibitors

These include **fluvastatin** (Lescol), **lovastatin** (Mevacor), **pravastatin** (Pravachol), and **simvastatin** (Zocor). This class of drugs has recently been shown to reduce the risk of dying, especially from coronary artery disease, and the risk of undergoing bypass surgery in patients with known heart disease (angina or previous heart attack) and high cholesterol. They cause a decrease in production and an increase in the breakdown of cholesterol, especially LDL cholesterol. HDL cholesterol is increased. These medications are generally well tolerated, with only 1 to 2 percent of people stopping medication due to side effects. Side effects include mild abdominal distress in about 5 percent of people; headaches in 9 percent. About 2 percent of people suffer an elevation of liver function greater than three times normal levels (after the medicine is stopped, tests return to normal). Liver enzymes should be checked before therapy and every six weeks for the first fifteen months of therapy. They may also cause cataracts. This class of medications should not be combined with niacin, gemfibrozil, or immunosuppressive drugs because of the potential for serious adverse effects.

Other Cholesterol-Lowering Drugs

Probucol (Lorelco) lowers cholesterol without lowering triglycerides, and lowers HDL cholesterol. It acts by increasing the breakdown of cholesterol and also slightly inhibits synthesis and absorption of cholesterol.

Psyllium (Metamucil and generic brands) works like oat bran, and has similar side effects.

EXAMPLES OF EFFICACY AND COSTS

Agent	*Percent cholesterol-lowering after 6 weeks of therapy*	*Cost/day*
Cholestyramine	5–20	$2.96 (4 scoops)
Colestipol	5–20	$2.40 (4 scoops)
Gemfibrozil	5–15	$1.90 (1,200 mg)
Lovastatin	20–32	$3.20 (40 mg)
Niacin	15–30	$0.60 (3,000 mg)
Oat bran*	10–20	$0.42 (1 cup)
Psyllium	5–10	$0.75 (3 teaspoons)
Probucol	10–15	$2.00 (1,000 mg)

*Based on consumption of ⅔ to 1½ cups dry weight oat bran/day.

My advice:

Your foundation for cholesterol-lowering therapy is a starch-based diet. If you need more help (and if there is no reason not to) you may begin by adding 2 ounces of oat bran daily to your foods, or eating an additional three ounces of oatmeal for breakfast. Take a clove of garlic or garlic preparations in the dosage recommended on the box. Take 2 g of vitamin C and 200–800 IU of a "dry" form of vitamin E a day. If the response is still not enough, try gugulipid, and then consider taking 8 g of activated charcoal three times daily (ugh!). If the "natural medications" aren't doing the job, then add prescription medications. I usually start with bile acid sequestering resin, then when necessary, go next to HMG-CoA reductase inhibitors. I rarely find anything else necessary. A combination of both types of medication is even more effective than either alone. For example, patients given both 20 mg of lovastatin and 10 g of colestipol twice a day had a 36 percent decrease in cholesterol (48 percent decrease in LDL cholesterol) in two months. Check cholesterol levels with laboratory tests every three weeks for progress. Your goal is less than 150 mg/dl.

Once you find a medication schedule that will lower your cholesterol to the ideal of 150 mg/dl (without significant side effects), I recommend that you stay on this dosage for six months. After six months you should try reducing one medication at a time and see if your cholesterol remains ideal. Your goal is to take as little medication as possible to achieve the desired effects.

Chest Pain (Angina)–Relieving Medications

Nitrates

Nitrates relax the smooth muscles of the blood vessels, especially the veins of the body. When the blood pools in the veins, return of the blood to the heart is reduced. The decrease of return of blood decreases the work of the heart, which usually relieves the chest pain. Work is also decreased by reducing the tone of the arteries, making it easier to pump the blood. The nitrates will not dilate diseased arteries filled with plaque; however, disease-free segments of the coronary arteries may dilate with some relief of pain.

Nitroglycerine pills administered under the tongue is the drug of choice for acute episodes of chest pain. Pills are swallowed in the form of isosorbide dinitrate. Patches and ointments of nitroglycerine are applied to the skin as an effective prolonged therapy.

Beta-Blockers

Beta-adrenoceptor blocking agents, known as beta-blockers, reduce the heart muscle's work and subsequent demand for blood and oxygen by blocking the action of heart-stimulating hormones (adrenaline). They have also been found to reduce the risk of death when given to patients after a heart attack. Many forms of these drugs will raise triglycerides and lower "good" HDL cholesterol.

Calcium Antagonists

Calcium antagonists, also known as calcium channel blockers, interfere with the entry of calcium into the muscle cells of the blood vessels, causing them to relax. When the blood vessels dilate, chest pain is often relieved and blood pressure lowered. Recent reports have found an increased risk of death from heart disease in patients on this class of medications. Constipation is a common side effect. Overgrowth to the gums (gingival hyperplasia) and surgical bleeding are recently reported complications.

Blood-Thinning Therapy

Anticoagulants are given to help prevent the formation of a blood clot (thrombus) in the coronary artery. Their use is very controversial. **Warfarin** (Coumadin) has been shown to reduce death rates slightly when given to patients after a heart attack, but the serious side effects (fatal hemorrhage) and costs have limited its use.

Antiplatelet therapy with aspirin has been shown to reduce the risk of death by 15 percent and nonfatal heart attacks by 30 percent. Because of the side effects only those people at a high risk of death from heart disease should be taking daily aspirin. This group includes those with a history of a heart attack, bypass surgery, and/or angioplasty. For most others the risk of bleeding and other side effects outweighs the benefits. The ideal dose is one baby aspirin or less daily (possibly as little as 30 mg/day).

Like the authors of an editorial that appeared in the March 1995 issue of the *Journal of the American Medical Association*, I much prefer using aspirin over warfarin because of costs and safety.

Thrombolytic Therapy

Soon after a heart attack, medication can be administered that will dissolve the blood clot (thrombosis), reducing the amount of heart damage and the risk of dying. Several different drugs are approved for use. They are administered through the vein into the bloodstream. The sooner these drugs are given, the better the results. Bleeding is the most common and potentially serious side effect. Aspirin has been added to this therapy. Because of the beneficial effects of aspirin on blood clotting, some doctors recommend that the patient take an aspirin as soon as a heart attack is suspected (while at home, before formal medical treatment is given). A reduced risk of dying has been found in those who have followed this advice.

It's in Your Power, and It's Never Too Late

Blood cholesterol is your clearest gauge to health, and it is largely under your control. You have a wide assortment of tools to control your cholesterol level and thereby promote your own good health. And remarkably, it's never too late to start. Just ask Ruth Caywood of Calistoga, California.

Ruth came to St. Helena at the age of 75. She had a chronic fibrillation and a cholesterol level of 235 mg/dl. She literally had had a lifetime of whole milk, eggs, and cheese. "Those were the foods I ate a lot of," she recalled recently. "I thought they were good for you." Ruth was getting tired and rundown, and her weak heart was increasingly restricting her activities.

In twelve days, we got Ruth's cholesterol level down to 170. Meanwhile, our exercise program, which we designed for people with heart problems, gradually increased her stamina and endurance. She went home from St. Helena committed to the program and it paid off. Today, at 81, Ruth is more active than she was at 75. In fact, one of her principal modes of transportation is her bicycle. It's no wonder she's a convert.

"I recommend the McDougall Program to everyone," she says. "It put me back on the right track."

13. Heart Surgery: When to Have It, and When to Say No

- *Each year, thousands of people undergo bypass surgery and balloon angioplasty needlessly.*
- *Bypass has many side effects, including brain damage.*
- *Bypass and balloon angioplasty are only temporary fixes. The underlying disease will come back, unless you change your ways.*
- *There are occasions when bypass surgery is appropriate, and should be done to save lives.*

The agonizing decision every candidate for coronary artery bypass surgery faces is not an abstraction to me, but a pain seared on my own heart. In May 1994, my father faced this very decision again. After suffering a major heart attack in 1981, my father had done splendidly on my diet and exercise program. He had been told that he needed a coronary bypass operation, the surgical replacement of one or more blood vessels leading to his heart. I disagreed with his doctors, based on the scientific evidence, and managed to get him out of the hospital and onto a healthy diet and exercise regimen right away. He was 59 at the time, but within a couple of months of eating grains, vegetables, and fruit, my father was youthful and vigorous once again. We dodged the bullet permanently, I thought. And to be perfectly truthful, I was not unduly proud that I had helped to pull him out of the quicksand. For the next thirteen years, he thrived. My sister Linda, a nurse, cooked for him and my mother. Linda was the key. She is an excellent cook and very knowledgeable about nutrition. Thus, she was able to combine flavor and quality, which made the food medicinal, though my father hardly knew it because he liked her cooking so much.

His cholesterol was initially over 300 mg/dl. After changing his diet his cholesterol fell to 180 to 200 mg/dl. Because it was still above the ideal level of 150 mg/dl I encouraged him to take cholesterol-lowering medications. He tried cholestyramine (Questran), which made him constipated. Then he tried lovastatin (Mevacor), which made his skin dry and worsened his insomnia. Finally he gave up, never being able to keep his cholesterol much below 210 mg/dl. When in the early winter of 1993 he gave up the large quantities of fruits and other simple sugars he consumed daily he was able to lower his cholesterol to about 170 mg/dl. Possibly if he would have been able to get his cholesterol below the ideal level—by following an even stricter diet, avoiding the simple sugars, and taking cholesterol-lowering medications—he would have delayed longer the deterioration in his health that followed.

In the late fall of 1993, my father's fortunes began to turn downward. My sister and her family had to move from Michigan to the West Coast, which meant that my father was losing an expert cook. My mother cooked McDougall food, but it just wasn't the same. Consequently, my father began eating out more frequently, and his compliance to the diet dropped enough to make a difference in his health. He had been having hip problems for the previous three or four years, which had gradually curtailed his walking and exercise. Eventually, it was decided that he needed hip replacement surgery. In preparation for the operation, my father gave a pint of blood in November 1993. Inexplicably, the loss of blood resulted in angina and fatigue. From that point onward, he suffered chronic chest pain. By the early part of 1994, my father's doctors wanted him to submit to a bypass operation. I opposed the surgery. Initial tests showed that my father had three coronary vessels that were significantly occluded. In addition, the function of his left ventricle, which is responsible for pumping blood to the general circulation, was not so severely impaired to indicate that bypass surgery would clearly benefit him. The question that our whole family struggled with was: Should Dad go ahead with the bypass? In order to get additional information, I had my father examined by a couple of the country's top cardiologists, both of whom agreed with me that he should not have the surgery.

Ironically, my experience worked against me here. I had prevented so many bypass operations at that point that I had almost grown used to being able to spare people from having to undergo the surgery. Experience had taught me that relying on the scientific studies would provide a reliable set of guidelines to determine who would benefit from bypass and who wouldn't. Over the years, I had lost track of the number of times I had been in this situation with other people, like Helmut Stonawski.

In 1990, Helmut was 50 years old and suffering with acute angina pectoris. His physicians recommended he undergo coronary bypass surgery. Tests showed that at least one of his coronary arteries was blocked with atherosclerosis. At that point, Helmut had been taking medication, including beta blockers, which made him feel like a "zombie."

"I was tired mentally and physically," said Helmut. He didn't want the surgery, but he didn't want to go on enduring the pain and fatigue brought on by his heart disease either.

After hearing me on one of my radio shows, Helmut considered his choices. "I could continue to take these pills and have chest pain," he said, "or I could go under the knife. Or I could give the McDougall diet a try. I decided I would try McDougall before I had the surgery."

That year, Helmut came to St. Helena Medical Center. Based on the scientific evidence, blockage of one coronary artery (often referred to as single-vessel disease) was not in itself an indication for bypass surgery. After examining Helmut, I told him that I felt confident that he could get rid of his chest pain and avoid bypass surgery if he followed the McDougall program to the letter. That's what he came for, he told me. During his first week at St. Helena, I took him off all medications. His cholesterol level, which was 250 mg/dl when he arrived at St. Helena, fell to 178 mg/dl. I didn't think that was low enough, so I put him on some cholesterol-lowering medications, which dropped his cholesterol even further to 135 mg/dl. Meanwhile, we got him on a daily exercise regimen, which he continues to follow to this day.

Gradually, he began to feel steady improvement in his health, and his chest pain began to diminish. Within a few months of starting the McDougall Program for a Healthy Heart, Helmut's angina had disappeared. To this day, he continues to be in good health. He is pain free, and he never did have bypass surgery.

"As soon as I stopped eating fat, my angina began to go away," Helmut said recently. "Today, I have no chest pain and I'm fairly strict. The program protects against a lot of problems, not just heart disease, but it really helped me with the problems of my heart. I definitely recommend the McDougall Program to people."

Helmut is just one of hundreds of people who have come to my program after doctors informed them that they needed coronary bypass surgery or balloon angioplasty, a treatment that uses a catheter tube and a balloon to enlarge and open one or more coronary arteries. After beginning the McDougall Program for a Healthy Heart, the vast majority of these people never needed either operation because their chest pain was relieved. In fact, their chest pain and other symptoms related to their heart disease either drastically diminished or completely disappeared.

In 1981, my father's own experience was not dissimilar to Helmut's. But in 1993, my father's case was different, and in the process he taught me a great lesson, namely that there are no absolutes when it comes to any medical therapy.

My father did not want to have the operation. Believing that his condition did not fulfill the standard criteria for bypass surgery, I supported him in his efforts to avoid the knife, which in retrospect probably was the wrong decision. In April, he had a massive heart attack and heart failure and nearly died. He underwent emergency bypass surgery that I believe saved his life. Since the operation, he has made a remarkable recovery, though he still has a few side effects from this latest heart attack and the surgery.

For me, the experience was a powerful, humbling lesson. The fact is that all the things I used to say about coronary bypass surgery—that most bypasses do not extend life and that many thousands of candidates for bypass would do better if they avoided the operation and adopted my program—are still true. The National Institutes of Health estimate that as many as 80 percent of bypass operations provide no extension of patients' life span beyond what they would have experienced had they treated their heart disease with medication alone. Among the hard realities of bypass surgery is that for many people it will shorten their lives, and for others it will cause irreparable brain damage that will change the quality of their lives forever. The fact is that there are far too many bypass operations done each year.

But that's only part of the truth. Just because the surgery is abused doesn't mean that it isn't essential for some people. For people with certain indications, bypass surgery may well be the right answer. Determining whether or not you fall into one of these categories is an easy thing to do; however, predicting the future—whether or not you'll actually benefit from the surgery—will be very difficult. If you were to die on the operating table, your relatives would say that you should have waited and enjoyed the years you had left to live. If you postpone the surgery and suffer a heart attack, you will probably guess that you should have had the surgery. This is the burden facing each patient and doctor, both of whom must live with the consequences of their decisions. I am going to sort through all of these issues with you in this chapter, to help you make the best decision for yourself, or your loved ones. I'll also discuss the pros and cons of balloon angioplasty.

Let's begin with the coronary artery bypass operation.

What Is Bypass Surgery?

Each year, approximately 380,000 people undergo coronary artery bypass surgery. Ironically, the number of bypass operations more than doubled during the 1980s, while the incidence of heart disease fell more than 30 percent during the same period.

Most of the bypass surgeries today are done to relieve angina pectoris, or chest pain. Angina is caused when people eat foods rich in fat and cholesterol. The resulting atherosclerosis blocks blood flow to the heart, thus depriving the heart muscle of adequate blood and oxygen, which causes chest pain when greater demand is placed on the heart.

The surgery entails taking vessels from one part of the body—usually the internal mammary artery, located in the chest, or the saphenous vein, located in the leg—and using them to *bypass* blocked sections of one or more clogged coronary arteries. Usually, the bypass vessels are grafted at one end to the aorta—the main artery carrying oxygen-rich blood away from the heart—and then attached to an unclogged part of the coronary artery at a place that's closest to the heart. In this way, the heart now receives an abundant supply of oxygen-rich blood flowing from the aorta.

The surgery is done by creating an incision in the skin of the chest, splitting open the breastbone with a bone saw, and then prying open the chest and rib cage. This exposes the pericardium, the sac that encloses and protects the heart. The pericardium is opened with a scalpel, which exposes the heart itself. A cold potassium solution is injected into the heart to cause it to stop beating.

A tube from the heart-lung machine is inserted into the right atrium—the right upper chamber of the heart—which channels the blood away from the heart and to the heart-lung machine. Inside the machine, the blood is oxygenated and returned to the body, via another tube that runs from the heart-lung machine to the aorta. Once in the aorta, the blood travels to

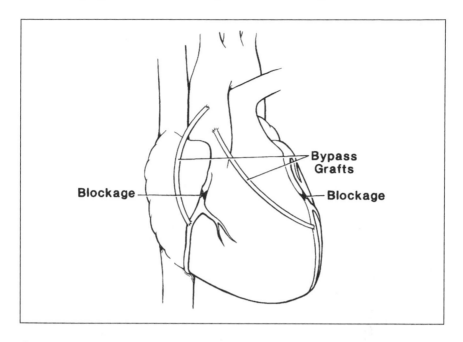

Labels on figure: Bypass Grafts, Blockage, Blockage

Bypass surgery is just what it sounds like. A blood vessel taken from an-
other part of the body is used to bypass a narrowing due to atherosclerosis
in the native heart artery. This is big-time surgery. Costs, risks, and side ef-
fects are substantial. Survival benefits are primarily limited to those patients
with severe narrowing of the left main coronary artery and those with dam-
age to the left ventricle (ejection fraction reduced to 35 percent to 50 per-
cent). Another benefit is relief of chest pain, which cannot be controlled with
a healthy diet and judicious use of medication (rare).

smaller arteries and capillaries and eventually to cells throughout the
body. During the operation, which will take several hours depending on
how many arteries need to be bypassed and the skill of the operating
team, the heart-lung machine will remove carbon dioxide from the
blood, infuse the blood with oxygen, and pump it back into the body.

Once the blood reaches the heart-lung machine, it is cooled. This cooled
blood enters the body itself and refrigerates it during the operation. When
the operation is complete, the blood is warmed by the heart-lung machine
and the body is brought back to its normal temperature.

A single artery bypass can cost anywhere from $28,000 to $40,000—
if all goes well. When complications occur, the cost increases and can
easily exceed $100,000.

Why Do Doctors Recommend Bypass Surgery?

In 1991, the American Heart Association published a set of guidelines designed to establish the conditions under which a physician should recommend bypass surgery and a patient should undergo it. The experts from the AHA and the American College of Cardiology came up with two basic reasons that justify bypass surgery. The first is to relieve severe and disabling chest pain that cannot be controlled with medication alone. This is often referred to as "incapacitating chest pain, unrelieved by good medical therapy." The second is to extend the patient's life.

All doctors and scientists concede that not everyone with angina actually needs surgery. Also, the surgery does not extend the lives of most of the people who undergo it. In fact, it will shorten the lives of many. In order to further define who will benefit from the surgery, scientists and physicians have established a further set of guidelines. As a rule, drug therapy should be used first, before surgery is considered. Only after drugs have failed to control the chest pain should surgery (bypass or balloon angioplasty) be used.

The generally accepted criteria for recommending bypass surgery are as follows:

1. The heart muscle has been severely weakened as a result of a heart attack or severe reduction of blood flow to the heart muscle. The key measurement for determining the strength of the heart is the efficiency with which the left ventricle can push out the blood from the chamber with each beat. This is called the *ejection fraction*. A heart is considered normal and healthy if the left ventricle can pump out at least 65 percent of the blood it contains in a single beat. The efficiency with which the left ventricle pumps blood is a critical indicator for whether or not a person needs bypass surgery. (Ejection fraction is measured by several tests, including an angiogram and blood pool imaging, all of which I described in Chapter 11.)

A heart with an ejection fraction of less than 65 percent is considered significantly weakened, but not necessarily in need of surgery. The upper cutoff point used to determine whether or not a person needs the operation is an ejection fraction of 50 percent, meaning that the ventricle can pump out only half of the blood it has received with each beat.

Studies have shown that people with ejection fractions of 35 to 50 percent tend to benefit from bypass surgery, especially if they also have at least three coronary arteries that are blocked with atherosclerosis. However, only a minority of heart disease patients have ejection fractions of less than 50 percent.

A landmark study compared how candidates for bypass surgery fared after ten years. The study compared those who chose bypass surgery with those who chose to have only drug therapy. Both groups had ejection fractions of 50 percent or less. The study found that there was an 18 percent greater chance of being alive after ten years if surgery was chosen. Sixty-one percent of the medication-only group survived after ten years, while 79 percent of the surgery group survived that length of time.

There are conditions in which the heart is so weak, however, that it may be best not to operate. People with ejection fractions of less than 30 percent are in this category. Because the left ventricle is so severely impaired, they have a very high risk of dying during or shortly after the surgery.

There is no question that ejection fraction is an independent and critical factor in determining whether or not a person should have bypass surgery. Also, ejection fraction should be taken into account when considering the importance of the other factors I list below.

2. Occlusion of the left main coronary artery. As I described in Chapter 2, the heart is nourished with blood and oxygen by two main coronary arteries, both of which originate in the aorta and then flow to the heart. Of the two central coronary arteries—the *right coronary artery* and the *left main coronary artery*—the left main is the larger. The left main coronary artery divides into two large branches: the *left anterior descending*, which flows down the center of the heart, and the *circumflex branch*, which runs along the extreme left side of the heart. From these large branches, of course, flow many other smaller vessels, which are also essential to the heart. When people refer to the three main coronary arteries, they're actually talking about the right coronary and the two branches of the left main.

The left main coronary artery is so large that its sudden closure could be fatal. People with significant occlusion (greater than 50 percent closure) fare better with the surgery. The greater the blockage of the artery, the worse the prognosis. Therefore, those with closure greater than 70 percent suffer even higher mortality rates if they forgo the surgery. However, recent long-term follow up of the CASS study found no survival benefit from surgery over medical care in patients with significant left main coronary artery disease if the left ventricle was still strong (ejection fraction equal to or greater than 50 percent). Therefore, *the condition of your left ventricle may be the only deciding issue* for predicting whether or not surgery will benefit you in terms of survival.

Fortunately, only 5 to 10 percent of patients who undergo angiograms actually have significant occlusion of the left main artery. That means that the vast majority of people undergoing bypass surgery do not fit this criterion.

3. Severe narrowing of all three main coronary vessels. When that happens, surgeons usually bypass all three vessels. However, the AHA guidelines suggest that such three-vessel disease should not be considered alone, but in light of the ejection fraction and the intractability of the angina. If three vessels are significantly occluded and the ejection fraction is 50 percent or lower, then surgery is probably the right choice. In this case, however, ejection fraction is an independent guide to the decision. As I will demonstrate shortly, people with normal ejection fractions and three-vessel disease don't live any longer with the surgery than those who avoid the operation and take medication for their disease.

4. The narrowing of the left anterior descending vessel. By narrowing, physicians usually mean a 50 percent closure of the vessel. As with the severe narrowing of the three coronary arteries, surgeons are supposed to take other factors, such as ejection fraction, into account before recommending a bypass for people with narrowing of the left anterior descending vessel.

Many bypasses are performed simply because the left anterior descending vessel is occluded. The research has demonstrated, however, that people who have bypass surgery for occlusion of the left anterior descending vessel, and whose ejection fractions are normal, do not live any longer than those who avoid the surgery and take medication.

Of these four standard criteria for bypass surgery, only two have been proved to consistently extend a patient's life, and thus are essential reasons for the operation:

1. An ejection fraction anywhere between 35 and 50 percent, which indicates a severely weakened heart that will, in all probability, benefit from bypass surgery

2. Significant occlusion of the left main coronary artery, as described under the second guideline (especially with a weakened heart)

Unfortunately, even though these criteria are standard and well accepted, many physicians encourage bypass surgery for people with far less severe disease. It's very common to hear of people who have had bypass surgery because they had angina, or because they had significant atherosclerosis in one or two of the coronary arteries (neither of which is the left main coronary). Some physicians will even argue for bypass surgery because an artery is 40 to 50 percent closed.

In order to give you a clearer picture of when to have bypass surgery, and when to avoid it, let's have a closer look at the evidence so that I can spell out for you a set of guidelines to assist you in your decision.

Before You Have a Bypass Operation
Get Answers to Four Questions

Before you decide whether or not to have a bypass operation, you should get complete and thorough answers to the following questions:

1. Do I have incapacitating angina unrelieved by medical therapy?
2. Have I taken full advantage of the pain-relieving benefits of medication and diet?
3. Do I fall into one or both of the categories that show that a bypass operation will improve my chances of survival?
4. What are the risks and side effects of the surgery?

By getting answers to these questions, you will clarify your condition and be in a position to make the right decision regarding whether or not to have the surgery. Let's examine each of these questions and their answers one at a time.

1. Do I have incapacitating angina unrelieved by medical therapy?

Whether or not chest pain is incapacitating can be a very subjective question. You may develop chest pain only while playing a singles tennis match and decide that you'd be satisfied with playing doubles. In this case, the chest pain is not incapacitating. Another person may regard playing singles as essential and therefore worth the surgery. Only you can determine whether the angina is indeed incapacitating and warrants surgery. In any case, you should understand that bypass surgery is not a permanent cure for your pain.

Bypass surgery does, in fact, improve or relieve chest pain in 85 percent of cases; however, that relief, very often, is only temporary. Studies have shown that between 8 and 12 percent of patients who undergo bypass surgery experience significant closure of their new vessels before they leave the hospital! A year after the surgery, 12 to 20 percent see their grafts close up. In fact, sometime during the first five years after surgery, about one-quarter of bypass patients experience what doctors call "ischemic events," meaning that they experience a recurrence of their angina, or have a heart attack, or suffer sudden death. By ten years, more than half will experience a recurrence of angina, or have a heart attack, or die suddenly. After fifteen years, 85 percent will have experienced one or more of these ischemic events. In my book, that makes bypass surgery a temporary approach, at best.

The reason for the rapid return of the disease is simple: Just because you have replaced the vessels doesn't mean you've treated—much less cured—the *cause* of the disease, which is atherosclerosis. The new vessels become clogged with cholesterol plaque just as the old ones did. And once that happens, angina pain returns and the risk of heart attack increases dramatically.

2.   Have I taken full advantage of the pain-relieving benefits of medication and diet?

Angina can be treated effectively by medication and/or diet and exercise. When patients are treated medically, that is, with drugs, the results are often just as good as when they are treated with bypass surgery. When patients are treated with appropriate diet and lifestyle, the results are almost miraculous. You will recall that I discussed in Chapter 4 the reversal of artery disease in the Lifestyle Heart Trial with a low-fat diet. In that study, a low-fat, no-cholesterol diet, coupled with a health-supporting lifestyle, also reduced the frequency of angina by 91 percent in twenty-four days.

Before you are considered a candidate for a bypass operation, you first must have tried to treat your angina medically, that is, with drugs or a program of diet and exercise, or both, and have failed with these methods. According to all the guidelines, bypass surgery is considered an option only after you've exhausted these methods.

Cure Angina Without Surgery

The same diet that reverses artery disease also relieves angina. As one recent study showed, the frequency of angina was reduced by 91 percent in less than a month on a low-fat, low-cholesterol diet. No form of medication can compare with those results for effectiveness. For the vast majority of people with angina, the best approach—and the only real cure—is a diet low in fat and absent of any cholesterol—in short, the McDougall Program for a Healthy Heart.

The McDougall Program for a Healthy Heart improves the circulation to the heart virtually overnight. Within hours of a change to a starch-based diet, fats no longer enter the bloodstream in such enormous quantities. The blood stops sludging, the oxygen content of the blood increases, overall blood flow improves, and the chest pain diminishes or disappears. (See Chapter 3, page 37.)

Finally, if the patient consistently follows it, the diet will reverse atherosclerosis, the underlying cause of heart disease, including angina pain. When the pain is significantly reduced or eliminated, the need for bypass and balloon angioplasty is removed. Following the dietary change, drugs that were intended to reduce chest pain may be reduced gradually in dosage and then discontinued entirely as soon as possible.

3.   Do I fall into one or both of the categories for which bypass improves my chances of survival?

Three major studies have compared the benefits of coronary artery bypass surgery with medical treatment designed to relieve chest pain: the Veterans Administration Cooperative Study Group, the European Coronary Surgery Study, and the Coronary Artery Surgery Study (CASS). In all three studies, long-term survival was essentially the same for the surgically treated groups and the medically treated groups.

In a landmark CASS study published in *Circulation*, researchers conducted a ten-year follow-up of 780 people, half of whom had had bypass surgery ten years prior to the follow-up report, while the other half took medication for their heart disease. The researchers found that there was no difference in survival between the two groups after ten years, nor was there any significant difference in the number of heart attacks experienced by each group. Of those who were treated with drugs, 79 percent were still alive after ten years. Of those who were treated with bypass surgery, 82 percent were alive after ten years. (The 3 percent difference was not considered statistically significant.)

The researchers who followed up on the participants of the study examined all the possible risk factors that might make bypass the treatment of choice. They looked at whether or not the patient had a history of heart failure or hypertension, at the number of vessels that were diseased, and even at the patient's age. None of these factors changed the outcome.

There was one factor, however, that did determine whether or not a person would benefit by the surgery: ejection fraction. If the patient's ejection fraction was 50 percent or greater, he stood a much better chance of avoiding a heart attack and living for ten years if he received medication only. Of those in the medication group with ejection fractions of 50 percent or greater, 75 percent had no heart attacks and survived ten years; of those with the same ejection fraction who underwent bypass surgery, only 68 percent had no heart attacks and survived.

When the researchers examined the population for survival alone, once again ejection fraction was the clear determinant for deciding whether or not to have bypass surgery. Patients with ejection fractions greater than 50 percent had a better chance of living ten years if they were treated with drugs as opposed to surgery. Those with an ejection fraction below 50 percent had a better chance of living ten years if they underwent bypass surgery.

People who had significant closure of one, two, or three coronary arteries and who had bypass surgery did not live any longer than those with the same degree of illness who were treated only with medication. An artery was considered "significantly" closed if it was at least 70 percent occluded. In addition, those with significant occlusion of the left anterior descending artery—50 percent or 70 percent closed—did not live any longer if they had bypass surgery than if they were treated only with medication.

The CASS Study showed that patients did not increase their chances of mortality if they postponed the bypass and opted for medication; in fact, bypass surgery may be harmful to people with ejection fractions greater than 50 percent. "A striking feature in CASS is the relatively low 10-year mortality of patients who had a normal ejection fraction, irrespective of the number of diseased coronary vessels," the authors stated.

For people in this situation, I believe the best chance of long-term survival and the avoidance of a heart attack is to treat their disease with medication and/or diet and lifestyle, as opposed to surgery. The researchers point out ominously that "For these [people with ejection fractions of 50 percent or higher], early bypass surgery was consistently associated with a greater frequency of [ischemic] events beyond 4–5 years."

Who doesn't benefit from bypass surgery?

1. People with single-, double-, and triple-vessel disease with normal ejection fraction
2. People with occlusion of the left anterior descending artery and normal ejection fraction
3. People who have no significant chest pain symptoms

Who benefits from bypass surgery?

1. People with ejection fractions of 35 to 50 percent
2. People with significant occlusion of the left main coronary artery (especially with a weakened heart)

What If You Say No to the Surgery?

Naturally, these studies point directly to the question of whether or not to avoid surgery. First, we should eliminate from consideration people who clearly benefit from the surgery, those with a low ejection fraction and those with left main coronary artery disease. Now, if you are not in one or both of these groups, it's likely you're asking yourself, What happens if I avoid the operation?

One study followed up on 150 patients who eight years before had decided not to undergo bypass surgery. The study, published in the *American Journal of Cardiology* reported that they did just fine. Researchers found that the annual death rate was 0 percent with one- and two-vessel disease, and 1.3 percent in patients with atherosclerosis in three vessels and those with occlusion in the left main coronary artery. Overall, 89 percent of those followed were still alive after eight years. There were fifteen heart attacks, of which twelve were not fatal. No patient with single-vessel disease suffered a heart attack. The authors concluded that patients who had had severe coronary artery disease who refused surgery had an excellent prognosis for survival.

Nevertheless, only 6 to 8 percent of patients actually refuse a bypass operation after their doctors sell them on the surgery. I wonder what that number would be if all heart disease patients knew all the facts about the surgery and its side effects, and knew that the underlying disease is reversible by diet and a daily walk? Unfortunately, many patients are told that they need a bypass operation while still recovering from a heart attack in the hospital. In that most vulnerable position, many doctors tell their patients that they will not live to reach the hospital doors if they do not have bypass surgery. What can a patient do, except hope that the doctor is giving him or her the best information.

4.   What are the risks and side effects of the surgery?

Before anyone goes into surgery, he or she should fully understand the risks of the procedure and the possible side effects. In the case of bypass surgery, both are significant.

The Risks

Most doctors will tell you that there is about a 1 percent risk of dying during a bypass operation. That's not really true. This figure refers to ideal patients and ideal settings. What you care about are the averages for *your* hospital, *your* surgeon, and *your* condition. Those numbers may be much different than the ideal.

Local community and university hospitals vary widely in their mortality rates for bypass surgery, from 4.9 percent death rates to greater than 10 percent. A recent University of Pennsylvania study showed that mortality rates in some hospitals can reach as high as 11.9 percent of the patients. In California, the mortality rate among people undergoing bypass surgery was 4.6 percent; for people over 65, it was 7.2 percent. A recent study of Medicare patients revealed that 10.5 percent never left the hospital after undergoing bypass surgery.

Surgeons themselves have varying rates of success, for many reasons. There are highly talented doctors who take on the worst cases and then there are doctors whose track records are simply subpar. Studies indicate that the success rates among surgeons vary from a 1.9 percent to 9.2 percent mortality. You have to make an effort to know how skilled your surgeon is. You can start by having a confidential talk with your general practitioner and other doctors around town. Physicians will not criticize other doctors, but they will praise those whose talents are well known and refer you to that surgeon. Another way to find out about the track records of surgeons is to ask a hospital nurse.

Mortality rates also vary according to sex and size of body. Women are particularly at risk. Studies have shown that women's death rate during bypass surgery is more than double that of men. Men of smaller stature also have higher mortality rates than men of normal size. These higher-than-average death rates for both men and women of smaller stature may be due to the smaller size of their hearts and vessels.

Side Effects

Shocking as it sounds, nearly all people who are kept alive during surgery by a heart-lung machine experience some degree of brain damage. Even worse, between 15 and 44 percent of people who have had bypass surgery suffer *permanent* brain damage. They can't remember names or numbers as they once did, experience sleep disturbances (including nightmares), suffer mood swings, and lose intellectual acuity. Approximately 30 percent of people suffer persistent depression and some even contemplate suicide.

In a study published in the *British Medical Journal*, 61 percent of patients who underwent bypass surgery showed signs of brain injury that was evident upon physical examination during the first week after the operation. Follow-up studies have shown that six months after surgery, more than half of those with initial symptoms still exhibited signs of brain damage.

The dark sides of bypass surgery are rarely discussed. The patient is released from the hospital, usually with the mildest warning that he or she may be a bit forgetful for a while. However, old friends and family members begin to notice strange abnormalities in behavior, as that mild forgetfulness, in fact, is accompanied by symptoms that are far more significant and disturbing.

How Does the Brain Damage Happen?

A heart-lung machine can introduce toxic gases, fat globules, and bits of plastic debris into the bloodstream of the patient under anesthesia. Once they are in the bloodstream, these particles migrate to the brain, where they can clog capillaries and prevent adequate amounts of blood and oxygen from flowing to the brain, thus damaging brain cells.

In addition, serious complications, such as strokes, heart attacks, kidney failure, internal bleeding, and infection occur in 13 percent of cases.

Recommending the Surgery for Inappropriate or Equivocal Reasons

Unless you arm yourself with this essential information, there's a good chance you will be operated on for inappropriate or questionable reasons. When scientists review the reasons people undergo bypass surgery, they find that this occurs in all too many cases.

In a landmark study published in the *Journal of the American Medical Association*, an expert panel of doctors assessed whether bypasses were being performed for appropriate or inappropriate reasons. After evaluating 386 cases of people who had undergone bypass surgery, the researchers concluded that only 56 percent were performed for "appropriate" reasons. The remainder of the surgeries—44 percent!—were performed for "inappropriate" or "equivocal" reasons.

Also in the *Journal of the American Medical Association*, a study done by Thomas Graboys, M.D., showed that 50 percent of people recommended for bypass surgery could have avoided the operation by getting a second opinion. In addition, none of those who were advised to avoid the surgery died during the study period of more than two years.

Remember, the two most appropriate reasons for having bypass surgery are:

1. To relieve chest pain that cannot be treated by good medical therapy
2. To save lives

If you're having the surgery before medical therapy has been given a chance to treat your angina, or if you do not fall into one of the categories for which bypass surgery has been proved to extend life, you are having the surgery for the wrong reason.

Only extraordinarily determined and well-informed patients question a doctor's recommendation, and very few have the will to seek a second opinion. But, obviously, such a decision can save your life. A second opinion can be your best safeguard against unwarranted surgery.

Treat the Underlying Problem

Changing your diet before you have bypass surgery will usually relieve the chest pain and begin the reversal of the underlying atherosclerosis. However, if you have already had the surgery, the McDougall Program for a Healthy Heart will slow and even halt the progress of the underlying disease, both in your original coronary arteries, and in the vessels that have been used in the bypass operation. A healthful diet will keep the angina from coming back, and keep you off the operating table for a second bypass.

Therefore, whatever your decision is regarding bypass surgery, keep in mind that the operation does not cure heart disease. As the authors of a ten-year follow-up study wrote in the *British Medical Journal*, "We should remember that surgery for degenerative disease never cures." In fact, it merely postpones the heart attack if we do not change our ways.

Recently, my father was asked if he followed the McDougall Program now, after his operation. "Are you kidding?" he said. "I have to follow the diet now, otherwise I'll be in trouble again."

My father had his hip replaced in October 1994. He is now healthier and happier than I could have imagined—putting in a full day of hard physical work, driving his car, and traveling whenever he has the chance. He follows the McDougall diet strickly (with very little sugar), walks daily, and takes enough cholesterol lowering medication to keep his levels ideal (below 150 mg/dl).

Balloon Angioplasty

Percutaneous transluminal coronary angioplasty (PTCA), more commonly referred to as balloon angioplasty, or simply angioplasty, is done by inserting a catheter into an artery, usually in the leg, and then threading it through

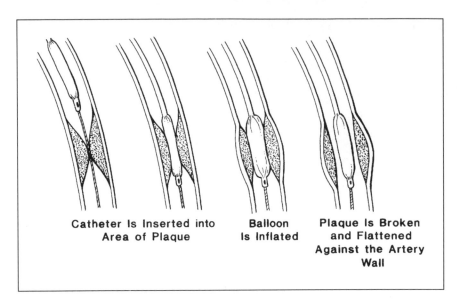

Catheter Is Inserted into   Balloon   Plaque Is Broken
      Area of Plaque   Is Inflated   and Flattened
                                                    Against the Artery
                                                          Wall

Angioplasty is performed over 300,000 times a year in the United States. If successful, chest pain is relieved and blood flow to the heart is improved. The Achilles' heel of this procedure is closure (restenosis), which occurs in 25 to 50 percent of cases within six months of the operation. Even with all this newfangled technology, an improved chance for survival has not been achieved with this surgery.

the body and into one of the coronary arteries that is clogged with atherosclerotic plaque. At the tip of the catheter is a balloon, which is positioned within the site of the plaque and then inflated, thus squeezing the plaque to either side of the artery and creating a larger opening.

Angioplasty is done on patients with one or more clogged coronary arteries who have chronic angina that has not responded to medication. It is also done on people who do not have angina, but do have proven and significant atherosclerosis of the coronary arteries.

The procedure is considered successful—which is to say, it manages to cut the size of the plaque in half—in 83 to 95 percent of cases. With the reduction in the size of the plaque, more blood is allowed to pass through the artery and on to the heart, thus reducing the ischemia and the angina. However, in 25 to 50 percent of all cases, these same vessels are blocked again within six months because of restenosis, or the formation of new atherosclerotic plaques. This occurs, in part, because the artery is injured during the procedure, causing platelets and blood-clotting proteins to form a thrombus over the wound, which can become large enough to close off the artery. The rate of restenosis is higher among people who had more than one angioplasty. The death rate during the operation is between 0.4 and 2.8 percent.

Each year, more than 300,000 people receive balloon angioplasties. The number has doubled between 1986 and 1990, years in which the rate of heart disease was declining, and is climbing rapidly.

At best, the procedure is a very temporary fix. *Angioplasty does not save lives.* Complications resulting from the procedure include a 1 percent chance of dying during the operation and a 10 percent chance of developing major complications—with a 5 percent risk of having a heart attack as a result of the procedure. Nevertheless, the procedure is not comparable to bypass surgery in its invasiveness, or its side effects, and therefore is considered the preferable treatment.

I consider angioplasty useful when the patient has chest pain that cannot be relieved by a good diet and judicious use of medication. It should never be sold to the patient as a way of prolonging life, since the studies are clear that this survival benefit has never been demonstrated.

My Advice to People with Angina

My advice to anyone who is having chest pain is to believe what your chest pain is trying to tell you: "You are on the verge of dying of a dietary disease. Help!" Your heart is pleading with every twinge of pain for relief from the lard you're shoveling into your belly three or more times a day. Have you noticed how the chest pains become worse after you've gulped down a fat-filled meal, or chomped on a thick, juicy steak? Change your life. Adopt this program. You'll feel better in every way, and with time you'll start to wonder how you ever ate all that fat in the first place.

In the few cases where changing diet is not enough, use drugs to relieve the chest pain. If the chest pain continues, you'll need further evaluation, which may require a treadmill stress test, thallium scan, and angiogram. You may elect to go ahead with bypass surgery if these tests reveal that you fall into one of the two categories for which surgery is beneficial for survival: significant occlusion of the left main coronary artery (especially with a weakened heart) and depressed ejection fraction. If you do not fall into one of these categories and you continue to have chest pain, then you may consider angioplasty for relief.

Regardless of what you choose to do, you still need to adopt a healthy diet and lifestyle in order to keep your disease from progressing.

Sometimes You Just Have to Say No

Bypass surgery is not for everyone. Consider all I have said and remember that you, like Gerrit Boerfyn, still have options.

In 1978 Gerrit Boerfyn, a 68-year-old minister, came to me after suffering from a partially obstructed artery in his neck due to atherosclerosis. He had tingling in his jaw (the result of the blocked blood vessel in his neck), mild symptoms of angina (from atherosclerosis in his coronary arteries), and tingling in his fingers. After following the diet for a short while, these symptoms disappeared.

For the next ten years, Gerrit followed the program off and on, but in 1988 he began to experience chest pains. He had an exercise treadmill stress test that showed that his heart did indeed suffer from ischemia. That test was followed by an angiogram, which discovered that his left main coronary artery was open; his left anterior descending artery was 100 percent occluded; his circumflex artery was 50 percent occluded; and one of the descending branches of the right coronary artery was 70 percent closed. His left ventricle ejection fraction was above 50 percent. Gerrit also had slightly high blood pressure that measured 160/80 mm Hg.

His doctors recommended that he have bypass surgery, but at age 78 Gerrit didn't want the surgery, nor did he believe he absolutely needed it.

That year, he came back to me and I placed him on the McDougall Program for a Healthy Heart, which rapidly brought his cholesterol level down from 230 mg/dl to 175 mg/dl. I put him on some cholesterol-lowering medication, which caused his cholesterol to fall below 150 mg/dl. Meanwhile, his blood pressure also fell to 142/80, barely in the normal range, it is true, but a big improvement nonetheless. Gerrit's chest pain subsided and he regained much of his old vitality.

Gerrit is doing great at 85. His most recent cholesterol level was 175, and he's still walking daily, without the chest pain. And he never had that bypass operation.

14. Controlling High Blood Pressure and Curing It Naturally

- *High blood pressure can be cured.*
- *Drugs can help, but they can also harm.*
- *Don't rush to take medication: You have time.*

Sixty million Americans have high blood pressure. The illness, also known as hypertension, is the most common reason people go to doctors. It's also the number one reason that medication is prescribed in the world today. More people are taking medication for hypertension than have ever taken medicine for any illness ever encountered in human history. High blood pressure is a plague!

Once you are diagnosed with high blood pressure, you are many times more vulnerable to a host of other illnesses and premature death. People with hypertension are seven times more likely to suffer a stroke, four times more likely to have a heart attack, and five times more likely to die of congestive heart failure.

Strictly speaking, high blood pressure is not a disease at all. It's an indicator of trouble in your circulatory system that results from a constellation of underlying problems affecting blood circulation. These underlying factors combine to raise blood pressure, sometimes to very dangerous levels. Yet, the disorder itself is merely a sign of underlying disease, just as fever is a sign of pneumonia, or swelling a sign of a broken bone.

High blood pressure is far more common among people who live in affluent nations than it is among people of the Third World. Among rich nations, such as the United States, blood pressure increases as we age. Half of Americans 65 and older are hypertensive. In many Third World countries, however, blood pressures remain within the healthy range throughout life. The people of New Guinea and many African nations—even their senior citizens—have blood pressures that resemble those of a healthy American teenager. There is no racial immunity for high blood pressure. If you were to take those same Africans and feed them the standard American diet, you would see their blood pressures skyrocket to levels that are typical of hypertensive Americans. That is precisely the case among African Americans, 28 percent of whom suffer from high blood pressure and are consuming the ideal diet for hypertension. The disorder attacks an estimated 16 to 18 percent of white Americans, as well as many Asians, Hispanics, Native Americans, and people of Middle Eastern descent.

If we back up and look at the worldwide distribution of hypertension, we get a very clear picture of who suffers from the illness, who doesn't, and why. That pattern points directly at the causes of the disorder, as well as at its prevention and cure. The cure is simple: a diet low in fat, cholesterol, salt, and refined foods, coupled with a lifestyle that includes moderate exercise and the maintenance of normal weight. That diet and lifestyle is the McDougall Program for a Healthy Heart. I put people on a diet and exercise program that closely resembles the simple eating and activity levels of traditional peoples, among whom cardiovascular diseases, including high blood pressure, are rare or nonexistent. Laboratory research has consistently shown that a healthy vegetarian diet, mild exercise, and weight loss not only reduce blood pressure, but normalize it and allow people to get off medication.

What Is Blood Pressure?

Blood pressure is the force exerted on the blood as it moves through your arteries. The force of the pumping heart muscle against the resistance of the blood vessels creates the pressure. Your blood pressure rises and falls naturally throughout the day. When you wake up, get out of bed, exercise, or experience stressful situations, your heart beats more rapidly to meet the increased demand for blood and oxygen from cells and tissues throughout the body. This increase in heart rate also increases your blood pressure during these particular times. Blood pressure falls while you rest, and especially while you sleep, because the demands on the heart are greatly diminished. In healthy people, blood pressure rises when heart rate increases, and drops into the normal ranges when the increased demand is relieved.

Blood pressure is expressed as a fraction, such as 110/75 (read one hundred and ten over seventy-five). Two numbers are used because there are two pressures being measured. The first pressure, called *systolic*, indicated by the top number, represents the phase when the heart contracts and pumps blood into the aorta, the body's main artery. As the blood is pushed into the arteries, they expand. The recoil of those arteries, or their contraction, creates the second type of blood pressure, called *diastolic*. This pressure occurs while the heart rests, the valves open, and the ventricles fill with blood. While the heart expands, the arteries contract and serve as a kind of second pumping action.

Diastolic pressure, therefore, indicates the relative flexibility of your arteries. The less flexible your arteries are the more pressure they will exert as they recoil or contract on the blood. It's a lot easier for the heart to pump blood through soft, flexible arteries than to pump blood through hard, inflexible vessels. The degree of inflexibility of those arteries tells us how much resistance the heart must overcome in order to pump the blood. Naturally, the harder the vessels, the harder the heart must work. Atherosclerosis makes these vessels get hard.

Blood pressure is measured as millimeters of mercury (mm Hg), which dates back to a time when the original blood pressure gauges used mercury in a glass tube to indicate how high or low the blood pressure was. Originally, the blood pressure gauge indicated how much pressure was necessary to move a column of mercury up a calibrated tube. Today, the gauge, called a sphygmomanometer, or a blood pressure cuff, uses air and a spring, and the test can be performed by just about anyone at home in a few seconds.

I urge people with high blood pressure, even if it's mild, to buy a cuff and check your pressure regularly at home because it will give you the most consistent and accurate reading. Blood pressure readings are usually higher when taken at a doctor's office. This phenomenon is called "white coat hypertension": You become hypertensive when faced with a stressful situation, such as having your blood pressure read by a doctor or nurse.

Recently, I went for a life insurance physical and had to have my blood pressure checked. Remarkably, I tested mildly hypertensive at

140/90. I was shocked. My blood pressure has always been excellent. How could I have high blood pressure? After the test, I drove home and had my wife, Mary, check my pressure. "If your blood pressure was any lower, you'd be dead," she said. What I had experienced was white coat hypertension. I do not test hypertensive at home, but like many people, I test hypertensive in a doctor's office. Lots of people have this experience, so I recommend that you test your blood pressure in a setting in which you feel safe. You may not get an accurate reading, otherwise.

BP Ranges: What the Numbers Mean

There is no line of demarcation separating a healthy from an unhealthy blood pressure. Rather, it's a small margin in which the ranges for health and illness vary somewhat, depending on the person and other risk factors. As we will see shortly, this margin is significant because it dictates how the illness is often treated.

An ideal blood pressure is 110/70 mm Hg or less *without* medication.

However, it is commonly agreed in medicine that a normal, resting blood pressure is 120/80 mm Hg. Blood pressure is considered high, or hypertensive, if either the top or bottom number is consistently above 140/90 mm Hg while the person is at rest.

There are varying degrees of high blood pressure. Most people with hypertension fall into the category of being mildly hypertensive, which is classified as having a diastolic pressure of between 90 and 104 mm Hg. Forty million Americans have diastolic pressures between 90 and 104 mm Hg, meaning a great many Americans are mildly hypertensive.

Moderate hypertension is a diastolic pressure that consistently falls between 105 and 114 mm Hg. Severe hypertension is a diastolic pressure that is consistently at 115 mm Hg or above. In a small number of cases, severe hypertension can accelerate into *malignant* hypertension, which is accompanied by hemorrhages of small blood vessels, headaches, vomiting, visual impairment (even blindness), convulsions, paralysis, and coma. The words mild and moderate can be misleading. Studies have shown that even modest elevations in blood pressure are associated with an increased risk of premature coronary heart disease.

Looking in All the Wrong Places

Between 90 and 95 percent of people with hypertension have the type of high blood pressure referred to by doctors as "essential" hypertension, which means that there is no definable or well-understood cause of the disorder. The problem, they say, is that too many systems are involved in the cause, which makes isolating any one cause difficult or impossible.

This approach is rather like giving a horse curare—a poison that paralyzes its victims—and then wondering whether the heart, lungs, or nervous system was paralyzed first and thus caused the horse's death. We could spend some time analyzing and discussing precisely which organ was the first to give out. We could even note that in certain horses, the heart goes first, but in others the nervous system is the first to go. But rather than discussing all these options, isn't it easier to say that the curare killed the horse and leave it at that? This solution would also give us some basis for treatment: Stop giving horses curare.

Medicine suffers from the same problem when it tries to figure out which system goes wrong and "causes" high blood pressure. The problem is that when you are looking at the systems involved in the cause of hypertension, you're not seeing the cause at all. You're only seeing the effects of the cause on certain biological systems. That cause, of course, is what you put in your mouth, which changes those systems and causes your blood pressure to rise. High blood pressure is actually the natural result of a diseased circulatory system. For many people with high blood pressure, the heart must work harder to pump the blood against the resistance in circulation—thus systolic pressure goes up—and the vessels themselves are narrow and rigid, which boosts diastolic pressure. Rather than stop our investigation with the problems of the heart and circulation, we should look deeper and investigate *why* the circulatory system is in such a diseased state, and how we can restore health.

Rounding Up the Usual Suspects

You learned the principles by which blood pressure is increased when you were a kid playing with a garden hose or water nozzle. One of the ways you could raise the pressure in the hose was simply by turning the water faucet on even further, which pumped more water into the hose. You could turn that hose into a powerful squirt gun if you turned up the volume and then placed your thumb partially over the hose's tip. This really got the pressure up because you increased the amount of water in the hose and you made the hose's opening smaller by placing your thumb partially over it. By placing your thumb over the end of the hose, you decrease the area through which the water can flow, which increases the amount of resistance to the flow and raises the pressure. In the body, squeezing all your little hoses—your blood vessels—increases resistance to flow, causing high blood pressure. This is called increased peripheral resistance.

Increasing Heart Rate Increases Pressure

As I said earlier, your blood pressure increases merely by getting out of bed or by exercising, simply because you have caused your heart to pump more blood per minute. This increases the pressure behind the blood. Caffeine is one of several drugs that will increase heart rate and drive up blood pressure, which explains why coffee drinkers often suffer from higher blood pressure and why doctors encourage people with hypertension to avoid caffeinated beverages.

Beware of Excesses of Sodium, Especially If You Are Sensitive

You can increase the volume within your circulation by eating excess amounts of sodium found in salt. Table salt is about 40 percent sodium. When eaten in excess amounts, sodium can draw fluid from your tissues into your bloodstream, which can increase the volume of fluid within the vessels. Once you've done that, you can easily increase the pressure behind the blood.

Not everyone who eats normal amounts of salt experiences elevations in blood pressure, however. About 30 percent of people with high blood pressure are considered "salt sensitive" and have elevated pressures as a result of sodium intake, according to an extensive review of the literature on sodium published in the *American Journal of Hypertension*. Studies have shown that when people with a salt sensitivity reduce their salt intake, their blood pressure returns to normal and they are able to go off medication.

If your blood pressure is elevated from sodium intake, you can lower it by reducing your salt consumption. Within a few days, your kidneys and skin should be able to eliminate the excess sodium and fluid from your body, and thus allow your blood pressure to return to normal. However, if you continue to eat unhealthy amounts of sodium, your blood pressure will remain elevated. People with sodium sensitivity must carefully monitor their sodium intake.

The body requires some salt to maintain both normal blood pressure and many biological systems. People consuming the standard high-fat, high-cholesterol diet typical of Western industrialized nations consume, on average, between 8 and 10 g per day, or about 1 to 2 teaspoons. The National Academy of Sciences recommends that healthy people eat no more than 2,400 mg of sodium per day, which is the equivalent of 6 g of salt, or about 1 teaspoon derived from all sources, including natural and packaged foods.

However, for the vast majority of people, sodium is not as damaging as fat and cholesterol. Studies of people following a vegetarian diet that includes generous amounts of salt show no elevations in blood pressure. The vegetarians studied (the diet was based on the principles of macrobiotics) avoided all dairy products, eggs, and meat. Consequently, their fat and cholesterol consumption was exceedingly low, but their sodium intake relatively high. On the McDougall Program for a Healthy Heart, you'll have no trouble keeping sodium intake at healthy levels, thus eliminating this cause of high blood pressure.

Fat: Still the Heart of Darkness

The third way to increase blood pressure, and clearly the most dangerous because it increases many other risk factors for heart disease, is by triggering several unhealthy changes in the circulatory system. When arteries are narrowed by atherosclerotic plaque, the caliber of the passageway becomes smaller, causing pressure to build behind the obstruction. Atherosclerosis does the same thing to your blood that pinching a water hose does: It increases the pressure.

Atherosclerotic plaque occurs in arteries of all sizes throughout the body. Big and small vessels may be pinched by plaque in the arms, legs, neck, chest, and around the heart. As we discussed in Chapters 2 and 3, the infiltration of fat and cholesterol into the artery makes the vessel less elastic, which prevents the arteries from expanding and thus accommodating the blood. The inability of vessels to expand forces the heart to work harder in order to pump blood through these vessels because these hard arteries create more resistance against which the heart must work. This extra work naturally raises systolic pressure, or the pressure exerted by the heart during its contraction. Elderly people exhibit the greatest elevations of systolic pressure, and, not coincidentally, have the most atherosclerosis.

Nevertheless, it isn't just the elderly who suffer from hypertension due to atherosclerosis. Forty percent of people with high blood pressure have cholesterol levels of 240 mg/dl or more. A cholesterol level of 240 mg/dl or higher will create rapid and profuse onset of atherosclerotic plaque throughout the body—what physicians routinely call "galloping atherosclerosis." These arterial plaques function the same way as a thumb covering the tip of a garden hose. When cholesterol is lowered through diet, people with hypertension often experience a drop in their blood pressure to normal levels.

Fat and cholesterol also affect blood chemistry in ways that promote the likelihood of hypertension. When high quantities of all types of fats—meaning saturated, polyunsaturated, and monounsaturated fats—are consumed, they cause blood cells to adhere to one another, or clump. These clumping cells can cause traffic jams in the medium-size and smaller vessels, and block blood flow entirely in the tiny capillaries, thus increasing resistance to flow and thereby increasing blood pressure. (See Chapter 3, page 38.)

The third change that increases peripheral resistance is the contraction of the muscular walls of the blood vessels. The rich foods we eat cause adverse changes in hormones known as prostaglandins, which trigger the blood vessels to contract and go into spasm. The clumping of platelets caused by animal fats also releases prostaglandins. The blockage, sludging, and spasm increase the resistance to blood flow, and the pressure goes up as expected. The heart works harder, and pressure is increased in order to maintain circulation to tissues.

Eliminating the Causes Normalizes BP

While cardiologists maintain that there is no known cause of high blood pressure, there is nevertheless a large body of evidence showing that high blood pressure normalizes when you eliminate the causes I've mentioned.

Blood Pressure Changes
(for entire group)

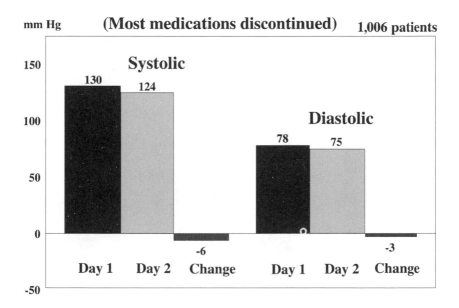

mm Hg   **(Most medications discontinued)**   1,006 patients

Systolic

150

130   124

100   Diastolic

78   75

50

0

-6   -3

Day 1   Day 2   Change   Day 1   Day 2   Change

-50

Blood pressure fell within hours of starting the McDougall Program. Twenty percent of the people were on blood pressure medication the day they began the program. In almost every case the medications were stopped that day. Yet the blood pressure dropped an average of 6/3 mm Hg by the second day. This data is from over 1,000 participants studied at the McDougall Program at St. Helena Hospital in the Napa Valley of California.

For example, in 1986 British researchers divided fifty-eight people with mild hypertension into two groups. One group was placed on a lacto-ovo-vegetarian diet, the other on a diet that included meat. Those who followed the vegetarian diet saw a drop of 5 mm Hg in their diastolic pressure. The authors concluded, "In untreated subjects with mild hypertension, changing to a vegetarian diet may bring about a worthwhile fall in diastolic blood pressure." It should be noted that a lacto-ovo-vegetarian diet contains plenty of fat, cholesterol, and sodium, which supports the underlying disease. But such a diet can be lower in fat and cholesterol than diets containing meats. Also, vegetarian diets are richer in fiber, which

Blood Pressure Changes
(with initial BP greater than 150/90)

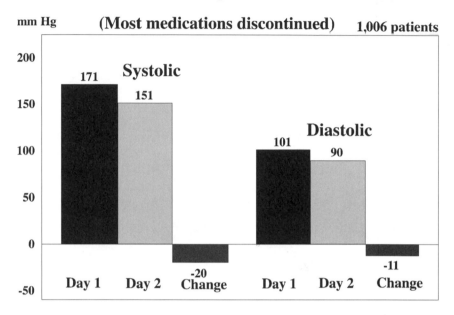

mm Hg   (Most medications discontinued)   1,006 patients

People starting the program with the highest blood pressures showed the greatest reductions in blood pressures. Patients with an initial blood pressure of 150/90 or greater had an average fall in pressure of 20/11 mm Hg overnight (and most medications are stopped). Decreasing salt, fat, caffeine, and psychological stresses had immediate beneficial effects on blood pressure. Medications must be reduced quickly in most people to avoid a dangerously low blood pressure. This data is from over 1,000 participants studied at the McDougall Program at St. Helena Hospital in the Napa Valley of California.

lowers cholesterol, and many vegetable foods that lower blood pressure. In general, both laboratory evidence and population studies have shown that vegetarian diets are associated with lower blood pressure.

British scientists investigated which of four approaches worked best for hypertensive people: a low-fat diet, a low-sodium diet, a high-fiber diet, or a diet that combined all three of these factors—low fat, low sodium, and high fiber. What they discovered was that none of the individual approaches worked as well as when all three were combined. The researchers examined 196 hypertensive people, all of whom were on hypertension medication. These people were divided into five groups: one group made no changes and served as controls; one adopted a low-fat diet; one adopted a low-sodium diet; one increased their fiber intake; and one adopted a diet low in fat and salt and high in fiber. It was the fifth group—the one that used all three dietary improvements—that showed the best results. Fifty-eight percent of those in the fifth group were able to stop taking their hypertension medication, and many of the rest were able to reduce their dosages by nearly two-thirds.

Weight Loss for Healthy BP

One of the most powerful treatments for high blood pressure is weight loss, and few programs, if any, reduce weight as effectively as the McDougall Program for a Healthy Heart (see *McDougall's Program for Maximum Weight Loss*). In numerous studies, weight loss by itself has been shown to reduce blood pressure and allow people to go off medication.

A study published in the *Archives of Internal Medicine* found that weight loss alone reduced blood pressure as effectively as drug therapy. The researchers compared the effects on diastolic pressure of weight loss versus drug treatment. After six months, people who lost at least 4.5 kilograms (nearly 10 pounds) had a drop in diastolic pressure of 11.6 mm Hg; the diastolic pressure of those who lost at least 2.25 kg (nearly five pounds) dropped by 7 mm Hg. These declines were compared to the effects of two drugs, 25 mg of chlorthalidone and 50 mg of atenolol, which brought about reductions of 11.1 mm Hg and 12.4 mm Hg, respectively, in diastolic pressure. The researchers concluded that "effective weight loss (greater than 4.5 kg) lowers blood pressure similarly to low-dose drug therapy."

In a study published in the *Journal of the American Medical Association*, researchers examined the effects of weight loss alone and weight loss plus salt restriction. They found that a modest weight reduction of 3.9 kg (about 8.5 pounds) resulted in a drop in diastolic pressure of 2.9 mm Hg. Reduction of sodium caused a diastolic drop of 0.9 mm Hg among those tested. When the researchers compared the effects on blood pressure of weight loss and sodium restriction to stress management alone and nutritional supplementation alone, they found that only weight loss and sodium restriction actually reduced blood pressure significantly.

Exercise: It Does Your BP Good

Another lifestyle approach to lower blood pressure that has consistently proved effective is moderate exercise. By moderate I mean taking a brisk thirty-minute walk, three or four times per week. You can get the equivalent exercise by doing any number of aerobic exercises, such as swimming, jogging, bicycling, aerobic dancing, and tennis. (See Chapter 6 for McDougall's exercise program for people with cardiovascular disease.)

In a review of the literature that examined the question of whether exercise reduced high blood pressure, researchers reported in the *Journal of Clinical Epidemiology* that "exercise appeared to be an effective strategy for reducing resting blood pressure in normotensive [people with normal blood pressure] and hypertensive participants."

When exercise is combined with weight loss and salt reduction, the effects on blood pressure are also positive—and impressive. Scientists studying the effects of a combined program of exercise, weight loss, and salt reduction on people (ages 65 to 80) with mild hypertension found that such a program was sufficient to eliminate hypertensive medication. "Our data indicate that a nonpharmacologic intervention [lifestyle therapy without drugs] will lower systolic and diastolic blood pressure in older people with borderline or mild elevations of diastolic pressure," wrote researcher William B. Applegate, M.D., and his colleagues in the *Archives of Internal Medicine*.

In study after study, exercise alone or in combination with salt restriction and weight loss effectively lowers blood pressure and often eliminates the need for medication.

It is important for people with high blood pressure to check with their physicians before starting an exercise program. Also, when you start to exercise, be sure that you do not overexert yourself. Walking is a safe and effective way to exercise and lower blood pressure. A simple way of testing whether you are overexerting is to make sure you can talk as you exercise. If you can't, you're working too hard. Slow down and resume a more moderate pace.

Weight Loss
(for entire group)

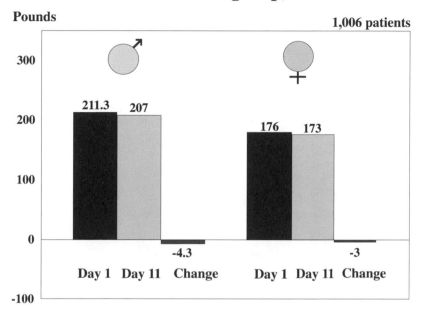

Pounds
300
200
100
0
-100

1,006 patients

211.3 207
176 173
-4.3
-3

Day 1 Day 11 Change   Day 1 Day 11 Change

Most weight loss programs fail because they ask you to fight one of your basic instincts for survival—hunger. The McDougall Program allows you to eat as much as you want of delicious foods. In eleven days men lost an average of 4.3 pounds, and women 3 pounds, while fully satisfying their hunger. This data is from over 1,000 participants studied at the McDougall Program at St. Helena Hospital in the Napa Valley of California.

The McDougall Program for a Healthy Heart:
Put All the Data Together in a Single Program

If you study the medical literature as closely as I do, you're able to see patterns that those who look only at individual studies may not see. But I must admit that it doesn't take a genius to figure out that if fat, cholesterol, salt, weight, and activity levels are all related to the cause and cure of hypertension, then perhaps the best approach to the illness is to create a lifestyle that addresses all these factors. And that's what I've done with the McDougall Program for a Healthy Heart.

Weight Loss
(for heavier people)

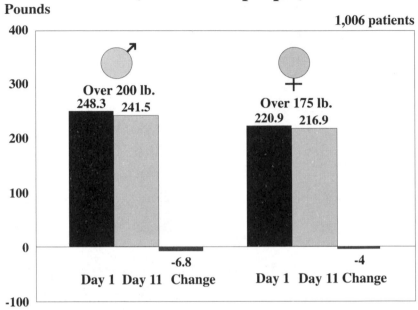

Pounds

1,006 patients

400

300

Over 200 lb.
248.3   241.5

Over 175 lb.
220.9   216.9

200

100

0

-6.8

-4

Day 1 Day 11 Change

Day 1 Day 11 Change

-100

Heavier people lose weight faster. Men starting at over 200 pounds lost nearly 7 pounds, and women starting at over 175 pounds lost 4 pounds, on the average, in eleven days, while fully satisfying their hunger. Weight loss continues when they leave the live-in program, often at a greater rate, because they no longer have a professional chef feeding them four-course meals three times a day. This data is from over 1,000 participants studied at the McDougall Program at St. Helena Hospital in the Napa Valley of California.

On my program, overweight people lose between 6 and 15 pounds per month, depending on how overweight they are. That kind of weight loss continues until they arrive at trim body weight, at which point the weight loss levels off and they have no trouble staying at their ideal weight.

Successful treatment of hypertension requires a healthy diet, lifestyle, and exercise. Most people can correct an elevated blood pressure within twenty-four to seventy-two hours. Once your blood pressure starts to fall, you must begin to lower the dosage of your medication quickly under your doctor's supervision.

Diseases That Often Increase Blood Pressure

Among the most common disorders that contribute to hypertension are diabetes mellitus and kidney disease.

Diabetes

Diabetes, a disease characterized by the body's inability to utilize blood sugar, dramatically increases your chances of contracting several cardiovascular diseases, including atherosclerosis, coronary heart disease, and hypertension. Diabetics have twice the risk of suffering a heart attack or stroke than nondiabetics. A diabetic man or woman is fifteen times more likely to lose a limb as a result of peripheral vascular disease. Diabetes contributes to the destruction of blood vessels throughout the system, and thereby increases the likelihood of suffering from kidney disease, blindness, and complications of childbearing. People with both diabetes and hypertension—a very common combination—are at greater risk of contracting many other illnesses.

There are two types of diabetes: type I (juvenile diabetes) and type II (adult-onset diabetes). Most people with diabetes have adult-onset, or type II; less than 10 percent of the 14 million diabetics have type I, or juvenile diabetes. The pancreas does not produce sufficient insulin to make blood sugar available to the cells of juvenile diabetics. Without sugar, cells lack fuel. People with type I diabetes must take insulin in order to survive. Type II diabetics, on the other hand, produce insulin, but their bodies are unable to efficiently utilize the natural insulin produced by the pancreas. Type II diabetics suffer from the same range of illnesses that threaten type I diabetics.

Excessive consumption of rich food loaded with fat and lacking complex carbohydrates and fiber prevents cells from utilizing the body's insulin, and is the major cause of adult-onset diabetes. These components of the food in the blood also create an array of other illnesses, among them atherosclerosis, peripheral vascular disease, kidney disorders, blindness, and hypertension.

Many people with type II diabetes can reverse the illness by adopting a diet low in fat and cholesterol, such as the McDougall Program for a Healthy Heart. Once blood levels of fat and cholesterol fall into the healthy ranges, the body's ability to utilize insulin returns to many type II diabetics.

Kidney Disease

The same factors that cause hypertension can also cause kidney disease, which in turn can further elevate blood pressure. The filtering unit within each kidney is called a nephron. These tiny structures extract waste products from the blood. The kidneys are highly vulnerable to our rich American diet, especially to the high quantities of fat, cholesterol, and protein. Fat and cholesterol can cause atherosclerotic plaques to form in the kidneys, thus blocking the arteries and diminishing the functional size of the organs. High-protein diets can also destroy kidney tissue. By restricting protein intake, people with degenerative kidney disease can dramatically slow the progression of the illness, and even experience remarkable improvement in kidney health.

Kidney damage can elevate blood pressure. When kidney function is diminished, the organs cannot adequately filter toxins and sodium from the blood, thus increasing the volume of fluid in the blood and raising blood pressure. Damaged kidneys also can produce greater than normal amounts of hormones like angiotension that can signal blood vessels to constrict and thus narrow the vessel's passageway, thereby elevating blood pressure.

Fat and protein levels are brought into healthful ranges, and kidney health is vastly improved, when you adopt the McDougall Program for a Healthy Heart.

Two Lives Back from the Brink

Before I delve deeper into hypertension and the problems associated with the standard treatment of the disease, let's look at two people with serious problems who adopted the McDougall Program for a Healthy Heart.

In the fall of 1992, Dave Machado, an environmental engineer living in the greater San Francisco area, was feeling "lousy." He was 49 years old and suffered from high blood pressure and adult-onset diabetes; he was overweight and had a cholesterol level that hovered between 280 and 300 mg/dl. He had been taking medication for his blood pressure for the past three years. Even on the drugs his blood pressure fluctuated but routinely stayed at 160/95—both numbers above normal. Dave had been on medication for his diabetes for the past eight years, with little positive effect. His doctor told him that Micronase, an oral medication for hyperglycemia, was not sufficient to control his diabetes and that he would soon have to go on insulin unless he made significant lifestyle changes. Among the recommendations his doctor made was for him to lose weight. In addition to the significant and even life-threatening problems he suffered from was the fact that he had little energy. "I only had energy for my work, and that was it," he recalled.

That fall, Dave and his wife, Lucy, started to look for a health program that might help Dave get back some semblance of his health. Numerous programs were available, "But we picked the McDougall Program and St. Helena because Dr. McDougall's program was the most stringent. I figured I'd go to St. Helena, get the information, and modify the diet for my own purposes after I got back." As it turned out, Dave and Lucy adopted the program in its entirety, and have been on it ever since. The reason they stayed on the program is simple: It worked.

When Dave and Lucy showed up at St. Helena, Dave's initial cholesterol level was 287 mg/dl. Two weeks later, his cholesterol level was 169 mg/dl—a drop of more than 100 points. When he got home, his cholesterol level fell even further to 144 mg/dl. During his two-week stay at St. Helena, both Dave's blood pressure and blood sugar returned to normal. Dave had spent three years on high blood pressure medication and eight years on drugs for diabetes, and both diseases were gone in just two weeks on the McDougall Program for a Healthy Heart. I took Dave off his medication for both diseases and he hasn't been on it since. In 1994 Dave reported that his blood pressure was 130/80; his blood sugar was also normal.

His energy levels have returned. Dave and Lucy walk daily and make time for a ten-kilometer walk every weekend. Dave works out on the StairMaster at his gym four days per week and lifts weights the other three days. Both Dave and Lucy have lost weight: 35 pounds for Dave, 30 for Lucy. "I want to lose another 20 pounds," says Dave, "but even on this vegetarian diet, I still eat a little too much. I still like the smell of steak and hamburgers, but when we got home from the program, we became dedicated vegetarians. We took the message to heart. We still have our feast days, like Thanksgiving and Christmas when I eat turkey or ham, but I am not tempted to eat those foods at any other times but during the holidays."

At 72 years of age, Tom Riley was considered long past recovery by his doctors. He had significant coronary heart disease, angina, and kidney damage. When he began to develop swelling in his legs caused by the failure of his kidneys, his doctors told him that he would have to begin regular kidney dialysis in order to remain alive. He consulted four local doctors who all concurred with the diagnosis and the recommendation that he submit to regular dialysis on the kidney machine. "These doctors thought I was doomed," Tom recalled. "I looked around and found the McDougall Program. Once I began the diet, my kidney function immediately improved to the point that I lost all the edema and the weakness in my legs. I never needed the kidney machine."

Tom has not only regained his health, but also resumed the activities that he has long enjoyed, including mountain climbing and windsurfing.

Medicine's Approach:
If It's Elevated, Shoot It Down

Because studies have shown that lowering blood pressure significantly reduces the risk of a stroke, American doctors have been quick to medicate virtually every individual who has a mildly elevated blood pressure. Physicians refer to this attitude as "aggressive treatment," which indeed it is. The policy among American physicians has been to prescribe blood pressure–lowering drugs for anyone with a diastolic pressure above 90 mm Hg.

But this is not an attitude shared by physicians elsewhere in the world, especially in Britain and Canada. After reviewing the U.S. medical approach to hypertension, one British physician said, "In the U.S., the threshold of diagnosis is the threshold for treatment. The question 'to treat or not to treat' need no longer be asked. A free-fire zone has been created above diastolic 90, in which we simply shoot everything that moves."

In other words, if you go to your doctor with a diastolic pressure above 90 mm Hg, the chances are very good he or she is going to give you medication. Around the world, the wisdom of this approach is seriously questioned, if not openly rebuked. In fact, the research simply does not support such an approach.

Before You Take a Drug, Ask a Few Simple Questions

Each patient on medication for high blood pressure should ask his or her doctor a few important questions: Does the medication save lives? Is there such a thing as being too aggressive with drugs? What are the side effects of the medication? Do any of the side effects increase my chances of having a heart attack? Can a healthy lifestyle substitute for drugs as a cure for high blood pressure?

No Proof of Clear Benefit

Among the studies of drug treatments for hypertension are nine large trials that examine the question of whether or not drug treatment is effective. These trials do not demonstrate any clear benefit from drug therapy for mild hypertension. When Norman Kaplan, M.D., reviewed these studies for *Heart Disease: A Textbook of Cardiovascular Medicine* (fourth edition), he reported that these studies revealed "the failure to show clear protection against coronary mortality by drug therapy in nine clinical trials involving more than 41,000 patients. . . . As a result of this apparent inability to protect against coronary disease, concerns have arisen about biochemical changes induced by the drugs." Though physicians continue to prescribe these drugs at unprecedented rates, many scientists are now questioning whether the benefit of drug therapy outweighs the side effects of the drugs.

British researchers reviewed these same studies and reported in the *British Medical Journal* that blood pressure–lowering medication had failed to demonstrate decreases in the number of heart attacks, strokes, and death. Based on the evidence, the authors concluded that only patients with malignant (or accelerated) hypertension need to be treated. For the vast majority of patients who have nonmalignant hypertension, there is no "cutoff" pressure above which treatment is mandatory.

The extent to which the evidence supports any treatment for nonmalignant hypertension suggests that treatment is only necessary when diastolic pressures exceed 115 to 120 mm Hg. Moreover, there will be no appreciable benefit to the patient when diastolic pressure is less than 100 mm Hg. Finally, there is no evidence that any particular level of systolic pressure should be treated; thus, there is no reason to treat patients with isolated systolic hypertension.

Indeed, as Dr. Kaplan points out in "Systemic Hypertension: Therapy," published in *Heart Disease: A Textbook of Cardiovascular Medicine*, the evidence clearly shows that patients with diastolic pressure between 90 and 95 mm Hg derive no benefit from medication. In fact, there is no proof that drug therapy for people with diastolic pressure between 90 and 100 mm Hg—a category that includes 40 million Americans with high blood pressure—is providing any benefit at all. Yet, doctors are prescribing medication every day for people who come into their offices with diastolic pressures of 90 to 100 mm Hg.

The evidence to date suggests that the current treatment for high blood pressure is largely a failure for the vast majority of patients. This means that millions of people are taking drugs that are doing them no good, costing them money, and subjecting them to potentially serious side effects. Clearly, "the emperor has no clothes": More people receive drug treatment for high blood pressure than for any other disease, but most of these people derive no benefit from these medications.

Why Do Drugs Fail?

The best explanation I can give is that drug therapy deals only with the *sign* of the disease and not the *cause*. Hypertension is the result of a "sick" circulatory system that is clogged up by atherosclerosis, sludged blood, and vessels that are in spasm. Drugs do nothing to improve the health of the blood vessel system; therefore, they fail to provide significant health benefits, just as treating a fever caused by an infected toe with an aspirin fails to save the toe.

Beware of "Aggressive" Treatment

The term "aggressive treatment" suggests an almost military conscientiousness, as if you and your doctor were struggling together to defeat a terrible enemy. Unfortunately, one of the side effects of aggressive treatment of hypertension is premature heart attacks and death.

In a study published in the *Journal of the American Medical Association*, researchers examined the effects of drug treatment on 1,765 people with mild to moderate hypertension (blood pressures equal to or greater than 160/95). After reviewing the effects of treatment, the researchers concluded, "An association was observed between myocardial infarctions [heart attacks] and both a large and a small fall [in blood pressure]. . . . Since both a large and small reduction in diastolic BP was associated with a higher incidence of myocardial infarction (relative to a moderate fall), perhaps a moderate reduction in diastolic BP should be the goal of treatment for mild and moderate hypertensives."

This finding was one of many studies that supports what is referred to in medicine as the "J-shaped curve of mortality." Studies have consistently shown that when blood pressure is severely elevated, heart attacks, strokes, and death rates increase. On the other hand, excessively *aggressive* treatment can bring down blood pressures too far, causing premature heart attacks. In other words, you lose at both ends.

If blood pressure is treated *with medication*, the pressure should not be brought down below 85 to 90 mm Hg. Otherwise, you will increase your risk of heart attack. In a review of the medical literature on the treatment of hypertension published in the *Journal of the American Medical Association*, researchers concluded that "low treated diastolic blood pressure levels, i.e., below 85 mm Hg, are associated with increased risk of cardiac events."

This review found that there is a point beyond which blood pressure reduction with medication is harmful. The authors state that "a reasonable current compromise is to be cautious in lowering blood pressure below 85 mm Hg in patients with known ischemic heart disease. The prudence of this tactic is accentuated by the conspicuous lack of evidence of benefit for therapeutic lowering of blood pressure levels beyond this threshold."

Don't worry if you are not on medication and your blood pressure is below 85 mm Hg. You are not at higher risk of having a heart attack. These numbers apply only to those people with high blood pressure who take medication. Remember, the ideal blood pressure is 110/70 mm Hg or lower *without* medication.

Why this J-shaped curve exists for people on medication is open to much speculation. One possible answer is that the heart requires a certain amount of blood and oxygen to survive. When blood pressure falls below 85 to

90 mm Hg as a result of drug therapy, the pressure may be insufficient to support the heart muscle and brings on a heart attack. In medical terminology, "profusion pressure" to the heart and other vital organs is decreased.

In any case, the risk of death is clearly increased by treatment that is too aggressive. Thus, many people with mild, moderate, and severe diastolic hypertension are being overmedicated, much to their detriment, when their doctor believes that the lower the blood pressure, the better.

Diabetics treated for high blood pressure have an exaggerated death rate compared to those not treated. For example, death from heart disease is nearly four times higher in patients treated for high blood pressure with diuretics compared to those left untreated.

The Pharmaceutical Menu: Is It Worth It?

Although many medications are used to treat hypertension, four categories of drugs are considered therapies of "first choice": beta receptor blockers, diuretics, calcium channel antagonists, and angiotension-converting enzyme inhibitors (also called ACE inhibitors). Let's have a look at the side effects of each of these drugs, bearing in mind what I said earlier: There is no proven benefit from drug therapy for people with "mild" hypertension.

Beta Receptor Blockers

Usually referred to simply as beta blockers, these drugs work by blocking the effects of adrenaline on certain receptor cells (called beta receptors) found in the heart, lungs, blood vessels, and other tissues. More adrenaline is released from the nervous system when you exercise or are excited or under stress. The beta receptors bind the adrenaline and trigger the heart to pump blood with greater force and speed. Beta receptors in the arteries cause them to expand to allow more blood to flow to the heart and other tissues; in the lungs, they open air passages and allow more oxygen to pass to tissues. Beta blockers prevent these natural physical reactions from occurring and consequently prevent the body from rising to meet the increased demands of heightened physical or emotional exertion. Many people who take beta blockers complain of chronic fatigue, feelings of weakness, and exhaustion, especially during exercise and excitement. An estimated 30 percent of people who take full doses of these drugs say they experience weakness in the legs and inability to hurry up stairs or hills. Other frequent side effects include dizziness, depression, bronchospasm (symptoms of asthma), nausea, vomiting, diarrhea, constipation, hallucinations, Raynaud's phenomenon (cold hands and feet), decreases in HDL cholesterol, and elevations in blood triglyceride levels.

Beta blockers also weaken the heart. In some people with heart disease, beta blockers can cause heart failure; heart function becomes so depressed that blood backs up in the lungs and the person drowns in his own body fluids. Finally, beta blockers can worsen asthma and increase blood sugar levels and triglycerides. They are commonly prescribed for numerous forms of heart disease, including angina, arrhythmia, and hypertension.

Diuretics

Diuretics cause the kidneys to excrete more water from the body, which lowers the fluid volume of the blood, and thereby lowers blood pressure. But these drugs are not without side effects.

In many clinical trials, diuretics have failed to show clear protection against coronary heart disease. Scientists are now suggesting darkly that perhaps the side effects of these drugs may be the reason for the high mortality rates among people treated with diuretics. As Dr. Kaplan notes in *Heart Disease: A Textbook of Cardiovascular Medicine*, "the presence of diuretic-induced biochemical derangements has been offered as a potential explanation of the lack of coronary protection."

And those "biochemical derangements" are numerous indeed. Diuretics can cause an excessive loss of potassium, resulting in weakness, confusion, palpitations, and dangerous arrhythmias. Studies have shown that a commonly prescribed diuretic (chlorthalidone) increases a patient's chances of dying of a heart attack. Some studies indicate that diuretics double the rate of sudden death.

The increases in mortality may occur because diuretics also cause elevations in blood sugar, uric acid levels, triglycerides, and cholesterol— all of which are risk factors associated with a person's chances of suffering a heart attack. Elevations in uric acid levels can give rise to gout, a type of arthritis, while higher than normal blood sugar can bring on diabetes, which contributes to atherosclerosis and heart disease. Mineral depletion can result in changes in heart rate and arrhythmias and bring on heart failure. To combat the loss of minerals, doctors often prescribe a type of potassium-sparing diuretic that preserves minerals to a limited extent, but it, too, can cause an array of side effects, such as enlargement of male breasts, diarrhea, and menstrual disorders.

In studies in which the effects of beta blockers were compared to those of diuretics for their protection against heart disease, neither drug demonstrated any clear protection against the illness.

Angiotension-Converting Enzyme Inhibitors

Also called ACE inhibitors, these drugs work by preventing the body from constricting blood vessels, thereby keeping the vessels dilated, or expanded. The list of potential side effects of these drugs is quite lengthy and should be a concern for anyone taking them. Most common are cough, shortness of breath, hypotension, dizziness, diarrhea, angioedema (swelling of the face, tongue, and airway), headache, vomiting, skin rashes, loss of taste, and kidney failure. White blood cell counts can drop, causing a decline in the strength of the immune system. ACE inhibitors are particularly useful in patients with heart and kidney failure, prolonging their survival.

Calcium Channel Antagonists

Calcium channel blockers prevent the uptake of calcium along electromagnetic channels within the cell. The diminution of calcium in the cells of blood vessels prevents those vessels from constricting. In this way they act like ACE inhibitors and cause the dilation of blood vessels. Like ACE inhibitors, calcium blockers can also cause a long list of side effects, including the onset of rapid heartbeat (sometimes reaching or exceeding 100 beats per minute), gastrointestinal disorders, excess potassium in the blood, headaches, edema, liver dysfunction, flushing, constipation, and heart block, a disorder in which the coordination between the atrium and ventricle is disrupted. They also cause overgrowth of gum tissue (gingival hyperplasia) and an increased chance of bleeding during surgery.

Studies have shown that between 20 and 40 percent of people who receive treatment for hypertension have adverse side effects from the medication. At the high end, that's nearly half of the people treated. However, these numbers may not be representative of the true picture. People do not always report the side effects of drugs. Some don't recognize them, others don't like to talk about side effects, especially if they involve sexual dysfunction. Many people take it upon themselves to reduce or stop the medication altogether without telling their doctors. Studies have shown that between 20 and 50 percent of patients fail to follow their doctor's instructions.

Given all the evidence, patients and doctors have to question whether the drugs are worth it, especially in light of their questionable efficacy and their effects on the quality of a patient's life.

You Have the Time to Be Cautious

A diagnosis of high blood pressure can be shocking. It can force a doctor to start a patient on medication immediately. However, it takes between ten and twenty years for high blood pressure to damage blood vessels severely enough to cause a heart attack or stroke. There is no need to prescribe medication on the first visit to the doctor's office, or even after several visits.

After reviewing the evidence, the World Health Organization now urges physicians to observe a patient with high blood pressure for three to six months before prescribing medication. If blood pressure is monitored over that period, chances are very good that it will fall into the normal ranges without any treatment at all. The studies have shown that diastolic pressures of 90 to 95 mm Hg will normalize within four months without treatment in most people. In fact, this was the case for 11 percent of the people in the Australian National Blood Pressure Study.

I recommend that people take their blood pressures at home, because many high readings are "white coat hypertension," and fall into the healthy ranges when the stressful situation passes. In any case, unless the blood pressure is very high the chances are excellent that diet and lifestyle treatments can bring down the pressure into the normal ranges. Today, scientists are asking doctors to reconsider their approach because the benefits of drug therapy have not been proved to outweigh their consequences in many cases.

My Policy Regarding Drugs

Fortunately, I rarely have to prescribe drugs. Most of my patients can easily lower their elevated blood pressure and stop their blood pressure medication shortly after adopting my diet and lifestyle recommendations. At my clinic in St. Helena Hospital, patients are able to lower their blood pressures 5 to 10 percent and stop all blood pressure medications within twelve days. (With very few exceptions, the drop in blood pressure takes place within twenty-four to thirty-six hours, and all drugs are then stopped, unless they are on beta blockers.)

However, if a person's diastolic blood pressure is consistently over 100 mm Hg after multiple readings, I cautiously use blood pressure–lowering medications in combination with diet and lifestyle changes. My target for diastolic blood pressure is 85 to 90 mm Hg. I do not let the pressure drop below 85 mm Hg.

Once the diet and exercise program begins to take effect, I start to wean my patients off their medication. I have patients stop their medication if they are taking only small amounts of the drugs. For patients taking large doses, I reduce the amounts over a period of days, while monitoring their blood pressure. Patients on beta blockers are slowly withdrawn, either under my supervision or another doctor's. Rapid withdrawal of beta blockers can cause chest pain and, in extremely rare cases, sudden death. Most patients tolerate reducing their medication in half every three to seven days until they are off all the beta blocker drugs.

No one should stop taking their medication unless they are being supervised by a physician.

Things to Avoid That Will Boost BP

In addition to rich foods high in fat, cholesterol, and sodium—and a sedentary lifestyle—that I've already talked about, several other substances affect blood pressure. Here are some other items to avoid.

Cigarette Smoking

Smoking a single cigarette can cause blood pressure to rise for thirty minutes to an hour. Smoking all day can cause blood pressure to remain elevated throughout the day. Smoking also raises (oxidized) LDL cholesterol and causes atherosclerosis, which is one of the risk factors associated with cardiovascular disease, including high blood pressure.

Alcohol

Studies have shown that moderate amounts of alcohol (1 to 1½ drinks per day) can lower blood pressure, but excessive drinking clearly elevates it. A study published in the *American Journal of Public Health* compared people who drank daily with those who drank once a week. The study showed that the daily imbibers had systolic pressures that were, on the average, 6.6 mm Hg higher, and diastolic pressures 4.7 mm Hg higher than those of people who drank once a week.

Caffeine

Caffeine has been associated with elevations in blood pressure. People with high blood pressure are therefore better off avoiding caffeinated beverages. This can be very important in controlling blood pressure, especially since so many of us take coffee and other caffeinated beverages for granted.

Foods and Nutrients That Lower BP

Potassium

Potassium intake has been shown to be directly related to drops in blood pressure. When potassium is lowered in the diets of healthy people, blood pressure often rises. In a study of twelve hypertensive people published in the *Annals of Internal Medicine*, eating potassium-rich foods—such as fruits, vegetables, and grains—lowered blood pressure, while systolic pressure rose an average of seven points, and diastolic pressure jumped by 6 mm Hg on a low-potassium diet. When salt was added to the low-potassium diet, blood pressure rose even more sharply. In another study published in the *Annals of Internal Medicine*, researchers found that more than one-third of patients who increased their potassium consumption (by increasing vegetables, beans, and fruit) experienced sharp declines in blood pressure and were able to stop all medication for their hypertension. Only 9 percent of controls were able to eliminate medication during the same period.

Garlic

Garlic may have a natural dilating effect on blood vessels, according to research conducted at the Tulane University Medical School, where scientists demonstrated that regular consumption of garlic lowered blood pressure significantly. (See Chapter 12 for more on garlic and other health-promoting herbs.) Garlic lowers cholesterol and boosts immune response.

People with high blood pressure should remember that hypertension is a sign of diseased blood vessels, and not a disease in itself. In this chapter, I've tried to demonstrate that the only rational way to treat hypertension is through diet and lifestyle. If drugs are used to treat the illness, they should only be seen as a secondary form of treatment. They are not a long-term answer, and they're certainly not a cure.

The McDougall Program for a Healthy Heart is a cure because it deals with the underlying cause of the illness. By combining diet and exercise, my program helps more than 90 percent of my patients lower their blood pressure, discontinue medication, and improve their overall health and vitality.

No drug can make that claim.

15. Women and Heart Disease

- *The medical business discriminates against women.*
- *Women of all ages have to protect themselves against heart disease.*
- *The McDougall Program for a Healthy Heart will defend you against the problems related to menopause.*
- *Hormones are delicate; upset their balance at your own risk.*
- *Pass safely through menopause and heart disease, cancer, and osteoporosis.*

Women Do Not Get Equal Treatment

Heart disease is now the most common cause of death for women in the United States. The incidence increases with age, rising rapidly after menopause. During their reproductive years, women are largely protected from heart disease by nature's design. However, heart disease is as common among women as among men after the age of 65. Unfortunately, the threat of heart disease for women is not taken as seriously as it is for men.

Women do not get the same treatment as men. Women take longer to get to the hospital than men, and they arrive with more serious disease. Once in the hospital, doctors are less likely to believe that a woman complaining of chest pain is having a heart attack; as a result, she is less likely to be sent to the coronary care unit and less likely to receive potentially lifesaving treatments such as thrombolysis (blood clot–dissolving drugs given soon after the onset of a heart attack). Although the incidence of chest pain is the same in both sexes, two to four times as many bypass surgeries are done on men. Women have twice the risk of dying during bypass surgery, possibly because when a woman finally gets to bypass surgery, she has more serious disease. After a heart attack doctors are less likely to prescribe drugs like aspirin and beta blockers that could lessen a woman's risk of another heart attack.

Overall, the prognosis for women is worse than for men, because our society tends to think of heart disease as a man's disease. This inequality needs to be remedied as soon as possible. We must not only face the facts concerning the incidence and treatment of heart disease, but must realize that the deadly diet served to most Americans does not discriminate between men and women.

Diet Can Save a Woman's Health

For women who eat the typical American diet, passing through menopause is like crossing a dangerous river. It's no picnic navigating the raging waters, and once you've managed to reach the other shore, you've got some very serious health issues staring you in the face. Among them are an increased risk of heart disease, osteoporosis, and breast and uterine cancers.

Most women don't realize it, but they've spent much of their lives laying the foundation for these diseases. The decline in estrogen production that accompanies menopause makes women more vulnerable to heart disease and osteoporosis, but the underlying factors that create these illnesses, as well as cancer, are already present. The drop in estrogen merely removes a form of protection against a lifestyle that makes heart disease and osteoporosis possible in the first place.

In an attempt to prevent heart attacks and bone fractures, women are counseled by their physicians to take hormone replacement therapy (HRT), which reduces the risk of heart disease and osteoporosis, but elevates the risk of getting breast and uterine cancers. When advising women on this momentous decision, doctors are encouraged to treat each situation individually, weighing the risks of illness against the possible benefits of the therapy. The problem is, however, that physicians see each of these illnesses as largely unrelated diseases. In the end, many simply lay out the odds of having a heart attack or contracting breast cancer, and then step back, leaving the woman to make a decision that will surely affect the rest of her life.

The situation a woman faces is this: If you take estrogens, your risk of heart attack and osteoporosis drops, but your chance of getting uterine (endometrial) cancers increase significantly. Long-term use of estrogens, which most women are expected to accept once they enter menopause, also increases your chances of getting breast cancer. To lower the risk of getting uterine cancer, doctors also prescribe progesterone (progestin), another female hormone, to be taken with estrogen. Progesterone seems to lower the risk of getting uterine cancer (no one is certain, yet) but it diminishes the protective benefits of estrogen against heart disease. In other words, by taking progesterone you are undermining one of the major reasons you started the estrogen program in the first place. By the time you're taking estrogen-progesterone hormones, you've come full circle: You began a drug program in part to protect yourself against heart disease, but because of the side effects of this drug (estrogen), you must take another drug (progestin) that essentially elevates your risk of getting heart disease. These added hormones also elevate your risk of getting breast cancer. Many women lament that the process itself is like rolling dice: Sometimes they roll a seven and escape the dangers; sometimes they roll snake eyes and find themselves facing illnesses that no one would want to deal with.

In addition to increasing the risk of illness, menopause presents other unpleasant side effects, but the degree of these symptoms is also related to a woman's lifestyle, especially to the foods she eats. In any case, it's no wonder women dread the approach of the so-called change of life. Serious disease becomes more likely; the choices are difficult; and the quality of life, especially while a woman is struggling with menopausal symptoms, is often diminished for years.

What the vast majority of women should understand is that it doesn't have to be this way. The key to understanding heart disease, cancer, osteoporosis, and a difficult menopause is to see all of these conditions as manifestations of the same underlying problem. One way to understand the threads that unify these diseases is to think of them all as lined up along the outside of a wheel. At the center of that wheel, put the following words: "The Standard American diet, rich in fat, cholesterol, protein, and refined foods." That diet is at the heart of all of these problems. A woman's therapeutic choices become problematical when she sees heart disease, osteoporosis, and cancer as unrelated problems that must be dealt with individually, each with its own approach.

My short answer to the questions surrounding these illnesses and menopause is this: First, understand that menopause itself is not a mistake of nature; menopause is as natural as birth, puberty, adulthood, and old age. Second, a woman must reduce or eliminate all the underlying causal factors that give rise to heart disease, cancer, osteoporosis, and a troublesome menopause; this is done by adhering to the McDougall Program for a Healthy Heart. Third, take hormones only under certain circumstances—which I discuss later in this chapter—and if you must take them, be sure to adopt the McDougall Program for a Healthy Heart, which will significantly reduce all the problems related to menopause and its related risks.

Dietary Diseases of Women

Diseases of the heart and arteries are the leading killers of women today, taking the lives of about 500,000 women each year. Heart attacks alone kill approximately 250,000 women annually. To put the latter number in its proper perspective, we should remember that breast cancer kills about 40,500 women each year, less than 10 percent of the heart disease deaths. Many women take immunity from heart disease for granted, in part because heart disease strikes more men than women, *up until the time a woman reaches menopause*. Then the relative rates of heart disease among men and women are the same. Women have no protection against heart disease after they've reached menopause.

Many women complain that they do not get the same treatment for heart disease that men do. Some women are angry about the sexism that seems built into science and medicine. I acknowledge the underlying truth of this criticism, but from my vantage point, as one who questions many of the common treatments being offered to heart patients today, I would say that there is a silver lining in this dark cloud. Sometimes men and women are better off avoiding many of the drugs and operations being offered. Sometimes, the best approach is to change your way of life rather than to surrender to the drugs and the surgeon's knife.

Where the Problems Begin

Estrogen, the sex hormone predominant in a woman's body, is created by the ovaries, adrenal glands, and fat cells. All forms of dietary fat (including oils) increase a woman's weight by boosting the fat in her cells. These fat cells are literally estrogen factories, producing substantial and unhealthy quantities.

Excess body fat is not the only diet-related factor that influences estrogen levels. The rich American diet, made up of refined foods, animal protein, and fat promotes the growth of intestinal bacteria (clostridia varieties) that have the ability to convert bile acids into estrogen-like hormones. The more fats you eat, the more bile acids your liver produces, to act as precursors for the production of hormones.

The Western diet also increases hormone stimulation from the hormones your own body synthesizes. Estrogens that your body produces are supposed to circulate through your system only once, stimulating your hormone-responsive organs, such as the breast and uterus, and then circulate to the liver, where they are combined with a nonabsorbable substance that prevents their reabsorption in the intestines. This nonabsorbable compound attached to the estrogens is your body's way of protecting itself from estrogens that would circulate over and over again, thus causing excessive levels of hormones. However, the rich American diet encourages the growth of certain intestinal bacteria that have the ability to free these estrogens from the nonabsorbable compound so that they can be reabsorbed into your body for another passage. The net effect is to substantially elevate your overall estrogen levels. (These same effects are also seen among men: The higher the fat content of a man's diet, the more estrogens and testosterone in his bloodstream.)

The best way to protect yourself from this unhealthy occurrence is to eat a diet rich in fiber and low in animal fat and protein. Such a diet prevents the growth of these hormone-releasing bacteria. Moreover, the fiber in a vegetable-based diet binds with estrogens and promotes their elimination through the intestines. Vegetarian women eliminate two to three times more estrogen in their feces than nonvegetarians, according to research published in the *New England Journal of Medicine* and elsewhere.

Hormone-Dependent Health Problems

Studies have shown that high levels of circulating estrogens are associated with:

   • Early menarche (first menstrual period), brought about by high levels of estrogen at an early age. Young girls who eat a low-fat diet experience menarche at approximately 16 years of age; girls on a high-fat diet have their first periods at 12 or earlier.

•   Irregular, heavy, and painful menstrual periods.

•   Late menopause, delayed because of the postponement of the natural decline in a woman's production of estrogen.

•   PMS, or premenstrual syndrome. First identified in 1931, PMS is associated with painful and irregular periods, irritability, and moodiness. The condition coincides with a woman's peak production of estrogen during her menstrual cycle.

•   Fibroids of the uterus. Excess production of estrogens overstimulate the muscle cells that make up the uterus. That stimulation results in the unregulated proliferation of clusters of these cells, causing a non-cancerous growth in the uterus. These growths vary in size from that of a pea to, in rare cases, the size of a basketball! Usually after menopause, when the ovaries shut down and estrogen production drops, these fibroids naturally shrink away.

•   Fibrocystic breast disease. For most women, the breasts become tender just before the onset of their menstrual periods, when female hormones reach their highest monthly levels. In approximately 10 percent of women the pain is described as severe. Overstimulation of the mammary tissues by higher than normal levels of estrogens causes the breasts to swell and become tender. After repeated bouts of inflammation, the breasts develop scar tissue in many places, and some of the milk ducts become plugged, forming cysts. Fibrocystic breast disease, not surprisingly, is associated with a higher risk of breast cancer (a disease promoted by estrogens).

•   Endometrial (uterine) cancer. Estrogens promote the growth of cells within the uterus (endometrium), increasing the risk of malignancy.

•   Breast and ovarian cancers. Like uterine cancer, breast cancer and ovarian cancers are hormone-related diseases. Studies consistently show that the higher a woman's estrogen levels, the more likely she is to contract these diseases.

Cancer and Estrogens

In the *American Journal of Clinical Nutrition*, David P. Rose, M.D., Ph.D., noted that research has now established that hormones are involved in promoting the development and progression of breast cancer. Studies have shown that malignant breast tumors are dependent upon the presence of female hormones. When estrogen levels are significantly reduced, the tumors regress. This has prompted scientists to begin using the drug tamoxifen to treat breast cancer, because it reduces the effects of estrogens on the body's cells. However, one of the best and fastest ways to lower estrogens in the blood is to change your diet, specifically by lowering fat and increasing fiber. The effects of such changes are dramatic.

Women who undergo HRT usually take estrogens orally. The consumption of estrogens causes the hormone-sensitive organs—the uterus, breasts, and ovaries—to be stimulated, often at higher than normal levels well beyond their "normal life," which is associated with numerous health problems, including the growth of tumors at these sites. The longer a woman takes estrogens—or the higher the dose she is exposed to—the greater her risk of developing cancer.

Studies have shown that the risk of contracting uterine cancer for women taking estrogens is five to fourteen times greater than for those who do not receive estrogens. This means that an additional forty to fifty cases of uterine cancer can be expected for every 1,000 women who take estrogen pills for fifteen years. Only five to ten cases of uterine cancer will appear in women who do not take estrogens. Studies have shown that when women stop taking estrogens, the risk of cancer decreases over the next three years.

The hormone progesterone is given to help counteract the cancer-producing effects of estrogen. Yet, despite the medically accepted protective benefits of progesterone, many women with an intact uterus are still taking estrogen alone.

The primary reason breast cancer rates are skyrocketing among American women is the enthusiastic consumption of the rich Western diet, abundant in dietary fat and lacking in dietary fiber. In the 1960s, a woman's chances of getting breast cancer were approximately 1 in 20. By the mid-1970s, her chances had increased to 1 in 14. By 1990, they had become 1 in 10, and today they are approximately 1 in 8. I predict that soon the chances of a woman developing breast cancer will be 1 in 5.

Research shows that taking estrogens for more than six years doubles the risk of contracting breast cancer; adding progesterone may further increase the risk. Many populations of people worldwide experience low breast cancer rates. Asian women not only have low rates of breast cancer, but also have lower levels of circulating estrogens in their bloodstreams. The same is true of Hispanic women, who eat diets richer in grains and beans than American women and thus have lower rates of breast cancer.

This situation is rapidly changing, however, as Asians and Hispanics enthusiastically adopt the rich Western diet. Studies have shown that when Asian women come to the United States and adopt a more Western-like diet, richer in fat and lower in fiber, their rates of breast cancer match those of other Americans. In other words, there's no "genetic" protection among these populations of women.

How Estrogen Affects Other Systems

Gallbladder disease occurs two to three times more frequently in women receiving estrogen therapy. Estrogen supplements have been found to cause or worsen diabetes and high blood pressure in some women. These hormones also increase the likelihood of a woman developing inflammation and blood clots in the veins that can lead to pulmonary embolism, in which blood clots travel to the lungs and can cause death.

Finally, women who take estrogens combined sequentially with progestins endure vaginal bleeding and a resumption of their menstrual periods, a condition many women find unsettling and unwelcome.

Breast Health Depends on Healthy Eating

The key to protecting yourself against breast cancer is to keep your estrogen level low. Scientists have calculated that a 17 percent reduction of estrogen in the blood could produce a fourfold to fivefold reduction in breast cancer incidence. Remarkably, when women with high estrogen levels are placed on a high-fiber, low-fat diet, their blood levels of estrogen drop precipitously. A group of postmenopausal women adopted a low-fat, high-fiber diet and found that, on average, their blood levels of estrogen dropped by 50 percent! That 50 percent reduction came after only twenty-two days on the diet! No woman today should take these words lightly. Anything that will reduce your chances of getting breast cancer so dramatically—with no adverse effects—is worth adopting immediately. And the McDougall Program for a Healthy Heart will do just that.

Heart Disease and Estrogen's Protective Benefits

The fact is that estrogen does provide women with some protection against both heart disease and osteoporosis. And the decline in estrogen levels after menopause is associated with an increased risk of both disorders.

On average, a woman's cholesterol level before age 45 is 220 mg/dl. The presence of estrogen in premenopausal women tends to increase blood levels of HDL cholesterol, while it lowers LDL. Even though a cholesterol level of 220 mg/dl is dangerously high, scientists argue that the positive ratio between HDL and LDL offers a significant degree of protection. And indeed, women do experience an exceptionally low incidence of heart disease prior to menopause. In fact, heart attacks are almost unheard of in otherwise healthy women who are still menstruating. This immunity to heart disease disappears after menopause. Once a woman reaches the ages of 45 to 55—the years during and after menopause—the average woman's cholesterol level ranges from 223 to 246 mg/dl. At the same time, women's rates of heart attacks quickly increase.

Ironically, the addition of progesterone diminishes estrogen's protective effect on the heart. Progesterone lowers HDL, which negatively impacts the balance between HDL and LDL. Progesterone also raises triglyceride levels, which causes the blood to sludge and increases the risk of coronary thrombosis, the main cause of heart attacks. Thus, progesterone in combination with estrogen increases a woman's risk of having a heart attack or stroke.

Scientists have begun to question the protective benefit of estrogens for heart disease. A study published in the *British Medical Journal* reviewed other studies designed to determine the effects of estrogen pills on heart disease in women. The studies showed that the women with the largest reduction in heart disease also had the largest reduction in cancer. Since estrogens increase a woman's chance of developing cancer, these findings point out that much of the benefit seen for heart disease is a consequence of a selection bias: Generally healthier women are more inclined to take estrogens after menopause. These healthier women have a smaller chance of developing cancer and heart disease—they are likely to avoid the illness with or without the hormone. In light of these facts, the researchers concluded, "universal preventive hormonal replacement therapy for postmenopausal women is unwarranted at present."

What every woman should understand is that heart disease is *not caused by an estrogen pill deficiency*, nor is it prevented by taking estrogen after menopause. Indeed, heart attacks among women increase dramatically after a woman reaches menopause, and a great percentage of women are taking estrogen by then. The cause of that increase in heart disease rates among women is the typical American diet. Manipulating women's hormone levels will not significantly change the fact that 500,000 women are dying of cardiovascular disease each year. Only by adopting a healthy diet and exercise program can women start to deal with the cause of their disease. Once this is done, a woman's health bounces back. I see this at my clinic almost every day.

Women vs. Men: The "Stats"

Between October 1986 and February 1994, 864 people attended the McDougall Program at St. Helena Hospital; 531 of them were women. Because they represent the vast majority of patients at the clinic, I would conclude that women are more interested in regaining good health. Based on the people I see in my clinic, women are just as sick as men.

The average cholesterol of women entering my program was nearly 9 mg/dl higher than that of men (approximately 224 vs. 215 mg/dl). On average, men experienced a 33 mg/dl drop in cholesterol (from 215 to 182 mg/dl); women experienced a 25 mg/dl drop (from 224 to 199 mg/dl). Women started the program with 12 mg/dl more HDL cholesterol than men (46 vs. 34 mg/dl), a fact that will doubtless protect them against heart attack.

The average triglycerides are lower in women than in men at the start of the program (171 vs. 203 mg/dl). However, men lowered their triglycerides from 203 to 187 mg/dl in twelve days. Women actually saw theirs go up 5 mg/dl (from 171 to 176 mg/dl).

The average blood pressure for men was 132/79, compared to 128/76 for women upon entry to my program. Upon leaving the program, men had an average blood pressure of 128/76; the average for women was 124/73. Both men and women showed a 4/3 mm Hg drop.

Men lost more weight (average loss, 4.8 pounds) than women (an average of 3.2 pounds). Not surprisingly, men came to the program significantly heavier than women (208.5 vs. 173 pounds).

Overall, the data on men and women in my program are very similar. Both are in poor health as a result of their diet and lifestyle and both respond favorably to good food and exercise.

Osteoporosis, Estrogens, and Diet

The body requires sex hormones—estrogen in women, testosterone in men—to maintain bone strength. When either of these hormones is diminished, bone loss is accelerated. Actually, hormones simply maintain normal production of bone. They do not accelerate or add new bone growth. Hence, HRT will only slow bone loss in postmenopausal women. It will not replenish lost bone. Women experience much higher rates of osteoporosis than men, simply because men do not lose testosterone at the same dramatic rate as postmenopausal women lose estrogen.

Both men and women reach their maximum bone density at around age 35. After that, all of us on the rich Western diet lose bone to some degree. The rate of bone loss after menopause varies. Many women experience only 2 percent loss; others lose as much as 4 or 5 percent. While the rate of bone loss is rapid for the first five years after menopause, it slows to about 1 percent per year after that five-year period. Nevertheless, a woman who eats an unhealthy diet and has a small skeleton can lose as much as 15 percent of her skeleton during those five years immediately after menopause. Even proponents of estrogen admit that the main benefits of HRT are in those first five years after menopause, when bone loss is at its peak.

Because estrogen provides some protection against osteoporosis, physicians almost universally prescribe HRT as a woman passes through menopause. They also recommend an increase in the consumption of calcium-rich foods, because the bones have a high calcium content. Hence, physicians encourage women to drink more milk and eat more dairy products because these foods are considered good sources of calcium.

Paradoxically, eating dairy foods, which are high in fat and cholesterol, increases your risk of dying of heart disease. As with heart disease, osteoporosis is caused not by an estrogen deficiency so much as by a diet that drains calcium from our bones.

Protein: A Little Is Good, a Lot Is Bone-Bad

The research has now firmly established that excess protein intake prevents the body from retaining calcium. In fact, protein has what is typically referred to as an "inverse relationship" with calcium: The more protein you eat, the more calcium your body excretes.

Dietary protein, especially from animal sources, is acidic. In the body this acid load must be buffered to maintain the closely guarded pH of the blood. The bones are one of the primary buffering systems of the body. To counteract an acid load from the diet, they dissolve to release calcium and phosphates. The alkaline phosphates neutralize the acids. Dietary protein has been referred to as the body's "equivalent of acid rain." In general, animal foods are acidic and vegetable foods are alkaline.

Excess animal protein causes another major change in the body that leads to osteoporosis—the kidneys lose large amounts of calcium that are not compensated for by intestinal absorption. Scientific research over the past four decades has uncovered several mechanisms by which animal protein causes the excretion of calcium into the urine (see *McDougall's Medicine: A Challenging Second Opinion*).

There is a growing body of evidence that demonstrates that excess animal protein consumption is the primary cause of osteoporosis. Hip fractures are more common in industrialized nations where animal protein is eaten in greater quantities than in less developed countries. When researchers examined where hip fractures are most common, they discovered a direct correlation among nations where people have a high animal protein intake. Nations where people rely on vegetables for their primary protein source have low hip fracture rates. China is a good case in point.

The Chinese consume mostly vegetable proteins. The average Chinese person eats only 64.1 g of protein per day, and 60 of those grams come from vegetable sources. The average American eats 90 to 120 g of protein, but only 27 g come from vegetable sources. At the same time, the average Chinese eats only small amounts of calcium—544 mg per day. Yet, the Chinese experience a very low incidence of osteoporosis. Americans, on the other hand, eat plenty of protein and are encouraged to eat lots of calcium—up to 1,500 mg a day—and suffer epidemic rates of osteoporosis.

Another example are African Bantu women, who consume an average of only 50 g of protein per day. That is less than half the protein intake of most American women. Yet the Bantu have low rates of osteoporosis. Other populations, in Africa, reveal the same patterns: relatively low-protein, low-calcium consumption and low rates of osteoporosis.

Americans have always had a love affair with protein, much to our detriment. We believe protein gives us strength and endurance, but the human body prefers carbohydrate as its source of energy.

In fact, an adult needs no more than 20 g of protein a day—about two-thirds of an ounce of pure protein—which are used by the body to replace and repair cells, produce hormones, and grow hair. The average American consumes 120 to 160 g or more of protein each day, however. That excess protein has a wide assortment of negative effects on the body, including the loss of calcium and other minerals from bone and tissues. Researchers estimate that doubling protein intake will increase the amount of calcium lost in the urine by 50 percent. Studies have shown that reducing protein consumption stops the loss of calcium from bones.

RECOMMENDATIONS AND VALUES OF CALCIUM CONSUMPTION FOR ADULTS FROM AROUND THE WORLD

Source	*Milligrams (mg)*
Minimum calcium need, determined by experiment	150–200
Worldwide calcium intake in most populations	300–500
World Health Organization recommendation for minimum intake	400–500
Food and Nutrition Board recommendation for the United States	800
Recent proposal for the United States by the National Institutes of Health	1,000–1,500

Osteoporosis and Protein

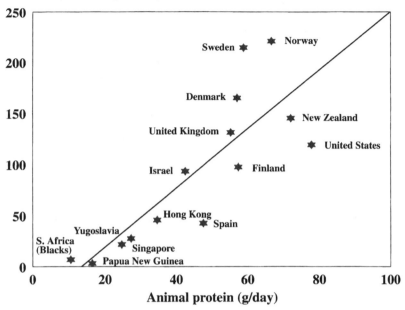

Fractures/100,000 person-years

Animal protein (g/day)

Worldwide, the incidence of osteoporosis is directly correlated with the amount of animal protein consumed. Animal protein presents the body with an acid load that is buffered by dissolving bone material. The excess animal protein also causes the kidneys to excrete large quantities of calcium, completing the process that leads to osteoporosis. (Population data from Calcif Tissue Int *50:14, 1992; further details in* McDougall's Medicine: A Challenging Second Opinion.

The Calcium Paradox

The Food and Nutrition Board of the National Academy of Sciences advises women to consume 1,000 to 1,500 mg of calcium a day. The message is music to the ears of the people at the National Dairy Council and the calcium supplement makers, who together have convinced women that they cannot get adequate calcium without eating dairy products and taking calcium pills. Ironically, on a nation-by-nation basis, people who

Osteoporosis and Calcium

Fractures/100,000 person-years

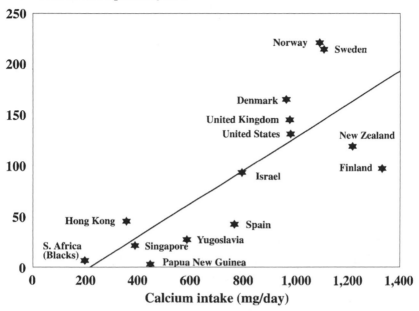

Worldwide, the incidence of osteoporosis is directly correlated with calcium intake. The more calcium consumed the more bone lost, not because calcium causes bone loss, but because most diets high in calcium are also high in animal protein. However, the higher calcium intakes seem to offer little protection from the ravages of a diet high in animal protein. (Population data from Calcif Tissue Int *50:14, 1992; further details in* McDougall's Medicine: A Challenging Second Opinion.*)*

consume the most calcium have the weakest bones and the highest rates of osteoporosis.

The primary source of calcium and other minerals is the soil. Plants absorb minerals from the soil and incorporate them into their roots, stems, leaves, flowers, and fruits. Animals, in turn, eat these plant parts and absorb their calcium. Humans have a highly efficient intestinal tract that, under almost every circumstance, will absorb the correct amount of calcium to meet the body's needs. The intestinal cells act as regulators for the amount of calcium that enters the body. When the calcium content of the diet is low, a relatively higher percentage of calcium will be absorbed from the foods. If the diet is high in calcium, a smaller percentage of the calcium will be absorbed. But the body's need is always the controlling factor regulating the entry of calcium into the cells of the intestinal wall.

A vegetable-based diet is rich in calcium and all the other nutrients the body needs. Let's not forget that the original source of all calcium is the earth, and plants make this mineral available to animals, including humans, in delicious, digestible packages. That's where all the animals get it and you can, too.

Studies have shown that an intake of 150 to 200 mg of calcium daily is adequate to meet the needs of most people, even during pregnancy and lactation. And in fact, most of the world's population ingests 300 to 500 mg of calcium each day. Calcium is so efficiently absorbed by the human intestine and so sufficient in diets of mankind, that calcium deficiency of dietary origin is unknown in human beings.

Only in those places where calcium and protein are eaten in relatively high quantities does a deficiency of bone calcium exist at such epidemic rates, due to an excess of animal protein.

Milk Fails to Protect You

Drinking milk does not protect against osteoporosis because of its high protein content. As I said earlier, excess protein causes the body to excrete calcium through the kidneys. In a study paid for by the dairy industry, postmenopausal women were fed three additional eight-ounce glasses of skim milk to provide a total of 1,500 mg of calcium daily. Nevertheless, these women were still in a negative-calcium balance at the end of a year. When compared to a control group of women who did not get additional milk, scientists discovered that the women who drank the milk actually lost more bone than those who did not drink it. (The data did not reach statistical significance, but the trend was clear.) According to the authors, "The protein content of the supplement (the skim milk) may have a negative effect on calcium balance, possibly through an increase in kidney losses of calcium or through a direct effect on bone reabsorption."

Women who are concerned about osteoporosis are, in fact, raising the risk of contracting the disease by consuming dairy products, including low-fat, skim-milk dairy foods. Common health problems from cow's milk include food allergy; anemia; atheroscelerosis leading to heart attacks and strokes; cancer of the breast, ovary, and uterus; diabetes; life-threatening infections from animal-born bacteria and viruses; and obesity.

Taking calcium supplements in the form of pills (including antacids) may provide slight benefits for bone health, but the evidence is controversial; however, taking these pills poses much less of a health hazard than drinking cow's milk. The calcium supplements will reduce your body's ability to absorb iron by 60 percent and may constipate some people.

Menopause: For American Women, the Dangerous Crossing

In its most finite terms, menopause means the end to menstruation. Typically referred to as "the change of life," it marks the time when a woman's ovaries stop producing eggs and significantly decrease their production of estrogen. It is during the two years prior to actual menopause, a period known as perimenopause, that many of the commonly known physical changes take place, among them irregular periods, hot flashes, night sweats, vaginal dryness, and thinning of the walls of the vagina.

Most women on the Western diet experience menopause between the ages of 50 and 51. Only 10 percent of women undergo "natural" menopause (as opposed to that brought on by surgery or other medical reasons) before the age of 38. By the age of 50, 90 percent of women have experienced menopause, and by age 58 virtually all have.

Estrogen pills will improve menopausal symptoms, such as hot flashes and night sweats. These symptoms occur more intensely with the sudden ending to the production of estrogens after surgical removal of the ovaries. Estrogens also prevent thinning and dryness of vaginal linings, which can make sexual intercourse painful.

Fat consumption increases estrogen production and slows the onset of menopause. Cigarette smoking, on the other hand, diminishes estrogen production by the ovaries, speeding up the arrival of menopause. Obesity delays menopause because of the estrogens produced by body fat; on average, very thin women enter menopause earlier.

For most postmenopausal women, estrogen is still being produced in small quantities by the adrenal glands (located just above the kidneys), by fat cells, and in very small amounts by the ovaries. Of course, women who have had surgery that removes the ovaries are the exception.

Because estrogens reduce menopausal symptoms, many physicians argue that estrogens should be taken, if for no other reason than to alleviate the discomfort. But taking estrogens isn't the only way to control these symptoms. Changing your way of eating will do a great deal toward reducing and even eliminating many of the most extreme symptoms.

A healthy diet has been found to relieve many of the symptoms of menopause. Plant foods contain compounds known as phytoestrogens (phyto = plant). These weak estrogens stimulate a woman's cells after menopause, providing an estrogen effect that relieves symptoms. (Phytoestrogens also protect the cells of premenopausal women by blocking overstimulation by stronger estrogens that are made in their ovaries, thus reducing the risk of breast and uterine cancers.)

Vickey Farrell experienced the power of diet to relieve her menopausal suffering. She suffered with extreme menopausal symptoms for years before adopting the McDougall Heart Program. Her menopause began at 45 and immediately she started suffering hot flashes, nightsweats, and depression. Because she had a long history of fibrocystic breast disease, she refused to begin estrogen therapy out of fear that the estrogens would trigger breast cancer. Instead, she endured such intense hot flashes that they caused her to become faint two or three times a day. "I called them my 'power surges,' " said Vickey. "I got fifteen to twenty of these power surges per day."

Vickey had been a believer in food's ability to improve health for the previous twenty-five years. Unfortunately, she had been following bad advice. "I ate lots of protein," she recalled. "I was a big believer in dairy—I drank milk and ate lots of cheese, and I thought it was good for me. I learned from experience that dairy was a big problem for my menopausal symptoms." Meanwhile, she had also been suffering from heart palpitations.

In the fall of 1993, Vickey, who owns a bed-and-breakfast hotel in Arizona, heard about my clinic at St. Helena Hospital in the Napa Valley, and decided to enroll herself for the two-week program.

"Right away, I started to feel better on Dr. McDougall's diet. After the first six days, my severe symptoms had been alleviated, and after twelve days, about 90 percent of the symptoms were gone." That included the "power surges" and the depression. "No more power surges. I feel great now. Even my breast lumps have diminished."

Since then, Vickey has learned to control all her symptoms with the program. "If I cheat on the diet one day, I feel it the next day. I'll get night sweats or a hot flash or something, but I have learned how to control them now with what I eat."

When to Take Estrogens

There are times when I do prescribe estrogens to patients fully informed of the potential benefits and adverse consequences. Women who have lost their ovaries through surgery or have had radiation or chemotherapy and, as a consequence, have lost the ability to produce estrogen in their ovaries before normal menopause benefit from estrogen therapy. Replacement hormones should be supplied until these women reach their early fifties, at which time their ovaries would naturally shut down.

I may prescribe estrogen if a woman has naturally or prematurely lost her ovaries and has a very thin skeleton. I will also prescribe estrogen if a woman has a dangerously high cholesterol level and other significant risk factors for heart disease (such as family history of heart disease), but is unwilling or unable to correct these problems with a healthy diet and lifestyle alone. However, as I said at the outset of this chapter, you must change your diet and lifestyle to protect yourself against heart disease and osteoporosis, with or without HRT.

You may want to take estrogens if, after changing your diet, you still suffer from intolerable menopausal symptoms—hot flashes, anxiety, or depression—due to decreasing estrogen levels. Small doses of natural conjugated estrogen (0.3 to 0.625 mg of Premarin) taken for a short time may be all that is necessary to provide relief. Conjugated estrogens, such as Premarin, are preferred over synthetic estrogens, such as Estrace, because the synthetic forms are found to elevate the risk for breast cancer, whereas users of the conjugated forms show little increase in the incidence of this disease. Lower doses administered over shorter periods of time are associated with lower risks of cancer for obvious reasons.

If vaginal dryness and thinning, leading to difficulty with sexual intercourse, are your primary concerns, then vaginal creams of conjugated estrogen will improve the condition of the vagina: half a gram used every two to four days. Even though a small amount of hormone is absorbed through the vagina, cancer has not been associated with this form of use. There are also moisturizing preparations, such as Replens, that can be used rather than, or in addition to, hormones to help women with vaginal dryness. You can make the choices that are right for you only if you are fully informed.

Many women today believe that when it comes to menopause, they face a series of no-win decisions: They must choose between hip fractures and some form of cancer. As we have seen, this just isn't so. All things considered, estrogen, even in combination with progesterone, is not the singular solution to the problems of heart disease or premature bone loss in postmenopausal women.

Many misconceptions drive a woman to taking HRT when such therapy is unnecessary. For example, many women fear that if they do not take estrogen their sex drives will diminish. But studies have shown that just because there is a change in the tissues of the vagina does not mean that women are less interested in sex after menopause. Sex drive continues for most women, and sex can be just as satisfying after menopause. Indeed, women generally report that the passage through menopause is liberating. In a study involving 2,300 women in Massachusetts, researchers found that only 3 percent regarded this phase of life with "regret," while most felt relief that concerns over menstruation, pregnancy, and contraception were now behind them. You will want to enjoy these golden years looking and feeling your best—and that is accomplished through the McDougall Program for a Healthy Heart.

Part IV

SHOPPING HELP, COOKING TIPS, AND THE RECIPES

16. Practical Preparation for the McDougall Program for a Healthy Heart

- *A well-educated shopper solves health problems.*
- *You can make food preparation as simple as opening a package.*
- *Start a McDougall oil embargo today with healthy cooking techniques.*
- *Familiar foods are your favorite foods*

Shopping Habits: Supermarkets and Natural Foods Stores

With the list you've made for the week's menu, start shopping at your local supermarket. Pick a market that is interested in supplying good fresh fruits and vegetables. Many of the upscale markets have health foods and speciality sections, too, where some of the unusual ingredients can be found. We shop in a natural foods store about once a month, stocking up on the items we cannot find in a supermarket. (A natural foods store puts emphasis on *foods*, not on vitamin and mineral supplements and protein powders.)

Reading Labels

The key to effective shopping is careful reading of labels. Ingredients are supposed to be listed in descending order of amounts in the package. Manufacturers can deceive you with the present food labels. Sometimes simple sugars like sucrose, corn syrup, fructose, and fruit concentrate can be listed individually, in order to remove "sugar" as the first ingredient on the list.

Manufacturers have found ways of hiding fats in ingredient lists by calling them "monoglycerides," or "diglycerides." You might recognize "triglyceride" as being a complex fat, but are likely to overlook the mono- and di- forms as some sort of additive, unrelated to fats. The chemical difference among these three is the number of chains of fatty acids attached to the backbone molecule (glycerol): 1 (mono), 2 (di), or 3 (tri). Lecithin is a fat you may not recognize as such. Most lecithin is made from soybeans and is no more effective at lowering cholesterol in the blood than is any other similar vegetable oil.

You want to avoid fat as much as possible. Look for oils that are listed as ingredients on the label and avoid these products. You will often find 1 g of fat listed on the label of an apparently no-added-fat product. This 1 g represents the total amount of fats in naturally low-fat vegetable foods.

The Food and Drug Administration is in the process of improving labels so that you will be able to better judge the contents of a package.

FIGURING PERCENT OF CALORIES

A little simple math will help you determine how much fat, protein, and carbohydrate is in a labeled food or packaged product.

Percent fat is calculated by multiplying the number of grams of fat by *9 calories per gram*, dividing the answer (the number of calories of fat) by the total calories, then multiplying by 100 percent. Your goal is less than 10 percent fat.

Percent protein is calculated by multiplying the number of grams of protein by *4 calories per gram* dividing the answer (the number of calories of protein) by the total calories, then multiplying by 100 percent. Your goal is 8 to 15 percent protein.

Percent carbohydrate is calculated by multiplying grams of carbohydrate by *4 calories per gram*, dividing the answer (the number of calories of carbohydrate) by the total calories, then multiplying by 100 percent. Your goal is more than 75 percent carbohydrate.

The ideal starch-based diet is:

5 to 10 percent fat
8 to 15 percent protein
75 to 87 percent carbohydrate

When you're buying packaged foods be sure to read the ingredient labels carefully. And then read them periodically again and again, to catch changes in manufacturing practices and advertising ploys.

HANDY THINGS TO HAVE ON HAND

Toppings and Seasonings
low-sodium, oil-free salad dressings
lemon juice (bottled)
vinegar (try balsamic vinegar as a salad dressing)
low-sodium ketchup
mustard
salsas (oil-free)
Tabasco sauce
pepper hot sauces
horseradish (oil-free)
low-sodium soy sauce
barbecue sauces (bottled; no oil)
spaghetti sauce (bottled; no oil)
salt-free vegetable seasonings and seasoning mixes

Handy Snacks
rice cakes and rice crackers
pretzels
whole wheat crackers (oil-free)
popcorn (Spice this up by sprinkling it with garlic, chili, curry, or onion powder, poultry seasoning, or diluted Tabasco sauce. If you're not salt-sensitive, spray soy sauce on it or moisten the popcorn with water and sprinkle it with table salt.)
sliced raw vegetables
seaweed
whole grain and sprouted wheat breads, whole wheat pita and bagels (oil-free)
instant oatmeal
baked potatoes (leftover; eaten cold or microwaved)
frozen hash brown potatoes
dry packaged or canned soups
canned beans
leftovers
herbal teas and other noncaffeinated hot drinks
soda water (low-sodium; flavored or unflavored) or mineral water

Making the Program Easy: Canned and Packaged Products by Brand Name

The work of the McDougall Program for a Healthy Heart can be cut drastically if you have canned and packaged products on hand. Having the following on hand in your kitchen will help you to adhere to the McDougall Program for a Healthy Heart and to enjoy the foods.

Acceptable canned and packaged products are free of added oils and animal products. However, many do contain salt, sugars, spices, and additives that some people cannot tolerate. Read the labels carefully before deciding to buy. Manufacturers will sometimes change the ingredients, so check labels periodically.

MCDOUGALL OK'D CANNED AND PACKAGED PRODUCTS

Manufacturer/Distributor	*Variety*

COLD CEREALS

Cold cereals are whole grain, low in salt, sugar, and additives, and contain no added fats or oils.

Nabisco	Shredded Wheat
Post	Grape-Nuts
Nature's Path Foods	Manna (Millet Rice Flakes, Multi-Grain Flakes)
	Fiber O's
	Corn Flakes
	Heritage O's, Heritage, Multigrain
	Millet Rice
Kolln	Oat Bran Crunch
Health Valley Foods	100% Natural Bran Cereal
	Oat Bran Flakes
	Oat Bran O's
	Blue Corn Flakes
	Stone Wheat Flakes
	Fiber 7 Flakes

Manufacturer/Distributor	Variety
U.S. Mills	Uncle Sam
	(Erewhon) Crispy Brown Rice
	(Erewhon) Wheat Flakes
	(Erewhon) Corn Flakes, Aztec
Barbara's Bakery	Breakfast O's
	Breakfast Biscuits
	Multigrain
	Shredded Spoonfuls
Kellogg Co.	Nutri-Grain (Corn, Wheat, Nuggets, etc.)
Weetabix Co.	Grainfields (Wheat Flakes, Corn Flakes)
	Wheetabix Whole Wheat Cereal
Arrowhead Mills	Wheat Flakes
	Bran Flakes
	Oat Bran Flakes
	Corn Flakes
	Puffed Wheat
	Puffed Rice
	Puffed Millet
	Puffed Corn
	Nature O's, Amaranth Flakes,
	Spelt Flakes, Kamut, Multigrain Flakes
New Morning	Super Bran
	Oatios
Alvarado St. Bakery	Organic Granola
Health Valley	Fat-Free Granola
Breadshop	Health Crunch

HOT CEREALS

Hot cereals are whole grain, low in salt, sugar, and additives, and contain no added fats or oils.

Mercantile Food Co.	American Prairie Organic Hot Cereals
Quaker Oats Co.	Quaker Oats
	Quick Quaker Oats
U.S. Mills (Erewhon)	Instant Oat Meal
	Barley Plus
	Brown Rice Cream

Manufacturer/Distributor	*Variety*
Stone-Buhr Milling	7-Grain Cereal
Golden Temple Bakery	Oat Bran
Barbara's Bakery	14 Grains
Kashi Company	Kashi (some sesame seeds)
Arrowhead Mills	Bear Mush
	Oat Bran
	Instant Oatmeal (Maple Apple Spice, Original Plain)
Maple Leaf Mills	Red River Cereal (Original, Creamy Wheat, and Bran)

FROZEN POTATOES

Frozen potatoes have no added fats, oils, or salt. Most have sugar (dextrose) and a preservative added. (Mr. Dell's are only potatoes.)

Ore-Ida Foods	Hash Browns
	Potatoes O'Brien
Bel-air	Hash Browns
Mr. Dell Foods	Hash Browns
J.R. Simplot Co.	Okray's Hash Brown Potato Patties
Pacific Valley Foods	French Fry Style Potatoes (fat-free)
Cascadian Farm	Country Style Potatoes

POPCORN

Unprocessed popcorn (with no added ingredients). You can pop any natural popcorn yourself in an air popper or in the microwave.

H.J. Heinz Co.	Weight Watchers (microwave popcorn)
Nature's Best	Nature's Cuisine (natural popcorn)
Energy Food Factory	Poprice
Lapidus Popcorn Co.	Lite-Corn
Specialty Grain Co.	Pop-Lite Microwave Popcorn
Country Grown Foods	Gourmet Popcorn

RICE CAKES

Rice with other whole grains and seasonings, no added fats or oils. Some have salt added.

Quaker Oats Co.	Rice Cakes (lightly salted)
	Corn Cakes

Manufacturer/Distributor	*Variety*
H.J. Heinz Co.	Chico San (Millet, Buckwheat, and more)
Hollywood Health Foods	Mini Rice Cakes (Teriyaki)
Pacific Rice Prod.	Mini Crispys (Italian Spice, Natural Sodium Free)
Westbrae Natural Foods	Teriyaki Rice Cakes
Lundberg Family Farms	Rice Cakes (Wild Rice, Wehani, Brown Rice)
	Organic Brown Rice Mini Rice Cakes

CRACKERS

Rice, wheat, rye, and other whole grains with seasonings, no added fats or oils. Some have salt added.

San-J International	Tamari Brown Rice Crackers
Westbrae Natural Foods	Brown Rice Wafers
Ralston Purina Co.	Natural Ry-Krisp
Edward & Sons Trading Co.	Baked Brown Rice Snaps
Parco Foods	(Hol-Grain) Brown Rice Lite Snack Thins, Whole Wheat Lite Snack Thins
O. Kavli A/S	Kavli Norwegian Crispbread
Barbara's Bakery	Crackle Snax
	Lightbread
Sandoz Nutrition Corp.	Wasa Crispbread (Lite Rye, Hearty Rye)
H.J. Heinz Co.	Weight Watchers Crispbread (Harvest Rice)
Shaffer, Clarke & Co.	Finn Crisp
Lifestream Natural Foods	Wheat & Rye Krispbread
Nabisco	Fat Free Premium Crackers
	Snack Wells Cracked Pepper Crackers
Baja Bakery	Rice & Bean Tortilla Bites
Edwards & Sons Trading Co.	Brown Rice Sembei
Snack Cracks	Organic Rice Crackers (tamari, lightly salted)
Soken Products	Sesame Wheels (brown rice)
Tree of Life	Fat Free Saltines
	Fat Free Crackers

Manufacturer/Distributor	*Variety*
Little Bear Organic	Bearitos Baked Harvest Snackers, Original
Auburn Farms Inc.	Fat Free 7 Grainers
	Spicy 7 Grainers (except Pizza)
	Fat Free Spud Bakes (Original only)
RW Frookies, Inc.	Fat Free Crackers
	Frisps
Pacific Grain	No Fries: Plain Potato, Tortilla Snacks
Stella D'Oro Biscuit Co.	Fat Free Bread Sticks
Venus Wafers, Inc.	Fat Free Crackers (Garden Vegetable, Toasted Onion)
Burns & Ricker	Fat Free Party Mix
	Fat Free Bagel Crisps
Trader Joe's	Mini Rice Cakes: Plain

PRETZELS

No added fats or oils. Most are high in salt, refined flours.

Laura Scudder's	Mini-Twist Pretzels
	Pretzel Sticks
	Bavarian Pretzels
Anderson Bakery Co.	Oat Bran Pretzels
Snyder's of Hanover	Sourdough Hard Pretzels (salted and unsalted)
Granny Goose Foods	Stick Pretzels 100% Natural
	Bavarian Pretzels (salted and unsalted)
J & J Snack Foods	Super Pretzels (frozen)
Barbara's Bakery	Barbara's Whole Wheat Bavarian Pretzels
	Organic Whole Wheat Pretzels (Honey Sweet, 9 Grain, Mini)
Frito-Lay Inc.	Baked Rold Gold Pretzels
Health Is Wealth Products	Soft Pretzel (frozen)

CHIPS

Guiltless Gourmet	Guiltless Gourmet No Oil Tortilla Chips
	White Corn No Oil Tortilla Chips

~~Manufacturer/Distri~~butor	*Variety*
Barbara's Bakery	Basically Baked Organic Tortilla Chips
Trader Joe's	Baked Tortilla Chips
Little Bear Organic Foods	Baked Tortilla Chips
Taco Works Inc.	Eva's Fat Free Potato Chips
American Speciality Foods	Smart Temptations Tortilla Chips
Mexi-Snax Inc.	Bake-itos Baked Tortilla Chips (Regular, Pico de Gallo, Blue Corn)
Garden of Eatin, Inc.	California Bakes Tortilla Chips
Frito-Lay, Inc.	Baked Tostitos
Barbara's Bakery	Amazing Bakes Tortilla Chips
R.W. Garcia Co.	Oven Baked Blue Corn Tortilla Chips
Louise's Inc.	Louise's Fat Free Potato Chips
Synergy Systems	Childers Natural Potato Chips
FitFoods	Baked Fat Free Potato Chips

BREADS

Any baked with whole wheat, sprouted wheat, rye, or other whole grains with no added oil or dairy products, such as whey. Low-sugar, low-sodium are desirable.

Cedarlane Foods	Whole Wheat Lavash Bread
	Fat Free Whole Wheat Tortillas
Lifestream Natural Foods	Essene Bread
Nature's Path Foods	Manna Bread
Grainaissance	Mochi (Plain, Mugwort, Organic)
International Baking Co.	Mr. Pita
Garden of Eatin', Inc.	Bible Bread (regular and salt-free)
	Thin-Thin Bread
Breads for Life	Sprouted 7-Grain Bread
	Sprouted Rye Bread
Interstate Brands	Pritikin Bread (Rye, Whole Wheat, Multi-Grain)
French Meadow Bakery	French Meadow Brown Rice Bread
New England Foods Co.	Whole Wheat Milldam Pouch Bread
Food For Life	Sprouted Grain Breads
Great Harvest Bread Co.	Great Harvest Bakery (Honey Wheat, 9-Grain, Rye Onion, Dill, Country Whole Wheat)

Manufacturer/Distributor	*Variety*
Brother Juniper's Bakery	Brother Juniper's Oil Free Breads (Cajun Three Pepper, Oreganato, Whole Wheat)
Alvarado St. Bakery	Alvarado St. Oil-Free Breads and Buns
Siljans Knacke	Siljans Knacke (Swedish Dark Rye Crispbread)
Norganic Foods Co.	Katenbrot (rye bread)
Ryvita	Ryvita Crisp Breads
Burns & Ricker	Crispini
Nokomis Farms	Country Loaf (Sourdough)
Snack Cracks	Pizza Crust (Organic Brown Rice)
Oasis Breads	Creative Crust Dinner Shells
Natural Ovens of Manitowoc	Soft Sandwich Bread
McCree Foods Int.	G. McCree's Crumpets
Afghan Gourmet Bakery	Kabuli Gourmet Pizza Bread
S.B. Thomas, Inc.	Sahara Pita Bread

SOUPS

Soups have no meat, dairy, no added fats and oils. Many are high in salt.

DRY PACKAGED

Nile Spice Foods	Cous-Cous (Tomato Minestrone, Lentil Curry)
	Chili'n Beans
	Lentil Soup, Black Bean Soup, Split Pea Soup
	Pack It Meals (Black Bean, Red Beans & Rice, Lentil Curry)
Westbrae Natural Foods	Ramen (Whole Wheat, Onion, Curry, Carrot, Miso, Seaweed, 5 Spice, Spinach, Mushroom, Buckwheat, Savory Szechuan, Oriental Vegetable, Golden Chinese)
	Instant Miso Soup (Mellow White, Hearty Red)
	Noodles Anytime (Country Style)
Sokensha Co.	Soken Ramen
Eden Foods	Buckwheat Ramen
	Whole Wheat Ramen

Manufacturer/Distributor	Variety
Wil-Pak Foods	Taste Adventure Soups (Black Bean, Curry Lentil, Split Pea Soup, Red Bean)
Fantastic Foods	Fantastic Soups (Fantastic Jumpin Black Beans, Fantastic Splittin' Peas, Pinto Beans & Rice Mexicana, Rice & Beans, Five Bean Soup, Cha-Cha Chili, Vegetable Barley, Couscous with Lentils, Country Lentil)
	Ramen Noodles (Chicken-Free, Tomato, Curry, Miso)
The Spice Hunter	Mediterranean Minestrone, Moroccan Couscous, Cantonese Noodle Soup, French Country Lentil, Kasba Curry, Mandarin Noodle Soup
Health Valley Foods	Fat Free Soup Cups
Pacific Foods of Oregon	Cajun Red Beans & Rice
	Curried Lentils & Rice
Sahara Natural Foods	Casbah Timeless Cuisine: Moroccan, La Fiesta, Pasta Fasul, Jambalaya, Hearty Harvest
San Francisco Spice Co.	Perfect Recipe Organics (Chicken Free Pasta, Salsa Black Bean, Minestrone, Minestrone Couscous, Salsa Beans & Rice, Vegie Vegan Couscous, Curry Beans & Rice)
W.J. Clark & Co.	Bean Cuisine Soup
Trader Joe's	Ramen Soup, Brown Rice Ramen, Soba Noodles

CANNED

Real Fresh	Andersen's Soup (Split Pea)
Health Valley Foods	Fat-Free Soups (5 Bean Vegetable, Country Corn and Vegetable, plus others)
	Organic Soups (Minestrone, Tomato, Black Bean, Mushroom Barley, Lentil, Split Pea, Potato Leek)

Manufacturer/Distributor	*Variety*
Hain Pure Food Co.	Fat Free Soup (Vegetarian Split Pea, Vegetarian Veggie Broth)
Mercantile Food Co.	American Prairie Vegetable Bean Soup
Trader Joe's	Mostly Unsplit Pea Soup, Bean & Vegetable Duet Soup, Tomato Vegetable Soup, Swabian Rice & Vegetable Soup
Little Bear Organic	Bearitos Fat Free Soups
Fair Exchange	Shari's Bistro Soups

BURGER MIXES/MEAT SUBSTITUTES

Mixes contain no added fats, oils, or dairy products. No soybean products added. Most tell you to fry in oil—DON'T. Cook on a nonstick griddle.

Fantastic Foods	Fantastic Falafil
	Nature's Burger (Barbecue Flavor)
Santa Fe Organics	Hickory Smoked Seitan and others
Arrowhead Mills	Seitan Quick Mix
Vegetarian Health Society	Vegetarian Hamburger Bits
Vegetarian Health	Vegetarian Beef Chunks
Sweet Earth Natural Foods	Seitan
WhiteWave Inc.	Seitan Fajita Strips
Yves Veggie Cuisine	Deli Slices, Veggie Pepperoni, Canadian Veggie Bacon, Veggie Wieners, Chili Dog, Original Bagel Dog, Chili Bagel Dog
Turtle Island Foods	Superburgers
Lightlife Foods, Inc.	Lightburgers
	Smart Deli Thin Slices
	Savory Seitan
	Smart Dogs
Knox Mountain Farm	Wheatballs, Chick'n Wheat, Not-So-Sausage
Boca Burger Co.	No Fat Meatless Boca Burger
Wildwood Natural Foods	Fat Free Wild Dogs
Worthington Foods	Natural Touch Fat Free Vegan Burger
	GranBurger
Fearn Natural Foods	Breakfast Patty Mix

Manufacturer/Distributor	*Variety*

EGG-FREE PASTAS

Pastas are egg-free with no added oils or fat. Most are made of flour and water, and are low-sodium.

Health Valley Foods	Spaghetti Pasta (Spinach, Whole Wheat, Amaranth, etc.)
Westbrae Natural Foods	Spaghetti Pasta (Spinach, Whole Wheat)
	Lasagna Noodles (Spinach, Whole Wheat)
	Whole Wheat Somen
DeBole's Nutritional Foods	Curly Lasagna, Elbows, Spaghetti Corn Pasta (Wheat-free)
Quinoa Corp.	Quinoa Spaghetti (Wheat-free)
Golden Grain Macaroni Co.	Spaghetti, Macaroni, Rotini, Lasagna, Manicotti
A. Zerega's Sons	Antoine's Pasta (Fusilli Tri Colori)
Eden Foods	Udon (Japanese Noodles)
	Soba (buckwheat)
	Eden Vegetable Pastas
	Vegetable Shells
Nanka Seimen Co.	Chow Mein Udon
Sokensha Co.	Soken Jinenjo Noodles
Health Foods	MI-del (Spaghetti, Macaroni, Alphabets)
Best Foods, CPC Int.	Muellers (Twist, Spaghetti, Linguine)
Borden	Creamette (Spaghetti, Fettuccine, Rotini, Shells)
Reese Finer Foods	Da Vinci Pasta
Ferrara Foods	Gnocchi with Potato
Ronzoni Foods Corp.	Radiatore
	Linguine
	Fusilli
	Rotelle
	Spaghetti
Pastariso Products	Pastariso (Brown Rice Pasta)
Food For Life Baking Co.	Wheat-Free Rice Elbows

Manufacturer/Distributor	*Variety*
Bertagni	Gnocchi di Palate
Mrs. Leepers, Inc.	Mrs. Leepers Pasta (Organic Vegetable, Organic Whole Wheat, Organic Kamut, Rice Pasta, Corn Pasta)
	Eddie's Organic Pasta (Spaghetti, Rotelli, Corkscrews, Bowties, Trumpets, Confetti, Radiatore, Shells, Orzo)
	Michelle's Natural 2 Minute Pasta
Purity Foods, Inc.	Vita Spelt Pasta
Garden Time Foods	Pasta (Spaghetti, Linguini, Rigatoni, Ribbons, Spirals, Bowties, Trumpets, Corkscrews)
Tuterri's	Pasta
Amway Corp.	Microwave Pasta Ribbons
New Hong Kong Noodle Co.	Pot Sticker Wraps
Emilia Foods	Gnocchi with Potato

PACKAGED GRAINS AND PASTAS

Packaged grains contain whole grains only; no added fats or oils.

Health Valley Foods	Oat Bran Pasta with Sauce (Fettucini Marinara, Fettucini Primavera)
Quinoa Corp.	Quinoa
Continental Mills	ala (cracked wheat bulgur)
Fantastic Foods	Brown Basmati Rice
	Whole Wheat Couscous
Arrowhead Mills	Wholegrain Teff
	Quick Brown Rice
	Wheat-Free Oatbran Muffin Mix
	Griddle Lite Pancake & Baking Mix
	Quick Brown Rice (Spanish Style, Vegetable Herb, and Wild Rice & Herbs)
Pritikin Systems	Pritikin Mexican Dinner Mix
	Pritikin Brown Rice Pilaf

Manufacturer/Distributor	*Variety*
Near East Food Prod.	Spanish Rice
	Wheat Pilaf
	Taboule
	Lentil Pilaf Mix
Nile Spice Foods	Nile Spice Whole Wheat Couscous
	Nile Spice Couscous Salad Mix
	Nile Spice Rozdali
Wil-Pak Foods	Taste Adventure (Black Bean)
	Flakes and Pinto Bean Flakes
J.A. Sharwood & Co.	Sharwood's India Pilau Rice
Texmati Rice	Basmati Brown Rice
Tipiak	Couscous
Liberty Imports	Instant Polenta
Trader Joe's	Sante Fe Rice, Creole Rice, Spanish Rice
Lundberg Farms	One-Step Entrees (Chili, Curry, Basil)
Sahara Natural Foods	Casbah Timeless Pilafs (Couscous, Casbah Whole Wheat Couscous, Lentil, Spanish, Bulgur)
San Francisco Spice Co.	Perfect Recipe Organics (Mediterranean Couscous)
Sorrenti Family Farms	Rising Star Ranch (Fiesta Rice, Harvest Rice, Pasta Roma)
The Food Merchants	Kamut Pasta Pilaf Southwestern Blend
W.J. Clark & Co.	Pasta & Beans
Melting Pot Foods	Po River Valley Risotto
Jerusalem Natural Foods	Jerusalem Tab-ooleh
Aurora Import & Dist.	Polenta
Berhanu International Ltd.	Authentic Olde World (Lentils Divine)

BEAN AND VEGETABLE DISHES (frozen or refrigerated)

Cascadian Farms	Three Rice Medley, Wild Tiger Stirfry
Trader Joe's	Spicy Black Bean Medley

SALAD DRESSINGS

Salad dressings are no dairy (whey, buttermilk, etc.), no fats, no oils added. Many state clearly "No-oil." Should also say low-sodium.

Manufacturer/Distributor	*Variety*
Pritikin Systems	Pritikin No-oil Dressing (Ranch, Tomato, Italian, Russian, Creamy Italian, etc.)
WM Reily & Co.	Herb Magic (All No-oil—Vinaigrette, Italian, Gypsy, Zesty Tomato, Creamy Cucumber)
American Health Products	El Molino Herbal Secrets (All No-oil—Herbs & Spices, etc.)
Kraft	Oil Free Italian (high salt)
H.J. Heinz Co.	Weight Watchers Dressing (Tomato Vinaigrette, French)
Cook's Classics	Cook's Classic Oil-Free Dressings (Italian Gusto, Country French, Garlic Gusto, Dijon, Dill)
St. Mary Glacier	St. Mary's Oil Free Salad Dressing (many flavors)
Trader Joe's	Trader Joe's (No Oil Dill & Garlic Dressing, Italian)
Nature's Harvest	Nature's Harvest (Oil-Free Vinaigrette, Oil-Free Herbal Splendor)
Nakano USA	Seasoned Rice Vinegar
Uncle Grant's Foods	Uncle Grant's Salute (Honey Mustard Tarragon Dressing)
S & W Fine Foods	Vintage Lites Oil-Free Dressing
Tres Classique	Grand Garlic, Tomato & Herb French
Rising Sun Farms	Oil Free Salad Vinaigrettes and Marinades (Raspberry Balsamic, Garlic Lovers, Dill with Lemon, Honey & Mustard Vinegars)
Hain Pure Food Co.	Fat Free Salad Dressing Mix (Italian, Herb)
Kozlowski Farms	Fat Free Dressings (Zesty Herb, Honey Mustard, South of the Border, Raspberry Poppy Seed)

Manufacturer/Distributor   *Variety*

Sweet Adelaide Enter.	Paula's No-Fat Dressing (Toasted Onion, Roasted Garlic, Garden Tomato)
	Paula's No Oil Dressing (Lime & Cilantro, Lemon Dill, etc.)

SPAGHETTI SAUCE

Spaghetti sauces contain no meat, dairy products, olive oil, or any other oils or fats.

Pure & Simple	Johnson's Spaghetti Sauce
Trader Joe's	Trader Giotto's Italian Garden Fresh Vegetable Spaghetti Sauce
	Organic Spaghetti Sauce (Fat Free)
Westbrae Natural Foods	Ci' Bella Pasta Sauce (No Salt, No Oil)
H.J. Heinz Co.	Weight Watchers Spaghetti Sauce with Mushrooms
Campbell Soup Co.	Campbell's Healthy Request Marinara Sauce
Pritikin Systems	Pritikin Spaghetti Sauce (Original, Chunky Garden Style)
Hunt-Wesson	Healthy Choice Spaghetti Sauce
Nature's Harvest	Rocket Pesto
Tree of Life	Fat-Free Pasta Sauce
Sierra Quality Foods	Muir Glen Fat Free Pasta Sauce
S & W Fine Foods	Simply Wonderful California Pasta Sauces
Organic Food Products	Millina's Finest Fat Free Pasta Sauces
Ventre Packing Co.	Enrico's Fat Free Pasta Sauce
Robbie's	Robbie's Fat Free Spaghetti Sauce

SOY SAUCES

Soy sauces contain no MSG (monosodium glutamate). They are all high in sodium, but some are salt-reduced.

Kikkoman Foods	Kikkoman Lite Soy Sauce
Westbrae Natural Foods	Mild Soy Sauce
San-J International	Tamari Wheat Free Soy Sauce
Live Food Products	Bragg Liquid Aminos
Edward & Sons Trading Co.	Ginger Tamari

Manufacturer/Distributor   *Variety*

OTHER SAUCES

Sauces contain no oils, fats, or MSG. Many have salt and preservatives. Most are very spicy and can burn.

Edward & Sons Trading Co.	Stir Krazy Vegetarian Worcestershire Sauce
New Morning	Corn Relish
Nabisco Brands	A.1 Steak Sauce
Lea & Perrins	Lea & Perrins Steak Sauce
San-J International	Teriyaki Sauce
St. Giles Foods Ltd.	Matured Worcestershire Sauce
McIlhenny Co.	Tabasco
Gourmet Foods	Cajun Sunshine
Durkee-French Foods	Red Hot Sauce
Baumer Foods	Crystal Hot Sauce
B.F. Trappey's Sons	Red Devil Louisiana Hot Sauce
J. Sosnick & Son	Kosher Horseradish
Reese Finer Foods	Prepared Horseradish
Annie Chun's Gourmet Foods	Fat Free Mushroom Sauce, Oil Free Teriyaki Sauce
Ayla's Organics	Salsa (Garlic, Tomatillo, Picante) Dressings (Oil Free) Sauces (Cajun, Curry, Szechwan, Thai)
Westbrae Natural Foods	Fat Free Barbeque Sauce (Original, Zesty)
Lang Naturals	Fat Free Sauces (Honey Mustard, Ginger)

SALSAS

Salsas contain vegetable ingredients only with no oils. Some have preservatives. Many contain sugar and/or salt.

Hain Pure Food Co.	Salsa
Pet	Old El Paso Salsa
Tree of Life	Salsa
Nabisco Brands	Ortega Green Chile Salsa
Pace Foods	Picante Sauce

Manufacturer/Distributor	Variety
La Victoria Foods	Chili Dip
	Salsas
Ventre Packing Co.	Enrico's Salsa
Guiltless Gourmet	Guiltless Gourmet Picante Sauce
Pritikin Systems	Pritikin Salsa
Trader Joe's	Salsa Authentica
	Salsa Verde
	Pineapple Salsa
	Raspberry Salsa
Nature's Harvest	Salsa
Garden of Eatin', Inc.	Organic Salsa & Dip
Organic Gourmet	Miso Paste (Honey, Apple)
S & D Foods, Inc.	Parrot Brand Enchilada Sauce, Salsas
Renfro Foods, Inc.	Sauces & Relishes

SALT-FREE SEASONING MIXES

Salt-free seasoning mixes are made with no added salt, but there is a small amount of natural sodium in them. They are made of dehydrated vegetables and spices, and they are low in sodium. Watch for added salt and oils in any seasoning mixes you buy.

Alberto-Culver Co.	Mrs. Dash (Low Pepper–No Garlic, Extra Spicy, Original Blend, etc.)
Modern Products	Vegit All-Purpose Seasoning
	Onion Magic
	Natural Seasoning
Maine Coast Sea Vegetables	Sea Seasonings (Dulse with Garlic, Nori with Ginger, etc.)
Estee Corp.	Seasoning Sense (Mexican, Italian)
Hain Pure Food Co.	Chili Seasoning Mix
Bernard Jensen Products	Broth or Seasoning Special Vegetable Mix

BAKING INGREDIENTS

Baking ingredients contain no aluminum and a minimum number of additives.

Manufacturer/Distributor	*Variety*
The Rumford Co.	Rumford Baking Powder
Sandoz Nutrition	Featherweight Baking Powder
Ener-G Foods	Egg Replacer (a binder for baking)
Eden Foods	Eden Kuzu Root Starch

ACCEPTABLE MILK SUBSTITUTES

Acceptable milks are dairy-free and low in natural vegetable fat. They are not to be used as beverages, but on cereals and in cooking.

Grainaissance	Amazake Rice Nectar
	Amazake Rice Drink
	Amazake Light
Eden Foods	Edensoy Vanilla Soy Milk
	Eden Rice Beverage
Sovex Natural Foods	Better Than Milk? Light
Health Valley Foods	Fat Free Soy Moo
Vitasoy U.S.A.	Vitasoy Light—Original 1%
Westbrae Natural Foods	West Soy Lite (1% fat) Plain
	Non Fat West Soy Milk
Pacific Foods of Oregon	Pacific Lite

HOT DRINKS

Drinks contain no caffeine or other strong herbs that you may be sensitive to.

Many manufacturers	Noncaffeinated teas
Modern Products	Sipp
Libby, McNeill & Libby	Pero
Worthington Foods	Kaffree Roma
Richter Bros.	Cafix
General Foods Corp.	Postum
Sundance Roasting Co.	Sundance Barley Brew
Bolt's Old World Grain Co.	Gaia's Cafe
Eden Foods	Yannoh
Adamba Imports Int.	Inka
Bioforce of America	Coffree

Manufacturer/Distributor	*Variety*

CANNED BEAN AND/OR VEGETABLE PRODUCTS

Canned products contain no added fats and oils. They should be low in sodium and preservatives. The cans are made of metals that leach into the foods unless they are coated. Glass jars, of course, have no metal.

Eden Foods	Great Northern Beans (glass jars)
	Pinto Beans (glass jars)
	Adzuki Beans (glass jars)
Whole Earth	Baked Beans
Health Valley Foods	Boston Baked Beans
	Fast Menu Vegetarian Cuisine (Western Black Bean & Veggies, Hearty Lentils & Vegetables)
Hain Pure Food Co.	Spicy Vegetarian Homestyle Chili
	Fat Free Vegetarian Refried Beans (Black & Pinto)
	Fat Free Bean Dips
Bush Bros. & Co.	Bush's Deluxe Vegetarian Beans
Brazos Products	Brazos Cajun Bean Dip
S & W Fine Foods	Deli-Style Bean Salad
	Mixed Bean Salad (glass jars)
	Dill Garden Salad
	Succotash
	Garden Style Pasta Salad
	Honey Mustard Baked Beans, Maple Sugar Baked Beans, Pinquitos, White Beans, Chili Beans with Chipotle Peppers
Del Monte Foods	Dennison's Chili Beans in Chili Gravy
Hunt-Wesson	Rosarita No Fat Refried Beans
Guiltless Gourmet	Bean Dips
Westbrae Natural Foods	Organic Canned Beans, Organic Mustard
Little Bear Organic	Bearitos Beans & Rice (Cuban Style, Cajun Style, Mexican Style)
	Bearitos Bean Dip (Black or Pinto)
	Bearitos Fat Free Refried Beans

Manufacturer/Distributor	Variety
	Bearitos Chili (Spicy, Original, Black Bean)
	Bearitos Fat Free Baked Beans
Trader Joe's	Kidney Bean Chili, Black Bean Chili
	Fat Free Pinto Bean Dips, Fat Free Black Bean Dips
Santa Cruz Fine Foods	Fat Free Bean Dips, Fat Free Guacamole Dip, Black Bean & Corn Salsa
Garden of Eatin', Inc.	Fat Free Bean Dips (Baja Black Bean, Smoky Chipotle)

CANNED TOMATO PRODUCTS

No-added-salt brands of tomato products can be found in many natural foods and grocery stores. Metals leach from cans unless specially coated.

Health Valley Foods	Tomato Sauce (coated lead-free can)
Del Monte USA	Tomato Sauce
	Tomato Paste
	Diced Tomatoes, Chunky Tomatoes, Stewed Tomatoes (Cajun Recipe, Mexican Recipe, Italian Recipe)
Hunt-Wesson	Tomato Paste
	Tomato Sauce
	Stewed Tomatoes
	Whole Tomatoes
Contadina Foods	Tomato Puree
	Tomato Paste
Pet	Progresso Tomato Paste
	Progresso Tomato Puree
	Progresso Tomatoes
Eden Foods	Crushed Tomatoes
Trader Joe's	Tomato Sauce
S & W Fine Foods	Ready-Cut Peeled Tomatoes
	Stewed Tomatoes (Cajun Recipe, Mexican Recipe, Italian Recipe)
	Salsa (with cilantro, with chipotle)
	Tomato Sauce (Thick & Chunky)

Manufacturer/Distributor	*Variety*
Ital Trade, USA	Pomi Strained Tomatoes, Pomi Chopped Tomatoes
Sierra Quality Canners	Muir Glen Organic Tomato Products

For an updated package list send a self-addressed, stamped envelope to:

The McDougalls
P.O. Box 14039
Santa Rosa, CA 95402

Choosing Cookware

An easy way to eliminate oil from your cooking is to use nonstick-coated pans. Acceptable materials for cookware include glass, stainless steel, iron, nonstick-coated pans and bakeware (such as Dupont's Silver-Stone or Teflon, or Mary's favorite, Millennium by Farberware), silicone-coated bakeware (such as Baker's Secret), and porcelain. A light oiling when you first get a Teflon or SilverStone implement will help to prevent sticking. Cast-iron pans and woks should be oiled before they're first used and then "seasoned" by heating.

When buying cookware you need to pay the most attention to the surface that your foods will contact, because some interaction always will cause your food to pick up molecules from the utensil's surface. Aluminum cookware should be avoided because of the association between aluminum ingestion and Alzheimer's disease. (If you're stuck with an aluminum pan or pot, put holes in the bottom, and plant flowers in it.) For cake pans, loaf pans, and baking sheets, you can use parchment paper between the metal and your food. Parchment paper also keeps food from sticking to the surface of the pans. You can find it in most grocery stores. Parchment can also be used under (or over) aluminum foil, in order to keep the aluminum from coming in contact with the food. Place a layer of parchment paper over the food in a baking dish, then cover with foil. Turn the edges over the pan to hold in the steam.

If vegetables stick while cooking in a pan or baking tray, let them cool for five to ten minutes and they will loosen easily. Cooling will also loosen muffins from the tins.

RECOMMENDED COOKWARE

(1) 2 qt. saucepan (stainless steel)
(1) 3 qt. saucepan (stainless steel)
(1) 4 qt. saucepan (stainless steel)
(1) 6 qt. stockpot (stainless steel)
(1) 8 qt. steamer/pasta cooker (stainless steel)
(1) 12 qt. stockpot (stainless steel)
(1) griddle (nonstick coating)
(1) large frying pan (nonstick coating)
(1) electric wok (nonstick coating)
(1) 9 1/4 × 5 1/4 in. loaf pan (silicone coated)
(1) 13 × 9 × 2 in. oblong baking pan (silicone coated)

(1) 8 × 8 × 2 in. square baking pan (silicone coated)
(1) muffin tin (silicone coated)
(2) baking trays (silicone coated)
(1) 2 qt. covered casserole dish (glass)
(1) 3 qt. covered casserole dish (glass)
(1) 6 qt. square covered casserole dish (glass)
(2) 13 × 9 oblong uncovered baking dishes (glass)
(1) 11 3/4 × 7 1/2 oblong uncovered baking dish (glass)

A Few Time-Saving Cooking Techniques

We realize that our readers are busy people and want to cut down on the time they spend preparing meals. The basic ingredients used in McDougall cooking can be shopped for in large quantities, saving you trips to the store. Many have long shelf lives, such as dried beans and rice, and others last long when refrigerated, such as fruits and vegetables.

You can also save time by cooking larger quantities of beans and rice and freezing the leftovers for use in another meal. You can also double a recipe and save half. Once cooked, the dishes themselves refrigerate and freeze well. Because there are no meat or dairy products, spoilage is much less of a problem. Your meatless, oil-free spaghetti sauce will taste fresh when thawed two months later.

Sautéing Without Oil

To sauté implies the use of butter or oil. But in McDougall cooking, oil is eliminated. Instead, we use other liquids to provide taste without the health hazards. Surprisingly, plain water makes an excellent sautéing liquid. It prevents foods from sticking to the pan, and still allows vegetables to brown and cook.

For additional flavor, try sautéing in:

soy sauce (Tamari)   tomato juice
red or white wine (alcoholic or   lemon or lime juice
   nonalcoholic)   Mexican salsa
sherry (alcoholic or nonalcoholic)   Worcestershire sauce
rice vinegar or balsamic vinegar

For even more taste, add herbs and spices, such as gingerroot, dry mustard, and garlic.

Browning Vegetables

Browned onions have an excellent flavor and can be used alone or mixed with other vegetables to make a dish with a distinctive taste. To achieve the color of browning, as well as to flavor your foods, place 1½ cups of chopped onions in a large nonstick frying pan with 1 cup of water. Cook over medium heat, stirring occasionally, until the liquid evaporates and the onions begin to stick to the bottom of the pan. Continue to stir for a minute, then add another ½ cup of water, loosening the browned bits from the bottom of the pan. Cook until the liquid evaporates again. Repeat this procedure one or two more times, until the onions are as browned as you like. You can also use this technique to brown carrots, green peppers, garlic, potatoes, shallots, zucchini, and many other vegetables, alone or mixed in a variety of combinations.

Baking Without Oil

To eliminate oil in baking is a real challenge because oil keeps the baked goods moist and soft. Replace the oil called for in the recipe with half the amount of another moist food, such as applesauce, mashed bananas, mashed potatoes, mashed pumpkin, tomato sauce, soft silken tofu, or soy yogurt (keep in mind that tofu and soy yogurt are high-fat foods).

There are a few new products that are specifically made to replace the fats in baked goods. These are usually made from plums. Two examples are Just Like Shortenin' (The Plumlife Co.) and Wonderslim (Natural Food Technologies).

Cakes and muffins made without oil usually come out a little heavier. For a lighter texture, use carbonated water instead of tap water in baking recipes. Be sure to test cakes and muffins at the end of the baking time by inserting a toothpick or cake tester in the center to see if it comes out clean. Sometimes oil-free cakes and muffins may need to be baked longer than the directions advise, depending on the weather or the altitude at which you live.

Microwave or Oven?

Since the introduction of microwave cooking some people have been suspicious of "nuked" foods. However, tests on these foods show excellent nutrient content and no significant increase in harmful by-products from microwave heating when compared to conventional oven cooking. We use a microwave mostly for boiling water, reheating leftovers, thawing vegetables, and cooking potatoes. Microwave ovens are fast and convenient. Sauces, stews, casseroles, and vegetables cook well in the microwave. Less liquid is needed and the cooking time is reduced, as compared to oven cooking. But you must stir or rotate foods often, and foods must be covered when microwaved to hold in steam and to cook faster without drying.

The greatest concern about the safety of microwave appliances is the potential leakage of radiation from damaged units. Inexpensive microwave testers are available in most department stores. Buy one and check your unit periodically.

Seasoning Foods

Use the recipes in this and other McDougall books as guidelines. You may want to add more or less spice. We learned about individual tastes through years of counseling people. One person would tell Mary, "Your food is so bland. Every time I make a dish I have to double the spice." The very next person would ask Mary why she used so much spice. Mary has tried to fla-

vor the foods to satisfy the average palate. (However, this moderate seasoning approach is subject to Mary's interpretation. For example, she happens
to love curry and I do not. Fortunately, over the years I have come to enjoy
many of Mary's Indian and Thai dishes.)

When deciding whether to use fresh herbs or dried ones, consider how
long the food is going to cook. Dried herbs fare better in longer cooking
times. For shorter cooking times, use fresh herbs, if available, to really
appreciate the flavors they can add. Generally, you need more fresh
herbs to equal the flavor of dried ones, because the dried herbs are more
concentrated. However, dried herbs lose their potency and their taste
when stored too long.

There are particular combinations of spices identified with ethnic
dishes. You can take advantage of these spices to vary recipes and create
new ones.

Mexican	*Asian*	*Indian*
Salsa	Soy sauce	Turmeric
Chili powder	Ginger	Pepper
Cumin	Dry mustard	Cilantro
Cilantro	Garlic	Cumin
Italian	*Greek*	
Parsley	Lemon juice	
Basil	Cinnamon	
Oregano	Cumin	
Garlic	Pepper	

Have Favorite Condiments on the Table

Having the right condiment or prepared sauce on the table can save the
meal for family members not yet ecstatic about the new dishes. If you
tolerate salt and/or sugar, these should be used sparingly on the surface
of the food. Take advantage of the enjoyment provided by traditional
sauces (make your own or choose your favorites from the McDougall
OK'd Canned and Packaged Products list on page 266).

It's Only a Matter of Time

The program can seem overwhelming when you first begin. However, in just a short time you will learn to prefer this kind of food and food preparation. Many people have told me they started to like to cook all over again once they made the change to healthy eating. The foods are more interesting and offer more colors, flavors, textures, and aromas than ever before. There is no disgusting animal flesh, fats, or oils to handle. Cleanup is much easier and quicker. Once you learn to cook and enjoy this kind of food you will realize that all you gave up was bad health and heart disease when you made the change. When people learn this new way they never look back.

17. Recipes for the McDougall Program for a Healthy Heart

BREAKFASTS

Breakfast Tortillas

SERVINGS: 4–6
PREPARATION TIME: 5 MINUTES (need cooked rice)
COOKING TIME: 20 MINUTES

2 cups frozen hash brown
  potatoes
1 cup cooked brown rice
¼ cup chopped green onions

⅓ cup salsa
⅓ cup frozen corn kernels
4–6 whole wheat tortillas

Cook the potatoes in a dry nonstick skillet, stirring frequently, until lightly browned, about 15 minutes. Add the remaining ingredients, except the tortillas, and cook another 5 minutes, stirring occasionally, until heated through. Spoon a line of the mixture down the center of each tortilla, roll up, and eat.

French Toast

SERVINGS: 8
PREPARATION TIME: 5 MINUTES
COOKING TIME: 5 MINUTES (in batches)

1½ cups nonfat soy milk   Pinch of turmeric
 2 teaspoons Egg Replacer   8 slices whole wheat bread
½ teaspoon soy sauce

Place the soy milk, Egg Replacer, soy sauce, and turmeric in a blender jar. Process until mixed. Pour into a bowl.

Preheat a nonstick griddle. Dip slices of the bread into the mixture and cook on a dry griddle until brown on both sides.

Griddle Crepes

SERVINGS: 8
PREPARATION TIME: 5 MINUTES
COOKING TIME: 10 MINUTES (in batches)

2 cups flour (unbleached white   2¼ cups carbonated water
   or whole wheat, rice flour,
   cornmeal, or a combination)

Mix the ingredients together using a wire whisk. Ladle about ¼ cup of the mixture into a small preheated nonstick frying pan. Swirl around to spread out. Bubbles will form immediately. Do not turn until the crepe has dried out slightly. Loosen gently and turn to cook the other side.

Hint: These crepes freeze well between layers of parchment paper.

Pancakes

SERVINGS: MAKES 8 PANCAKES
PREPARATION TIME: 15 MINUTES
COOKING TIME: 10 MINUTES (in batches)

1 **cup unbleached white or
whole wheat flour (or use a
combination of the two)**
1 **cup nonfat soy milk**
1 **teaspoon vanilla**

½ **teaspoon baking powder**
½ **teaspoon baking soda**
1 **teaspoon Egg Replacer
mixed with 2 tablespoons
water**

Combine the flour, soy milk, vanilla, baking powder, and baking soda in a bowl. In a separate bowl, beat the Egg Replacer and water until very frothy and peaks almost form. Add the Egg Replacer mixture to the batter and mix well.

Preheat a nonstick griddle. Pour a 4-inch circle of batter into the griddle and bake until done, turning once when bubbles form.

Cooked Cereal

SERVINGS: 2
PREPARATION TIME: 1 MINUTE
COOKING TIME: 5–7 MINUTES

2 **cups water**
1 **cup cereal grains (oatmeal, cracked wheat, etc.)**

Bring the water to a boil in a saucepan. Slowly stir in the cereal grains. Reduce the heat to low, cover, and cook for 5 to 7 minutes, stirring occasionally.

Rice Milk

SERVINGS: MAKES 4 CUPS
PREPARATION TIME: 5 MINUTES
COOKING TIME: NONE (cooked rice needed)

1 **cup cooked brown rice**
4 **cups water**

1 **teaspoon vanilla extract**
   (optional)

Place the rice in the blender with the water and vanilla (if desired) and process until thoroughly liquefied. Strain, if desired.

SALADS AND DRESSINGS

Italian Broccoli Salad

SERVINGS: 8
PREPARATION TIME: 25 MINUTES
COOKING TIME: 15 MINUTES
CHILLING TIME: 1 HOUR

2 cups water
1 cup barley
2 cups chopped broccoli
2 large tomatoes, chopped
1 carrot, shredded

¼ cup chopped onion
¼ chopped green bell pepper
1 4-ounce jar chopped
  pimientos
¾ cup oil-free Italian dressing

Place the water and barley in a small saucepan. Bring to a boil, cover, reduce the heat, and cook for about 15 minutes, until the barley is tender and the water is absorbed. Remove from the heat and set aside. Combine the remaining ingredients, except the Italian dressing, in a bowl. Add the barley and mix. Pour the Italian dressing over the salad and toss again to mix. Chill for at least 1 hour before serving.

Curried Corn Salad

SERVINGS: 4
PREPARATION TIME: 20 MINUTES
CHILLING TIME: 1 HOUR

3 cups frozen corn kernels,
  thawed and drained
1 red bell pepper, chopped
1 small cucumber, chopped
½ cup chopped green onions
½ teaspoon curry powder

Dash of Tabasco sauce
½ cup Fast Salad Dressing
  (page 301)
1 cup loosely packed fresh
  spinach leaves

Combine the corn, bell pepper, cucumber, and green onions in a bowl. Set aside. Using a wire whisk, mix the curry powder and Tabasco sauce into the salad dressing. Pour over the vegetables and toss to mix. Chill for at least 1 hour.

Serve over the spinach leaves.

Black Bean and Orzo Salad

SERVINGS: 6
PREPARATION TIME: 20 MINUTES (need cooked orzo)
CHILLING TIME: 1 HOUR

4 cups cooked orzo (rice-shaped pasta)
1 15-ounce can black beans, drained and rinsed
1 red bell pepper, chopped
1 cup frozen corn kernels, thawed and drained

½ cup chopped red onion
½ cup chopped fresh parsley
¼ cup chopped fresh basil
½ cup Spicy Salad Dressing (page 300) or other oil-free dressing

Combine the orzo, beans, bell pepper, corn, onion, parsley, and basil in a bowl. Pour the dressing over the salad and toss to mix. Chill for at least 1 hour before serving.

Couscous Salad

SERVINGS: 6
PREPARATION TIME: 20 MINUTES
COOKING TIME: 5 MINUTES
CHILLING TIME: 1 HOUR

1¼ cups Vegetable Broth (page 308)
¾ cup uncooked couscous
2 tomatoes, chopped
1 red bell pepper, chopped
1 stalk celery, chopped

½ cup chopped cucumber
¼ cup chopped green onions
¼ cup chopped fresh parsley or cilantro
½ cup Fast Salad Dressing (page 301)

Bring the vegetable broth to a boil in a small saucepan. Add the couscous and stir to mix. Cover, remove from the heat, and let stand for 5 minutes. Uncover and fluff with a fork. Let stand for 10 minutes.

Combine the vegetables and parsley in a bowl. Add the couscous and toss to mix. Pour the dressing over the salad and toss again. Chill for 1 hour before serving.

South of the Border Salad

SERVINGS: 6–8
PREPARATION TIME: 20 MINUTES
CHILLING TIME: 6 HOURS

2 15½-ounce cans kidney beans, drained and rinsed
1 small red onion, chopped
6 stalks celery, chopped
1 green bell pepper, chopped
1 cup baby corn, cut into 1-inch pieces
1 cup roasted red bell peppers, sliced
1 14- or 15-ounce can water-packed hearts of palm, drained and sliced into ½-inch pieces
1 15- or 16-ounce can water-packed artichoke hearts, drained and cut in halves
¼ cup chopped fresh cilantro
1 teaspoon finely chopped canned jalapeño peppers (or to taste)
1 large tomato, seeded and chopped
1 bottle Kozlowski Farms Fat Free No Oil South of the Border Salad Dressing

Combine all ingredients. Cover and refrigerate for at least 6 hours.

Garbanzo Salad

SERVINGS: 6
PREPARATION TIME: 20 MINUTES
CHILLING TIME: 2 HOURS

2 15-ounce cans garbanzo
   beans, drained and rinsed
1 7-ounce jar roasted sweet
   red peppers, drained and
   chopped
½ cup chopped green onions
½ cup chopped celery

2 tablespoons capers
½ cup oil-free dressing
1 clove garlic, minced
3 tablespoons chopped fresh
   mint
Freshly ground pepper to
   taste

Combine the garbanzos, peppers, green onions, celery, and capers in a large bowl. Using a wire whisk, combine the oil-free dressing, garlic, and mint. Pour over the vegetables. Toss well to mix. Season with freshly ground pepper. Cover and chill for at least 2 hours before serving.

Italian Potato Salad

SERVINGS: 8
PREPARATION TIME: 25 MINUTES
COOKING TIME: 25 MINUTES

1½ pounds small red potatoes
 2 cups green beans, cut into
   1-inch lengths
 2 cups yellow wax beans, cut
   into 1-inch lengths

1 large red bell pepper,
   chopped
½ cup finely chopped red onion
½ cup fat-free Italian dressing
   Freshly ground pepper to
   taste

Cook the potatoes in water to cover until just tender. Drain and cut into chunks. Cook the beans in water until just tender, about 15 to 20 minutes. Drain.

Combine all the vegetables in a large bowl. Pour the dressing over the salad and toss to mix. Season with freshly ground pepper.

Serve warm, at room temperature, or chilled.

Burman's Perfect Salad

SERVINGS: 4
PREPARATION TIME: 20 MINUTES

1 head lettuce
2 large cucumbers, peeled and
   sliced
2 large tomatoes, cut into
   wedges
2 large carrots, shredded

1 red onion, sliced into rings
1 4-ounce jar capers, drained
½ cup red wine vinegar
1 teaspoon powdered mustard
1 teaspoon oregano
1 teaspoon soy sauce

Shred the lettuce and place it in a large bowl. Add the cucumbers, tomatoes, carrots, onion, and capers. Toss to mix.

Place the vinegar, mustard, oregano, and soy sauce in a blender jar and process until blended. Pour over the salad and toss well. As the dressing is absorbed, the volume of the salad will reduce considerably.

Southwest Salad

SERVINGS: 6
PREPARATION TIME: 20 MINUTES
CHILLING TIME: 1 HOUR

2 15-ounce cans black beans,
   drained and rinsed
3 cups frozen corn kernels,
   thawed and drained
1 teaspoon minced garlic
½ cup finely chopped red
   onion

1 medium red bell pepper,
   chopped
½ cup chopped fresh parsley
½ cup chopped fresh cilantro
¾ cup oil-free dressing
2 teaspoons ground cumin

Mix the beans, corn, garlic, onion, bell pepper, parsley, and cilantro together in a large bowl. Using a wire whisk, combine the oil-free dressing with the cumin. Pour the dressing over the salad and mix well. Chill for at least 1 hour before serving.

Hot Coleslaw

SERVINGS: 6
PREPARATION TIME: 15 MINUTES
COOKING TIME: 15–20 MINUTES

1 small head cabbage,   ¼ cup chopped pimientos
  shredded   4 tablespoons vinegar
¼ cup chopped green bell   1 teaspoon prepared
  pepper   horseradish mustard

Place the cabbage and green pepper in a medium pot with a small amount of water, about ¼ cup. Cook over medium heat, stirring constantly, until the cabbage begins to turn clear, about 8 to 10 minutes. Add more water if necessary to keep the vegetables from sticking to the pot. Add the remaining ingredients, mix, cover, reduce the heat, and cook for 5 to 6 minutes. Serve hot.

Spicy Salad Dressing

SERVINGS: MAKES ½ CUP
PREPARATION TIME: 5 MINUTES
CHILLING TIME: 30 MINUTES

4 tablespoons rice vinegar   2 teaspoons chili powder
4 tablespoons lemon juice   2 teaspoons ground cumin
4 tablespoons cider vinegar   1 teaspoon ground
1 clove garlic, minced   coriander
2 teaspoons soy sauce   ¼–½ teaspoon crushed red
                                 pepper

Place all ingredients in a blender jar and process until blended. Pour into a jar and chill before using.

Fast Salad Dressing

SERVINGS: MAKES ½ CUP
PREPARATION TIME: 3 MINUTES
CHILLING TIME: 30 MINUTES

½ **cup rice or balsamic vinegar**
2 **teaspoons Dijon-style mustard**

1 **clove garlic, minced**

Place all ingredients in a blender jar and process until blended. Pour into a jar and chill before using.

DIPS AND SPREADS

Corn Butter

SERVINGS: MAKES 1½ CUPS
PREPARATION TIME: 5 MINUTES
COOKING TIME: 30 MINUTES FOR CORNMEAL

1 **cup cooked cornmeal**
½ **cup water**
1–2 **teaspoons lemon juice**

1 **teaspoon no-salt seasoning blend**

Place all ingredients in blender jar and process until smooth. Add more water, if necessary, to reach desired spreading consistency. Refrigerate to keep fresh. Use as a spread on bread, muffins, or rolls.

To cook cornmeal, place ½ cup cornmeal in a pan. Add 2 cups water. Cook, stirring occasionally, until smooth and thick.

Caponata

SERVINGS: MAKES ABOUT 6 CUPS
PREPARATION TIME: 30 MINUTES
COOKING TIME: 20 MINUTES

½ **cup water**
4 **cups peeled and diced eggplant**
½ **pound fresh mushrooms, chopped**
1 **onion, chopped**
1 **green bell pepper, chopped**
2 **cloves garlic, chopped**
3 **tablespoons chopped fresh basil**
1½ **tablespoons chopped fresh oregano**

1 **14½-ounce can chopped tomatoes and their juice**
1 **8-ounce can tomato sauce**
1 **4-ounce jar chopped pimientos**
¼ **cup balsamic vinegar**
Several dashes of Tabasco sauce
Lots of freshly ground pepper

Place the water in a large pot. Add the eggplant, mushrooms, onion, green pepper, garlic, basil, and oregano. Cook, stirring occasionally, for 10 minutes. Add the tomatoes and juice and tomato sauce. Cook for another 10 minutes. Add the remaining ingredients, mix, and heat through. Serve warm or cold.

Hints: Use as a dip for bread, crackers, or vegetables. It is also good tossed with small cooked pasta shells, or other small shapes.

Kit's Mock Guacamole

SERVINGS: MAKES ABOUT 2 CUPS
PREPARATION TIME: 20 MINUTES
CHILLING TIME: 1 HOUR

1 **potato, boiled and peeled**	1 **teaspoon ground cumin**
1 **15-ounce can garbanzo beans, drained and rinsed**	**Freshly ground pepper to taste**
¼ **lemon, peeled and seeded**	1 **tomato, finely chopped**
2 **cloves garlic, chopped**	2 **tablespoons finely chopped red onion**
½ **cup chopped fresh parsley**	
½ **cup salsa**	2 **tablespoons chopped green chilies**
⅓ **cup chopped fresh cilantro**	
¼ **cup nonfat soy or rice milk**	

Place all ingredients, except the tomato, onion, and chilies, into a food processor. Process until almost smooth, then place in a bowl. Stir in the remaining vegetables. Chill for at least 1 hour before serving. Serve with oil-free baked tortilla chips.

Aram Spread

SERVINGS: MAKES 1½ CUPS
PREPARATION TIME: 10 MINUTES
CHILLING TIME: 1 HOUR

1 15½-ounce can garbanzo
   beans, drained and rinsed
2 green onions, chopped
1 tablespoon soy sauce
3 teaspoons grated fresh
   gingerroot

½ teaspoon minced garlic
1 teaspoon rice vinegar
   Dash of Tabasco sauce
½ teaspoon honey (optional)

Combine all ingredients in a food processor and blend until smooth. Refrigerate at least 1 hour before using.

Use as a spread on bread or crackers, or roll up in a tortilla.

Hint: To make Aram Rolls, spread Aram Spread on the bottom of a large whole wheat tortilla. Follow with a layer of grated carrots, grated red cabbage, a few alfalfa sprouts, and some julienned green onions. Roll up like a log, then slice into thick slices, 1 to 2 inches. These are a wonderful appetizer, great to take to a potluck or picnic.

"Cheese" Spread

SERVINGS: MAKES 2 CUPS
PREPARATION TIME: 10 MINUTES
CHILLING TIME: 1–2 HOURS

1 15½-ounce can Great
   Northern or navy beans,
   drained and rinsed
¼ cup chopped pimientos
6 tablespoons nutritional
   yeast

2 tablespoons lemon juice
2 tablespoons water
½ tablespoon soy sauce
½ teaspoon onion powder
½ teaspoon prepared mustard
¼ teaspoon salt (optional)

Place all ingredients in a food processor and blend until very smooth. Refrigerate before serving.

Hints: Use on crackers, sandwiches, or baked potatoes. Thin slightly with some water, heat gently, and use as a sauce over vegetables or on enchiladas or tortillas. Make into a fondue with some nonalcoholic white wine and dip bread chunks into it.

Spinach Cilantro Dip

SERVINGS: MAKES ABOUT 1½ CUPS
PREPARATION TIME: 15 MINUTES
CHILLING TIME: 1 HOUR

3 cups finely chopped spinach
½ cup chopped fresh cilantro
2 cloves garlic, crushed
4 green onions, chopped
2 tablespoons lemon juice

Combine all ingredients. Refrigerate at least 1 hour to blend flavors.
Hints: Use a food processor to save time chopping. If you don't like cilantro, use parsley instead. This dip is excellent with oil-free tortillas.

Garbanzo Spread

SERVINGS: MAKES 2 CUPS
PREPARATION TIME: 15 MINUTES
CHILLING TIME: 1 HOUR

1 15½-ounce can garbanzo
  beans, drained and rinsed
1 stalk celery, chopped
¼ cup finely chopped onion
¼ cup finely chopped green
  onions
2 tablespoons oil-free salad
  dressing
Freshly ground pepper to
  taste

Mash the beans with a bean masher—do not use a food processor. Stir in the remaining ingredients and mix well. Chill for 1 hour to blend the flavors.

Stuff into pita bread, use as a dip for oil-free chips, or use as a sandwich spread.

Pinto Bean Spread

SERVINGS: MAKES 2 CUPS
PREPARATION TIME: 5 MINUTES

2 cups cooked pinto beans
¼ cup chopped onion
2 tablespoons sweet pickle
   relish

½ tablespoon prepared
   mustard
½ tablespoon ketchup or
   barbecue sauce

Place all ingredients in a food processor and blend until smooth. Use as a spread on sandwiches or crackers.

Hint: To make the spread into bean burgers, stir in about ¾ cup quick-cooking oatmeal. Form into patties and bake at 350°F for 30 minutes, turning over once in the middle of baking.

Caramelized Roasted Garlic

SERVINGS: VARIABLE
PREPARATION TIME: 5 MINUTES
COOKING TIME: 2½ HOURS

5 heads garlic
¾ cup Vegetable Broth
   (page 308)

2 teaspoons soy sauce

Preheat the oven to 300°F.

Peel some of the loose papery skin from the garlic heads, leaving the whole head intact. Slice a thin strip off the top of the garlic head so that most of the cloves are exposed. Place the heads, sliced side up, in a baking dish. Drizzle ½ cup of the vegetable broth over the garlic heads, making sure that each one is coated with the broth. Using a pastry brush, baste each head with half of the soy sauce. Cover and bake for about 2½ hours, or until the cloves are very soft. (Test by piercing with a fork.) Uncover and check several times during the baking process to make sure there is still some broth in the bottom of the baking dish. Drizzle the remaining ¼ cup of the vegetable broth over the garlic heads. Brush the garlic with the remaining soy sauce about halfway through the baking time. When the baking process is complete, there should be no broth in the bottom of the baking dish, only a brown film. This is the process that caramelizes the garlic, giving it an absolutely wonderful, mild flavor. Squeeze the garlic cloves out of the head and spread on crackers or bread, or just eat them plain.

Hint: This roasted garlic makes a wonderful addition to mashed potatoes, soups and stews, salad dressings, and many main dishes. Spread it on pancakes or French toast.

Spicy White Bean Spread

SERVINGS: MAKES 1½ CUPS
PREPARATION TIME: 10 MINUTES

1 **15-ounce can cannellini beans, drained and rinsed**
½ **cup chopped fresh parsley**
½ **cup chopped fresh cilantro**
¼ **cup chopped green onions**
1 **clove garlic, crushed**

2 **tablespoons lemon juice**
½ **teaspoon chili powder**
½ **teaspoon ground cumin**
¼ **teaspoon ground coriander**
   Several twists of freshly ground pepper

Place all ingredients in a food processor and process until smooth.
Hints: This makes an excellent sandwich spread. Use it as a dip for fat-free tortilla chips or crackers.

SOUPS

Vegetable Broth

SERVINGS: MAKES ABOUT 6 QUARTS
PREPARATION TIME: 20 MINUTES
COOKING TIME: 2–3 HOURS

5 quarts water
2 large onions, quartered
4 stalks celery, halved
4 carrots, halved
2 leeks, white part only,
   coarsely chopped
4 ears corn, cut in large pieces

Several sprigs of fresh
   parsley
1 bay leaf
10 whole peppercorns
1 sprig fresh thyme
1 sprig fresh marjoram

Place all ingredients in a large soup pot. Bring to a boil, cover, reduce the heat, and cook over low heat for 2 to 3 hours. Strain and discard the vegetables.

Refrigerate the broth until ready to use, up to 1 week, or freeze in small containers to use in recipes calling for vegetable broth.

Creole Gumbo

SERVINGS: 6–8
PREPARATION TIME: 30 MINUTES (need cooked rice)
COOKING TIME: 30 MINUTES

6 cups Vegetable Broth
   (recipe above)
2 large onions, chopped
4 stalks celery, chopped
2 green bell peppers,
   chopped
3 cloves garlic, minced
1 tablespoon Creole seasoning
   mix

1 15-ounce can black beans,
   drained and rinsed
1 15-ounce can black-eyed
   peas, drained and rinsed
1 cup frozen corn kernels,
   thawed
¼ cup chopped fresh parsley
Several dashes of Tabasco
   sauce

**Several twists of freshly
ground black pepper
Pinch of crushed red pepper
(optional)**

**1½ cups frozen chopped okra,
thawed
1 cup cooked brown rice**

Place 1 cup of the broth in a large pot. Add the onions, celery, green peppers, garlic, and Creole seasoning mix. Cook, stirring frequently, for 10 minutes. Add the remaining 5 cups of vegetable broth, the beans, black-eyed peas, corn, parsley, Tabasco, black pepper, and red pepper, if using. Cover, reduce the heat, and cook for 15 minutes. Add the okra and rice. Cook an additional 5 minutes until heated through.

Corn Chowder

Saffron gives this soup a unique flavor and a beautiful yellow color.

SERVINGS: 6
PREPARATION TIME: 10 MINUTES
COOKING TIME: 30 MINUTES

**3 cups Vegetable Broth
(page 308)
1 leek, cut in half lengthwise,
then sliced
1 medium red bell pepper,
chopped
1 cup sliced fresh mushrooms
3 cups frozen hash brown
potatoes**

**1½ cups frozen corn kernels,
thawed
1 cup frozen baby lima
beans, thawed
2 cups nonfat soy or rice milk
A pinch of powdered
saffron
Freshly ground pepper to
taste**

Place the broth in a large pot with the leek, bell pepper, mushrooms, and potatoes. Bring to a boil, reduce the heat to medium, and cook for 10 minutes. Add the corn and lima beans, reduce the heat to low, and continue to cook an additional 15 minutes. Stir in the soy or rice milk, saffron, and pepper. Cook until heated through, about 2 minutes.

Lima Orzo Soup

SERVINGS: 6
PREPARATION TIME: 25 MINUTES
COOKING TIME: 1½ HOURS

1 cup dried baby lima beans
6 cups water
2 leeks, cut in half and thinly
  sliced
2 cloves garlic, minced
2 stalks celery, sliced
2 medium potatoes, peeled
  and diced
½ pound fresh mushrooms,
  sliced

½ cup orzo pasta
1 bay leaf
¼ cup packed chopped fresh
  dill weed
1 tablespoon soy sauce
¼ teaspoon freshly ground
  pepper

Place the beans and water in a large pot. Soak overnight, or bring to a boil, boil for 2 minutes, remove from the heat, and let rest for 1 hour.

Bring the beans and water to a boil, cover, reduce the heat, and simmer for 30 minutes. Add the leeks, garlic, celery, and potatoes. Cook an additional 30 minutes. Add the mushrooms. Cook for another 20 minutes. Add the remaining ingredients. Cook for another 10 minutes, or until the orzo is tender.

Note: This may also be made with rice or barley instead of the orzo. Add the grain when you add the mushrooms.

Quick Bean and Vegetable Chowder

SERVINGS: 4
PREPARATION TIME: 10 MINUTES
COOKING TIME: 1 HOUR

1 cup Quick Bean Mixture
  (recipe follows)
4 cups vegetable broth or
  water
1 leek, thinly sliced

1 cup frozen diced hash
  brown potatoes
½ cup frozen corn kernels
1 bay leaf
1 tablespoon soy sauce

½ teaspoon dried marjoram
½ teaspoon dried thyme
½ teaspoon rubbed sage

¼ teaspoon freshly ground
pepper

Combine all ingredients in a medium soup pot. Mix well, cover, bring to a boil, reduce the heat, and simmer for 1 hour, stirring occasionally.

Quick Bean Mixture

1 cup split green peas
1 cup split yellow peas
1 cup brown lentils
1 cup red lentils

1 cup barley
1 cup orzo pasta (or other small pasta)

Combine well. Store in a covered jar.

Chard and Squash Soup

SERVINGS: 6–8
PREPARATION TIME: 30 MINUTES
COOKING TIME: 4 HOURS, 35 MINUTES (see note)

1½ cups dried garbanzo beans
8 cups water
4 cups Vegetable Broth
(page 308)
2 leeks, thinly sliced
2 cloves garlic, minced
2 medium yams, peeled and
chopped
2 cups peeled and chopped
winter squash

1 tablespoon soy sauce
½ teaspoon grated fresh
gingerroot
1 teaspoon dried oregano
½ teaspoon dried rosemary
¼ teaspoon freshly ground
pepper
2 cups tightly packed,
coarsely chopped Swiss
chard

Place the beans and water in a large soup pot. Cover and cook over medium heat for 4 hours. (Most of the liquid will be used up during this process.) Add the vegetable broth and the remaining ingredients, except the Swiss chard. Simmer, covered, over low heat until the vegetables are tender, about 30 minutes. Stir in the Swiss chard. Cook for another 3 to 5 minutes, until the chard softens.

Note: To save time, cook the garbanzos overnight in a slow cooker. Drain off most of the remaining liquid and proceed as directed. Canned garbanzos do not do justice to this delicious soup.

Mulligatawny Soup

SERVINGS: 8
PREPARATION TIME: 15 MINUTES (cooked rice needed)
COOKING TIME: 50 MINUTES

½ **cup water**
1 **medium onion, chopped**
2 **carrots, chopped**
2 **stalks celery, chopped**
1 **medium green bell pepper, chopped**
1 **medium green apple, chopped**
6 **cups Vegetable Broth (page 308)**

1 **15½-ounce can chopped tomatoes**
1 **tablespoon curry powder**
½ **teaspoon grated nutmeg**
¼ **teaspoon ground cloves Dash of cayenne pepper (optional)**
3 **cups cooked brown rice**

Place the water, onion, carrots, celery, green pepper, and apple in a large soup pot. Cook, stirring occasionally, until the vegetables are tender, about 15 minutes. Add the broth, tomatoes, and seasonings. Mix well, cover, and cook over low heat for 30 minutes. Stir in the rice, heat through, and serve.

Tortilla Soup

SERVINGS: 6–8
PREPARATION TIME: 20 MINUTES
COOKING TIME: 38 MINUTES

5–6 **soft corn tortillas, cut into strips**
1 **large onion, chopped**
1–2 **cloves garlic, crushed**
⅓ **cup water**
1 **28-ounce can chopped tomatoes**
1 **16-ounce can garbanzo beans, rinsed and drained**
1 **16-ounce can kidney beans, rinsed and drained**

4 **cups water**
1 **4-ounce can chopped green chilies**
4 **small zucchini, chopped**
1 **cup frozen corn kernels**
½ **cup chopped scallions**
1 **tablespoon chili powder**
½ **teaspoon dried oregano**
½ **teaspoon ground cumin**

Preheat the oven to 350°F.

Place the corn tortillas on a dry baking sheet. Bake for 10 minutes, until crispy. Remove and set aside.

Meanwhile, sauté the onion and garlic in the ⅓ cup water for 5 minutes. Add the remaining ingredients. Cover, bring to a boil, reduce the heat, and simmer for 30 minutes, stirring occasionally. Add the tortilla strips, stir, and continue to cook gently for 3 minutes, until the tortillas soften slightly.

Minestrone Casalinga

SERVINGS: 8–10
PREPARATION TIME: 35 MINUTES
COOKING TIME: 2½ HOURS

1 cup dried flageolets or white beans
10 cups water or vegetable broth
1 onion, coarsely chopped
2 cloves garlic, minced
2 leeks, sliced
2 carrots, sliced
2 stalks celery, sliced
2 large potatoes, peeled and chunked
½ pound fresh mushrooms, thickly sliced
2 zucchini, cut in half lengthwise, then thickly sliced

1 cup green beans, cut in 1-inch pieces
1 15-ounce can Italian stewed tomatoes
1 tablespoon parsley flakes
1 teaspoon dried basil
½ teaspoon dried rosemary
¼ teaspoon dried sage
1 cup shredded cabbage
½ cup frozen peas
½ cup small pasta, such as orzo
Freshly ground pepper to taste

Soak the beans overnight in water to cover. Drain and place the beans and water or broth in a large soup pot with the onion and garlic. Bring to a boil, cover, and cook over low heat for 1 hour. Add the leeks, carrots, celery, potatoes, mushrooms, zucchini, green beans, tomatoes, and seasonings. Continue to cook for another hour. Add the cabbage and peas. Cook for 20 minutes. Add the pasta and cook for another 10 minutes. Sprinkle with freshly ground pepper before serving.

Hint: This soup is even better when it is reheated. It also freezes well. The vegetables may be varied to suit your own tastes or to use what you have available.

Gourmet Cream of Mushroom Soup

SERVINGS: 4
PREPARATION TIME: 20 MINUTES
COOKING TIME: 30 MINUTES

2 leeks, sliced	½ teaspoon dried thyme
1 cup chopped fresh oyster mushrooms	½ teaspoon dried marjoram
1 cup chopped fresh shiitake mushrooms	½ teaspoon dried rosemary
1 large fresh portobello mushroom	¼ teaspoon dried sage
	⅛ teaspoon dried oregano
	⅛ teaspoon dried basil
1 cup sliced fresh button mushrooms	Several twists of freshly ground pepper
3½ cups water	2 tablespoons unbleached white flour
3–4 tablespoons soy sauce	1½ cups nonfat soy milk

Clean the leeks and use the white part and a little of the light green part. Remove the stems of the oyster, shiitake, and portobello mushrooms. Save for future use or discard. Using a teaspoon, remove the black gills of the portobello. Chop the portobello into bite-size pieces.

Place the leeks and mushrooms in a soup pot with ½ cup of the water. Cook, stirring frequently, for 5 minutes. Add the remaining 3 cups of water and the seasonings. Slowly bring to a boil while stirring. Sprinkle very small amounts of the flour over the soup while stirring. When all the flour has been stirred in (do not hurry this step) and the soup is boiling, reduce the heat to low and cook for 20 minutes. Slowly add the milk while stirring. Heat through and serve.

Hint: To make this into a creamy mushroom sauce, mix 3 tablespoons of cornstarch into ⅓ cup cold water. Add to the mixture while stirring. Cook and stir until thickened. This is excellent over baked potatoes or pasta.

Three Potato Chowder

SERVINGS: 6
PREPARATION TIME: 20 MINUTES
COOKING TIME: 45 MINUTES

½ cup water
1 cup halved and sliced leeks, cut in half
¾ cup chopped celery
½ cup sliced carrots
1–2 cloves garlic, minced
4 cups Vegetable Broth (page 308)

1 cup *each* chopped and unpeeled purple, red, and yellow potatoes
1 tablespoon parsley flakes
1 bay leaf
½ tablespoon soy sauce
Freshly ground pepper to taste

Place the water, leeks, celery, carrots, and garlic in a soup pot. Cook, stirring occasionally, for 5 minutes. Add the broth, potatoes, and seasonings. Bring to a boil, reduce the heat, cover, and cook over low heat for 40 minutes. Remove the bay leaf. Serve hot with fresh bread.

Note: This chowder may be made with only 1 kind of potato, but using a variety adds a lot of flavor and color.

Craig's Favorite Noodle Soup

SERVINGS: 4
PREPARATION TIME: 10 MINUTES
COOKING TIME: 22 MINUTES

4 cups Vegetable Broth (page 308)
½ cup finely chopped onion
½ cup finely chopped celery
¼ teaspoon dried marjoram

¼ teaspoon dried thyme
¼ teaspoon dried sage
⅛ teaspoon poultry seasoning
Dash of soy sauce
2 cups uncooked flat noodles

Place the broth, vegetables, and seasonings in a large saucepan. Bring to a boil, cover, and simmer over low heat for 15 minutes. Add the noodles and cook gently for 7 to 8 minutes, until the noodles are tender.

Creamy Vegetable Soup

SERVINGS: 6
PREPARATION TIME: 20 MINUTES
COOKING TIME: 25 MINUTES

1 small onion, finely chopped
1 stalk celery, finely chopped
1 small carrot, finely chopped
½ cup finely chopped green or red bell pepper
½ cup finely chopped broccoli
½ cup finely chopped zucchini
2 cups frozen chopped hash brown potatoes

1 cup frozen corn kernels
4 cups Vegetable Broth (page 308)
2 cups nonfat soy milk
⅓ cup unbleached white flour
1 tablespoon soy sauce
⅛ teaspoon white pepper

Place the vegetables and broth in a large soup pot. Cover and cook over medium low heat for 20 minutes

Mix the soy milk and flour together and set aside.

Add the soy sauce and pepper to the soup. Mix well, then add the milk mixture. Cook over low heat, stirring frequently, for about 5 minutes.

Speckled Orange Soup

SERVINGS: 8
PREPARATION TIME: 15 MINUTES
COOKING TIME: 40 MINUTES

1½ cups red lentils
6 cups water
1 15½-ounce can chopped tomatoes
1 onion, chopped
1 red bell pepper, chopped
1 cup grated carrots
2 cloves garlic, crushed
1 6-ounce can V8 Picante juice

2 tablespoons soy sauce
2 teaspoons grated fresh gingerroot
2 bay leaves
2 teaspoons ground cumin
2 teaspoons ground coriander
Freshly ground pepper to taste

Combine all ingredients in a large soup pot. Cover and cook over low heat until the lentils and vegetables are tender, about 40 minutes. Remove the bay leaves before serving.

Portuguese Bean Soup

SERVINGS: 6
PREPARATION TIME: 15 MINUTES
COOKING TIME: 30 MINUTES

½ cup water
1 onion, chopped
1 clove garlic, chopped
1 red bell pepper, chopped
1 cup frozen chopped hash brown potatoes
2 cups Vegetable Broth (page 308)
1 15½-ounce can undrained white beans
2 tablespoons sherry

1 tablespoon soy sauce
1 tablespoon lemon juice
1 tablespoon parsley flakes
½ teaspoon fennel seeds
¼ teaspoon Worcestershire sauce
Freshly ground pepper to taste
2–3 no-fat, no-meat hot dogs (Yves Veggie Chili Dogs), sliced

Place the water, onion, garlic, and bell pepper in a large saucepan. Cook, stirring occasionally, over medium heat for 5 minutes. Add the remaining ingredients, except the hot dogs. Cook over low heat for 10 minutes. Add the hot dogs and cook for another 15 minutes.

Mexican Corn Soup

SERVINGS: 6
PREPARATION TIME: 10 MINUTES
COOKING TIME: 25 MINUTES

⅓ cup water
1 green bell pepper, chopped
1 bunch green onions, chopped
1 clove garlic, minced

4 cups Vegetable Broth (page 308)
1½ cups mild salsa
¼ teaspoon dried oregano

3 cups frozen shredded
   potatoes (no fat added)
1½ cups frozen corn kernels

Chopped fresh cilantro for
garnish (optional)

Place the water in a large soup pot with the green pepper, green onions, and garlic. Cook, stirring occasionally, for 5 minutes. Add the remaining ingredients, except the cilantro, and cook over medium low heat for 20 minutes. Garnish with chopped cilantro before serving, if desired.

Vegetable Soup

SERVINGS: 4–5
PREPARATION TIME: 15 MINUTES
COOKING TIME: 40 MINUTES

3 cups Vegetable Broth (page
   308)
1 15½-ounce can chopped
   tomatoes
½ cup chopped onion
½ cup frozen chopped hash
   brown potatoes
½ cup frozen corn kernels
½ cup frozen baby lima beans

¼ cup chopped carrot
¼ cup chopped celery
¼ cup chopped green bell
   pepper
1 bay leaf
½ tablespoon soy sauce
½ teaspoon dried basil
¼ cup alphabet noodle pasta
   (or other small pasta)

Place all ingredients, except the pasta, in a large soup pot. Cover and cook over medium heat for 30 minutes. Add the pasta and cook an additional 10 minutes.

Hearty Bean Soup

SERVINGS: 4
PREPARATION TIME: 15 MINUTES
COOKING TIME: 35 MINUTES

⅓ cup water
1 medium onion, chopped
2 celery stalks, chopped
2 carrots, chopped
1 medium zucchini, chopped
2 15½-ounce cans cannellini
  beans, drained and rinsed

1 15½-ounce can stewed
  tomatoes
2 cups vegetable broth or
  water
½ teaspoon dried basil
  Freshly ground pepper
1 cup packed chopped fresh
  spinach

Place the water, onion, celery, carrots, and zucchini in a large soup pot. Cook, stirring occasionally, until the vegetables are fairly tender, about 15 minutes.

Take one of the cans of beans and mash until fairly smooth. Add to the soup pot along with the tomatoes, the whole beans from the second can, vegetable broth, basil, and pepper to taste. Reduce the heat to low, cover, and cook for 15 minutes. Add the spinach and cook an additional 5 minutes.

Dilled Broccoli Soup

SERVINGS: 8
PREPARATION TIME: 30 MINUTES
COOKING TIME: 40 MINUTES

1 medium onion, chopped
¼ cup water
5 cups Vegetable Broth
  (page 308)
3 cups peeled, chopped potatoes

6 cups chopped broccoli
4 cups small broccoli florets
  (bite-size)
3 cups nonfat soy or rice milk
1 teaspoon dried dill weed

Sauté the onion in the water in a large soup pot for 5 minutes. Add the vegetable broth, potatoes, and chopped broccoli. Cover, bring to a boil, reduce the heat, and simmer for 30 minutes, until the potatoes and broccoli are tender.

Meanwhile, place the broccoli florets in a saucepan with water to cover. Bring to a boil, cover, and cook over low heat for 5 minutes. Remove from the heat, drain, and set aside.

Blend the soup in batches in a blender until smooth and creamy. Return it to the pan. Add the cooked broccoli florets, soy or rice milk, and dill weed. Heat through. Serve at once.

Hint: Use frozen chopped hash brown potatoes to save chopping time. Use prepared chopped broccoli if available.

Potato and Cabbage Soup

SERVINGS: 4
PREPARATION TIME: 10 MINUTES
COOKING TIME: 25 MINUTES

3 cups Vegetable Broth (page 308)	2 tablespoons soy sauce
1 cup water	½ tablespoon caraway seed
2½ cups frozen chopped hash brown potatoes	½ teaspoon paprika
1 leek, thinly sliced	½ cup nonfat soy milk (optional)
4 cups shredded cabbage	Freshly ground pepper
2 cups sliced fresh mushrooms	

Place the vegetable broth, water, and frozen potatoes in a large soup pot. Bring to a boil, reduce the heat, then add the leek, cabbage, mushrooms, soy sauce, caraway seed, and paprika. Cover and cook about 20 minutes. Remove from the heat. Stir in the soy milk, if desired, and the ground pepper to taste.

Your Kids Will Love This Soup

SERVINGS: 4
PREPARATION TIME: 5 MINUTES
COOKING TIME: 12–13 MINUTES

¼ finely chopped onion
¼ cup water
2 16-ounce cans no-fat
  refried beans
1¾ cups vegetable broth or
  water

2 cups frozen corn kernels
⅓ cup mild salsa
½ teaspoon ground cumin
  Chopped fresh cilantro for
  garnish (optional)

Place the onion and water in a medium saucepan. Cook and stir until the onion is tender and the water has evaporated. Add the remaining ingredients, except the cilantro, mix well, and cook over very low heat for 10 minutes. Garnish with cilantro, if desired.

SAUCES

Melty "Cheese" Sauce

SERVINGS: MAKES 2 CUPS
PREPARATION TIME: 10 MINUTES
COOKING TIME: 10 MINUTES

¼ **cup cooked, peeled potatoes**
2 **cups water**
1 **4-ounce jar pimentos**
½ **teaspoon onion powder**

¼ **cup nutritional yeast**
3 **tablespoons cornstarch**
2 **tablespoons lemon juice**
   Salt, if desired

Blend the potatoes with a small amount of the water in a blender jar. Add remaining ingredients and blend until very smooth, with no flecks of pimento remaining. Pour into a saucepan, and cook and stir until smooth and thick, about 7–8 minutes.

Serve at once. Will set when cool. May be reheated. Serve over vegetables or baked potatoes. Hint: Makes a delicious "nacho" topping for tortilla chips.

Red, White, and Green Sauce

SERVINGS: 4
PREPARATION TIME: 15 MINUTES
COOKING TIME: 15 MINUTES

¼ **cup water**
1 **leek, cut in half and thinly sliced**
1 **stalk celery, sliced**
1 **red bell pepper, chopped**
2 **cups nonfat soy or rice milk**
¼ **cup unbleached white flour**

1 **cup frozen corn kernels, thawed**
½ **cup frozen baby lima beans, thawed**
2 **tablespoons minced fresh dill weed**
¼ **teaspoon salt (optional)**
¼ **teaspoon freshly ground pepper**

Place the water, leek, celery, and red pepper in a saucepan. Cook over low heat for about 7 minutes, stirring occasionally.

Mix the milk and flour together. Add to the vegetables with the remaining ingredients. Cook over low heat, stirring often, until the sauce has thickened slightly and the vegetables are tender, about 7 to 8 minutes. Serve over whole grains, potatoes, or toast.

Golden Kanieski Sauce

SERVINGS: 8
PREPARATION TIME: 25 MINUTES
COOKING TIME: 3 HOURS FOR BEANS, 35 MINUTES FOR SAUCE

2 **cups dried garbanzo beans**	4 **tablespoons cornstarch**
6½ **cups water**	**mixed in ½ cup cold water**
4 **carrots, sliced**	1 **tablespoon soy sauce**
2 **onions, sliced**	1 **cup chopped fresh**
2 **tablespoons minced fresh**	**parsley**
gingerroot	

Soak the garbanzos overnight in water to cover. Drain and place in a large pot with 6 cups of the water. Cook over medium heat until tender, about 3 hours. Remove from the heat and set aside. Place the carrots, onions, and gingerroot in a large pot with the remaining ½ cup water. Cook, stirring frequently, until almost tender, about 20 minutes.

Remove 3 cups of the cooked garbanzos from the cooking pot and puree in a food processor. Place the pureed garbanzos, the remaining whole garbanzos, and their cooking liquid into the pot with the vegetables. Cook for 10 minutes. Add the cornstarch mixture and stir until thickened. Add the soy sauce and parsley. Continue to cook for a few minutes longer, stirring frequently. Serve over brown rice or couscous.

Spaghetti Sauce

SERVINGS: MAKES 2 QUARTS
PREPARATION TIME: 10 MINUTES
COOKING TIME: 1½ HOURS

2 cups finely chopped onion
4 cloves garlic, crushed
2 teaspoons dried basil
1½ teaspoons dried oregano
1 bay leaf
3 1-pound, 12-ounce cans
Progresso Italian tomatoes
with basil

2 8-ounce cans Progresso
tomato sauce
¼ teaspoon freshly ground
pepper
4 tablespoons chopped fresh
parsley

In a large pot, heat the onion, garlic, basil, oregano, bay leaf, toma-toes, tomato sauce, pepper, and parsley. Mix well, mashing the tomatoes with a fork. Bring to a boil, reduce the heat, and simmer, uncovered, stir-ring occasionally, for 1½ hours.

Serve over whole wheat pasta.

Garbanzo/Broccoli Sauce

SERVINGS: 4
PREPARATION TIME: 15 MINUTES
COOKING TIME: 10 MINUTES

1 medium onion, cut in half
and thinly sliced
2 cloves garlic, minced
¼ cup water
1 bunch fresh broccoli,
cut into bite-size
florets

2 cups Vegetable Broth
(page 308)
1 15½-ounce can garbanzo
beans, drained and rinsed
1½ tablespoons soy sauce
2½ tablespoons cornstarch
mixed in ⅓ cup cold water

Place the onion and garlic in a pot with the water. Cook and stir until the onion is translucent, about 3 minutes. Add the broccoli, broth, beans, and soy sauce. Cook over low heat about 7 minutes until the broccoli is crisp-tender. Add the cornstarch mixture, and cook and stir until thickened. Serve over pasta or potatoes.

Creamy Mushroom Sauce

SERVINGS: 4–6
PREPARATION TIME: 15 MINUTES
COOKING TIME: 20 MINUTES

½ pound fresh mushrooms, sliced
1 small onion, chopped
1 stalk celery, chopped
¾ cup water

2 cups nonfat soy or rice milk
2 tablespoons soy sauce
Freshly ground pepper
3 tablespoons cornstarch

Place the mushrooms, onion, and celery in a pot with ½ cup of the water. Bring to a boil, cover, and cook over low heat until the mushrooms are tender, about 10 minutes. Add the milk and slowly bring back to a boil. Add the soy sauce and freshly ground pepper to taste. Mix the cornstarch in the remaining ¼ cup water. Stir into the mushroom mixture. Cook and stir until thickened.

Excellent served over baked potatoes.

Beefless à la Queen Sauce

SERVINGS: 6
PREPARATION TIME: 15 MINUTES
COOKING TIME: 20 MINUTES

1 onion, chopped
1 red or green bell pepper, chopped
¾ pound fresh mushrooms, chopped
½ cup water
½ cup frozen peas
4 cups Vegetable Broth (page 308)

¼ cup soy sauce
¼ cup diced pimientos
1 tablespoon parsley flakes
1 teaspoon dried basil
Freshly ground pepper
4–5 tablespoons cornstarch mixed in ½ cup cold water

Sauté the onion, bell pepper, and mushrooms in the water for 5 minutes. Add the peas and cook another 5 minutes. Add the remaining ingredients except for the cornstarch mixture. Bring to a boil, reduce the heat, and simmer for 5 minutes. Add the cornstarch mixture, and cook and stir until the mixture thickens. Serve over toast, whole grains, or potatoes.

Vegetable/Bean Pasta Sauce

SERVINGS: 6–8
PREPARATION TIME: 15 MINUTES
COOKING TIME: 25 MINUTES

½ cup water
1 small onion, chopped
½ pound fresh mushrooms, sliced
2 medium zucchini, cut in half, then sliced

1 red bell pepper, cut into thin strips
1 26-ounce jar fat-free pasta sauce
1 15½-ounce can garbanzo or navy beans, drained and rinsed

Place the water, onion, mushrooms, zucchini, and bell pepper in a large pot. Cook, stirring occasionally, until the vegetables are fairly tender, about 15 minutes. Add the pasta sauce and beans. Cook an additional 10 minutes. Serve over pasta.

Fast Chili Topping

SERVINGS: 4–6
PREPARATION TIME: 10 MINUTES
COOKING TIME: 15 MINUTES

1 medium onion, chopped
¼ cup water
2 14½-ounce cans Cajun-style stewed tomatoes
1 15-ounce can kidney beans, drained and rinsed

1 15-ounce can black beans, drained and rinsed
1 cup frozen corn kernels, thawed
½ teaspoon chili powder

Place the onion and water in a medium saucepan and cook over low heat, stirring frequently, until the onion softens slightly, about 4 minutes. Add the remaining ingredients. Cook for 10 minutes until the flavors are well blended. Serve over toast, potatoes, whole grains, or griddle cakes.

Hint: For a thicker topping, thicken with a mixture of 2 tablespoons of cornstarch mixed in ⅓ cup cold water. Add to the chili and cook and stir until thickened.

Rich Brown Gravy

SERVINGS: MAKES 6 CUPS
PREPARATION TIME: 20 MINUTES
COOKING TIME: 20 MINUTES

5¾ **cups water**   ½ **cup soy sauce**
 1 **onion, chopped**   **Freshly ground pepper**
 1 **cup whole wheat flour**

Place ¼ cup of the water and onion in a medium sauce pan. Cook, stirring occasionally, until the onion softens, about 5 minutes. Add the flour and mix in well. Continue to cook for another 3 minutes, stirring constantly. (This will toast the flour and give it a rich flavor.) The flour and onion will clump together. Add the remaining 5½ cups water and soy sauce. Cook for another 5 minutes, stirring frequently. Remove from the heat. Blend in batches in a blender jar until smooth. Place in a clean pan. Cook over medium heat, stirring frequently, until the gravy thickens, about 10 to 15 minutes. Season with freshly ground pepper to taste.

Hint: If the gravy fails to thicken to your satisfaction, you may want to add an extra thickener to it. Use a mixture of 2 tablespoons cornstarch mixed in ¼ cup cold water. Add a small amount to the gravy while stirring until it is thick enough for serving.

MAIN DISHES

Basque Paella

SERVINGS: 8
PREPARATION TIME: 30 MINUTES
COOKING TIME: 40 MINUTES

1 cup uncooked brown rice
2 cups boiling water
¼ cup water
1 onion, chopped
2 cloves garlic, minced
1 small green bell pepper, sliced
1 small red bell pepper, sliced
2 small red potatoes, sliced
1 small tomato, chopped

2 cups hot Vegetable Broth (page 308)
1 teaspoon soy sauce
1 teaspoon ground oregano
   Pinch of powdered saffron
1 small can water-packed artichoke hearts (about 6), cut in half
1 cup frozen peas

Place the rice and boiling water in a bowl. Cover and let stand for 20 minutes. Pour off the water and set aside.

Place ¼ cup water in a large pot. Add the onion and garlic. Cook and stir over medium heat about 2 minutes, until the onion softens. Add the bell peppers, potatoes, and tomato. Cook and stir for another 3 minutes. Add the rice and hot broth. Bring to a boil. Stir in the soy sauce, oregano, and saffron. Reduce the heat, cover, and cook for 30 minutes. Add the artichokes and peas. Cook for another 5 minutes

Risotto Primavera

SERVINGS: 4–6
PREPARATION TIME: 30 MINUTES
COOKING TIME: 15 MINUTES FOR RICE,
12 MINUTES FOR VEGETABLES

3½ cups Vegetable Broth
　　(page 308)
1 cup uncooked arborio rice
⅓ cup water
2 stalks celery, cut in
　　matchstick strips
2 carrots, cut in matchstick
　　strips
1 large leek, white part only,
　　thinly sliced

1 cup french-cut green beans
1 red bell pepper, cut into
　　matchstick strips
1 zucchini, cut into matchstick
　　strips
½ cup frozen peas, thawed
2 tablespoons chopped fresh
　　basil
　　Freshly ground pepper to
　　taste

Place the vegetable broth in a saucepan and bring to a boil. Stir in the rice, reduce the heat, and cook over low heat, stirring frequently, until the rice is tender and the broth is absorbed.

Meanwhile, place the water in another saucepan and bring to a boil. Add all vegetables, except the peas. Cook, stirring frequently, for 10 minutes until the vegetables are crisp-tender. Stir in the peas and cook for 2 minutes longer. Remove from the heat.

Combine the rice and vegetables. Stir in the basil and freshly ground pepper. Serve at once.

Greek Spinach Rice

SERVINGS: 4–6
PREPARATION TIME: 30 MINUTES
COOKING TIME: 60 MINUTES

¼ cup water
2 pounds fresh spinach,
　　washed, trimmed, and torn
　　into pieces

1 onion, sliced into
　　rings
1 28-ounce can chopped
　　tomatoes and juice

3 cups Vegetable Broth
  (page 308)
2 teaspoons soy sauce
  Several twists of freshly
  ground pepper

1 small bunch fresh dill weed,
  chopped
1 cup uncooked brown rice

Place the water in a large pot with the spinach and onion. Cook and stir until the spinach wilts. Add the tomatoes, broth, soy sauce, pepper, and dill. Bring to a boil. Add the rice, cover, reduce the heat, and cook over low heat for about 50 minutes, stirring occasionally.

Serve lukewarm.

Kelly's Manicotti

SERVINGS: 8
PREPARATION TIME: 25 MINUTES
COOKING TIME: 60 MINUTES

1 bottle fat-free pasta sauce
2 cups Creamy Mashed
  Potatoes (page 361)
1 tablespoon Italian seasoning
  mixture

1 box manicotti shells
  (12 shells), uncooked

Preheat the oven to 350°F.

Spread a small amount of the pasta sauce in the bottom of a 12 × 9-inch baking dish. Mix the potatoes, ¼ cup of the pasta sauce, and the Italian seasoning together. Stuff the potato mixture into the manicotti shells and place side by side in the baking dish. Pour the remaining sauce over the shells. Cover with parchment paper and then seal with a sheet of foil. Bake for 60 minutes.

Variation: Stir 1 cup finely chopped fresh spinach into the potato mixture before stuffing the manicotti.

Goulash

SERVINGS: 4
PREPARATION TIME: 15 MINUTES (need cooked pasta)
COOKING TIME: 18 MINUTES

½ cup water
1 large onion, chopped
1 large green bell pepper, chopped
1 medium red bell pepper, chopped
1 clove garlic, crushed
1 tablespoon soy sauce

1 tablespoon parsley flakes
½ teaspoon paprika
⅛ teaspoon black pepper
1 28-ounce can stewed tomatoes
4 cups cooked elbow macaroni

Place the water in a large pot. Add the onion, green and red peppers, and garlic. Cook and stir for several minutes, until the vegetables soften slightly. Add the seasonings and continue to cook over low heat for several more minutes. Add the tomatoes and macaroni. Mix well. Heat over low heat for another 10 minutes to blend the flavors.

Italian Vegetable Risotto

SERVINGS: 4
PREPARATION TIME: 30 MINUTES
COOKING TIME: 25 MINUTES

¼ cup water
1 small onion, chopped
1 small leek, cut in half and thinly sliced
1 clove garlic, minced
1 cup of uncooked arborio rice
Several twists of freshly ground pepper
4 cups Vegetable Broth (page 308)

¼ cup chopped sun-dried tomatoes
1 cup sliced fresh mushrooms
¾ cup green beans, cut into 1-inch pieces
¼ cup chopped fresh basil
1–2 tablespoons soy Parmesan-style cheese (optional)

Place the water, onion, leek, and garlic in a large saucepan. Cook and stir for 2 minutes until the onion softens slightly. Add the rice and pepper. Cook and stir for another 2 minutes. Add the vegetable broth and tomatoes. Bring to a boil, reduce the heat, and simmer for 5 minutes. Add the remaining ingredients, except the soy cheese, and simmer for an additional 15 minutes. Stir in the soy Parmesan-style cheese, if desired.

Hints: Use kitchen shears to chop sun-dried tomatoes. Shears also work well for chopping fresh basil. Risotto is best eaten fresh. The rice becomes sticky when reheated.

Southwest Kasha Bake

SERVINGS: 6–8
PREPARATION TIME: 20 MINUTES (need cooked grains)
COOKING TIME: 1 HOUR, 15 MINUTES

½ **cup water**
1 **medium onion, chopped**
¼ **cup diced celery**
½ **cup diced carrot**
2 **cloves garlic, minced**
1 **tablespoon canned chopped green chilies**
1½ **teaspoons ground cumin**
1½ **teaspoons ground coriander**
1 **teaspoon chili powder**

2½ **cups cooked kasha (or other whole grain)**
1 **cup cooked kidney beans**
1 **tomato, chopped**
¼ **cup frozen corn kernels, thawed**
2 **tablespoons chopped fresh parsley**
2 **tablespoons chopped fresh cilantro**
1 **cup salsa**

Preheat the oven to 350°F.

Put the water in a large saucepan with the onion, celery, carrot, garlic, and chilies. Cook, stirring occasionally, until the vegetables are tender, about 15 minutes. Add more water if necessary to keep the vegetables from sticking to the pan. Remove from the heat and stir in the remaining ingredients. Spread into a 13 × 9-inch baking dish and bake for 1 hour.

Fried Rice

SERVINGS: 3
PREPARATION TIME: 20 MINUTES
COOKING TIME: 15 MINUTES (need cooked rice)

⅓ cup water
1 tablespoon soy sauce
½ teaspoon minced garlic
½ teaspoon minced gingerroot
1 bunch green onions, sliced
1 red bell pepper, chopped
1 stalk celery, diagonally
  sliced
1 cup sliced fresh
  mushrooms

1 teaspoon chopped fresh
  basil
¼ teaspoon paprika
1 cup packed chopped fresh
  spinach
Several twists of freshly
  ground black pepper
Pinch of crushed red pepper
3 cups cooked brown rice
1 tablespoon soy sauce

Place the water in a nonstick frying pan with the soy sauce, garlic, and gingerroot. Heat, then add the green onions, bell pepper, celery, and mushrooms. Cook, stirring frequently, for 10 minutes. Add the basil, paprika, spinach, black and red peppers, brown rice, and soy sauce. Cook over low heat, stirring frequently, for 5 minutes until heated through.

Tomato Spinach Risotto

SERVINGS: 4
PREPARATION TIME: 20 MINUTES
COOKING TIME: 25 MINUTES

¼ cup water
1 onion, chopped
1 red bell pepper, chopped
1–2 cloves garlic, minced
⅛ cup chopped sun-dried
  tomatoes
⅛ cup chopped dried porcini
  mushrooms

1 cup chopped fresh tomatoes
1 cup uncooked arborio rice
4 cups Vegetable Broth
  (page 308)
1 cup frozen corn kernels
1 tablespoon soy sauce
2 packed cups chopped fresh
  spinach

Place the water, onion, bell pepper, and garlic in a medium saucepan. Cook, stirring frequently, until the onion softens, about 3 minutes. Add the remaining ingredients, except the spinach. Bring to a boil, reduce the heat, and simmer for 15 minutes, stirring every few minutes. Add the spinach and continue to cook for 5 minutes, until the water is absorbed.

Spinach Rice

SERVINGS: 4
PREPARATION TIME: 15 MINUTES
COOKING TIME: 50 MINUTES

1 small onion, chopped
1 small green bell pepper, chopped
½ cup chopped green onion
1 clove garlic, minced
⅓ cup water
1 cup uncooked long-grain brown rice
2 cups vegetable broth or water
1 4-ounce jar chopped green chilies
1 4-ounce jar chopped pimientos
1¼ cups corn kernels
1 tablespoon parsley flakes
1 teaspoon ground cumin
2 cups packed chopped fresh spinach
¼ cup chopped fresh cilantro
Freshly ground pepper to taste

Place the onion, bell pepper, green onion, and garlic in a medium saucepan with the water. Cook over medium heat for 3 minutes, until the vegetables soften slightly and the water has evaporated. Add the rice, broth, green chilies, pimientos, corn, parsley, and cumin. Cover and cook over low heat for 45 minutes. Stir in the remaining ingredients and cook for 2 minutes longer. Serve at once.

Southwest Jambalaya

SERVINGS: 4
PREPARATION TIME: 10 MINUTES
COOKING TIME: 20 MINUTES

1 onion, cut in half, sliced, and separated into rings
1 green bell pepper, chopped
1 carrot, cut in half lengthwise, then sliced
1 clove garlic, crushed
½ cup water
1 bunch green onions, cut into 1-inch pieces
1½ cups sliced napa cabbage
1 tablespoon soy sauce
1 teaspoon chili powder
1 teaspoon dried basil

2 cups chopped plum tomatoes
2 cups packed chopped fresh spinach
2 15-ounce cans black beans, drained and rinsed
½ cup salsa
Several dashes of Tabasco sauce
Freshly ground pepper to taste
1–2 tablespoons chopped fresh cilantro

Place the onion, bell pepper, carrot, and garlic in a large pot with the ½ cup water. Cook and stir over medium heat until the onion softens slightly, about 4 to 5 minutes. Add the green onions, cabbage, soy sauce, chili powder, and basil. Cook, stirring occasionally, for 10 minutes. Stir in the remaining ingredients, except the cilantro, and cook for 5 minutes. Add the cilantro just before serving, and stir to mix. Serve in a bowl, over baked potatoes, or rolled up in a tortilla.

Michelle's India Casserole

SERVINGS: 8–10
PREPARATION TIME: 30 MINUTES
COOKING TIME 1 HOUR, 15 MINUTES

4 slices whole wheat bread, torn into pieces
2¼ cups water

1 10-ounce box frozen spinach, thawed and drained

1 10-ounce box frozen turnip greens, thawed and drained

1 10-ounce box frozen broccoli, thawed and drained

1½ cups frozen chopped hash brown potatoes

1 4-ounce can chopped green chilies

½ cup chopped onion

½ cup chopped fresh mushrooms

1 tablespoon soy sauce

2 teaspoons minced fresh gingerroot

2 teaspoons Garam Masala (recipe follows)

2 teaspoons paprika

1 teaspoon ground cumin

1 teaspoon ground coriander

½ teaspoon ground turmeric

Place the bread in a food processor and process into crumbs. Set aside.

Put 2 cups of the water into a large pot. Add the spinach, turnip greens, broccoli, potatoes, and chilies. Bring to a boil, cover, reduce the heat, and cook over low heat for 30 minutes. Drain and transfer to a food processor. Process until pureed. Set aside.

Place the remaining ¼ cup water in another pan. Add the onion and mushrooms. Cook, stirring constantly, for 2 minutes. Add the seasonings and cook another 3 minutes. Remove from the heat and set aside. Preheat the oven to 350°F.

Combine the pureed vegetables and the mushroom mixture. Sprinkle half of the bread crumbs on the bottom of a nonstick 13 × 9-inch baking dish. Spread the vegetable mixture over the bread crumbs and sprinkle the remaining crumbs over the top. Bake for 45 minutes.

Garam Masala

4 teaspoons ground coriander

2 teaspoons ground cumin

1 teaspoon ground cloves

1 teaspoon ground cinnamon

1 teaspoon ground black pepper

Combine all ingredients in a tightly covered jar.

French Bean Casserole

This reminds us of the old creamy green bean and mushroom casserole that Mom used to make when we were kids.

SERVINGS: 6
PREPARATION TIME: 30 MINUTES
COOKING TIME: 45 MINUTES

2 **medium potatoes, peeled and chopped**
1 **carrot, chopped**
1 **small onion, chopped**
2¼ **cups water**
5 **ounces tofu**
⅓ **cup nutritional yeast**
1 **tablespoon lemon juice**
⅛ **teaspoon garlic powder**

¼ **teaspoon salt (optional)**
1¼ **cups uncooked instant brown rice**
2 **10-ounce packages frozen french-cut green beans, thawed**
1 **(4½-ounce drained weight) jar sliced mushrooms**

Preheat the oven to 350°F.

Place the potatoes, carrot, and onions in a small saucepan with 1½ cups of the water. Bring to a boil, reduce the heat, cover, and cook until tender, about 10 minutes.

Place the tofu, yeast, lemon juice, and garlic in a blender jar. Add the cooked vegetables and water. Blend until smooth and very creamy. Add salt, if desired. Pour into a 3-quart casserole dish. Add the remaining ingredients. Mix well. Bake for 45 minutes.

Southwest Vegetable Stew

SERVINGS: 4
PREPARATION TIME: 10 MINUTES
COOKING TIME: 35 MINUTES

1 **large onion, chopped**
⅓ **cup water**
1 **28-ounce can chopped tomatoes**

1 **4-ounce can chopped green chilies**
2 **cups frozen baby lima beans**
2 **cups frozen corn kernels**

2 teaspoons ground cumin   ¼ cup chopped fresh cilantro
1 teaspoon chili powder

Place the onion and water in a large saucepan. Cook, stirring occasionally, for 5 minutes. Add the remaining ingredients, except the cilantro. Bring to a boil, reduce the heat, cover, and cook over low heat for 25 minutes. Add the cilantro and cook another 5 minutes. Serve over brown rice or potatoes.

Oriental Noodle Scramble

SERVINGS: 6
PREPARATION TIME: 30 MINUTES
COOKING TIME: 15 MINUTES

⅓ cup plus ¾ cup water
3 tablespoons soy sauce
2–3 cloves garlic, crushed
1 tablespoon grated fresh
  gingerroot
1 carrot, sliced
2 stalks celery, sliced
1 red bell pepper, cut into
  thin strips
½ pound fresh mushrooms,
  sliced
1 baby bok choy, sliced
1 bunch green onions, cut in
  1-inch pieces

1 leek, thinly sliced
1 5-ounce can water
  chestnuts, sliced
1 cup shredded cabbage
1 cup mung bean sprouts
1 cup frozen green peas
8 ounces uncooked fettuccine
  or spaghetti
¼ cup soy sauce
2 tablespoons cornstarch
2 teaspoons "chicken-style"
  seasoning mix

Heat the ⅓ cup water, 3 tablespoons soy sauce, garlic, and gingerroot in a large pan or wok. Add the carrot and celery and cook, stirring occasionally, for 3 minutes. Add the remaining vegetables and continue to cook, stirring occasionally, for 7 minutes.

Meanwhile, cook the pasta in boiling water until tender. Drain, place in a large bowl, and set aside. Mix the ¾ cup water, ¼ cup soy sauce, and cornstarch together. Add to the vegetable mixture while stirring. Stir until thickened. Sprinkle the seasoning mix over the top and mix in well. Pour the vegetable mixture over the pasta and toss well to mix. Serve at once.

Hint: Vegetarian "chicken-style" seasoning mix is sold at most natural foods stores, usually in the bulk foods section.

Quick Goulash

SERVINGS: 6
PREPARATION TIME: 15 MINUTES
COOKING TIME: 25 MINUTES

2 cups uncooked elbow macaroni
1 medium onion, chopped
1 green bell pepper, chopped
1–2 cloves garlic, minced
½ cup water
1 tablespoon chili powder

½ teaspoon ground cumin
1 15½-ounce can chopped tomatoes
1 15 ½-ounce can kidney beans, drained and rinsed
1 17-ounce can corn, drained
1 tablespoon canned chopped green chilies

Cook the macaroni in boiling water until just tender. Remove from the heat and set aside.

Meanwhile, sauté the onion, green pepper, and garlic in the water for 5 minutes. Sprinkle on the chili powder and cumin. Cook and stir for another 2 to 3 minutes. Add the remaining ingredients and cook for 15 minutes. Add the cooked macaroni, and heat through for about 2 minutes. Serve as is, or rolled up in a tortilla or stuffed into a pita bread.

Tex-Mex Spaghetti

SERVINGS: 4
PREPARATION TIME: 15 MINUTES
COOKING TIME: 20 MINUTES

1 15½-ounce can Mexican-style stewed tomatoes

1 15½-ounce can kidney beans, drained and rinsed

1 4-ounce can chopped green
   chilies
1 tablespoon chili powder
1 teaspoon paprika
1 teaspoon ground cumin
½ teaspoon dried oregano
½ cup water
¼ cup sherry

1 large onion, sliced
½ pound fresh mushrooms,
   sliced
1 tablespoon cornstarch
   mixed in ¼ cup cold water
¾ pound uncooked spaghetti
   or linguine

Combine the stewed tomatoes, kidney beans, chilies, chili powder, paprika, cumin, and oregano in a bowl. Set aside.

Place the water and sherry in a medium saucepan. Add the onion and mushrooms and cook, stirring frequently, until the liquid has evaporated and the onion is softened, about 15 minutes. Add the reserved tomato mixture and cook over low heat until heated through, about 5 minutes. Add the cornstarch mixture, cook, and stir until thickened.

Meanwhile, cook the spaghetti according to directions. Drain. Pour the tomato-vegetable mixture over the spaghetti and toss gently to mix. Serve at once.

Spicy Potato Stew

SERVINGS: 6
PREPARATION TIME: 15 MINUTES (need cooked red potatoes)
COOKING TIME: 25 MINUTES

1   medium onion, chopped
1   medium red or green bell
     pepper, chopped
1–2 cloves garlic, minced
⅓   cup water
1   fresh tomato, chopped
1   14½-ounce can Mexican-
     style stewed tomatoes
¼   cup salsa

1 tablespoon parsley flakes
½ teaspoon ground cumin
2 14½-ounce cans garbanzo
   beans, drained and rinsed
2 cups cooked red potatoes,
   cut into chunks
   Freshly ground pepper to
   taste

Place the onion, bell pepper, garlic, and water in a large pot. Cook, stirring occasionally, for 5 minutes. Add the fresh tomato and cook for 2 minutes; then add the stewed tomatoes, salsa, parsley flakes, and cumin. Cook for another 2 minutes, then add the remaining ingredients. Cover and cook over low heat for 15 minutes. Serve over rice or other whole grains.

Mexican Vegetable Stew

SERVINGS: 8
PREPARATION TIME: 30 MINUTES
COOKING TIME: 3 HOURS

1½ cups dried pinto beans
9 cups water
1 onion, chopped
1 red bell pepper, chopped
1 stalk celery, sliced
1 carrot, sliced
1 bunch green onions, chopped
2 small zucchini, chopped
1½ cups chopped broccoli

1 4-ounce can chopped green chilies
1½ cups frozen corn kernels
2 teaspoons ground cumin
1 teaspoon ground coriander
1 teaspoon chili powder
   Dash of cayenne pepper
3 tablespoons cornstarch mixed in ¼ cup cold water

Place the beans, water, and onion in a large pot. Bring to a boil, cover, and reduce the heat. Cook for 1¼ hours. Add the red bell pepper, celery, and carrot. Continue to cook for another hour. Add the remaining ingredients, except the cornstarch mixture. Cook until the beans and vegetables are tender, about 45 minutes. Add the cornstarch mixture. Cook and stir until thickened. Serve at once.

Steidley's Meatless Loaf

SERVINGS: 8–10
PREPARATION TIME: 25 MINUTES
COOKING TIME: 1½ HOURS

1 15-ounce can kidney beans, drained and rinsed
2 cups quick-cooking oatmeal flakes
1 onion, chopped

1 green pepper, chopped
1 stalk celery, chopped
½ pound fresh mushrooms, chopped
1 small potato, peeled and grated

1 15-ounce can tomato
  sauce
1 4-ounce can chopped green
  chilies
2 cloves garlic, minced

1 teaspoon dried sage
1 teaspoon Egg Replacer,
  mixed in 2 tablespoons water
  and beaten until fluffy
¼ cup ketchup or barbecue sauce

Mash the beans and mix with the oatmeal. Set aside and let rest for 20 minutes.

Preheat the oven to 350°F.

Add the remaining ingredients, except the ketchup or barbecue sauce. Mix well. Transfer to a nonstick loaf pan (or line the bottom of the pan with parchment paper). Spread the ketchup or barbecue sauce over the top. Bake for 1½ hours.

Remove from the pan and slice to serve.

Southwest Vegetable Griddle Cakes

SERVINGS: MAKES 7–8 GRIDDLE CAKES
PREPARATION TIME: 15 MINUTES
COOKING TIME: 15 MINUTES

1 cup whole wheat flour
1 cup unbleached white flour
1 teaspoon baking powder
½ teaspoon salt (optional)
2 cups frozen corn kernels,
  thawed and drained
4 green onions, chopped

3 tablespoons canned
  chopped green chilies
2 tablespoons chopped fresh
  cilantro
1½ cups nonfat soy or rice
  milk

Combine the flours, baking powder, and salt (if using), in a bowl. Combine the corn, green onions, chilies, cilantro, and soy milk in a separate bowl. Mix wet and dry ingredients together. The batter will be very thick.

Preheat a nonstick griddle until hot. (Sprinkle a few drops of water on the griddle; if they bounce, it's ready.) Spread the mixture on the griddle in the size and shape you prefer, about ⅓ inch thick. Cook about 3 minutes on each side, until lightly browned. Serve with a sauce to spoon over the top, such as Fast Chili Topping (page 327), Red, White, and Green Sauce (page 323) or any savory gravy. They're also good with salsa.

Pinto Bean Loaf

SERVINGS: 8–10
PREPARATION TIME: 15 MINUTES (need cooked beans)
COOKING TIME: 45 MINUTES

3 cups cooked pinto beans, mashed
1 cup tomato sauce
1 cup bread crumbs, finely ground
¼ cup minced onion
¼ cup quick-cooking oatmeal

3 teaspoons Egg Replacer mixed with 4 tablespoons water, beaten until frothy
Freshly ground pepper to taste
¼ cup ketchup or barbecue sauce

Preheat the oven to 350°F.

Combine all ingredients, except the ketchup or barbecue sauce, in a large bowl. Mix well. Transfer to a nonstick 9¼ × 5¼ × 3-inch loaf pan, and flatten. Spread the ketchup or barbecue sauce over the top. Bake for 45 minutes.

Hint: Makes a good sandwich spread when cold.

Healthy Heart Burgers

SERVINGS: MAKES 12 BURGERS
PREPARATION TIME: 50 MINUTES
COOKING TIME: 40 MINUTES

2 cups frozen hash brown potatoes
4¼ cups water
1 cup lentils
¼ cup chopped onion
½ cup quick-cooking oatmeal
½ teaspoon dried sage

½ teaspoon dried thyme
½ teaspoon dried marjoram
¼ teaspoon poultry seasoning
Freshly ground pepper
Dash or two of Tabasco sauce (optional)

Place the potatoes in a small saucepan with 2 cups water. Cook, uncovered, over medium heat until the potatoes are soft and the water has evaporated, about 20 minutes. Remove from the heat and set aside.

Place the lentils in another saucepan with 2 cups water. Cook, covered, over medium heat until the lentils are very soft and the water is absorbed, about 40 minutes. Remove from the heat and set aside. Place the onion in a small frying pan with the remaining ¼ cup water. Cook, stirring occasionally, until the onion is soft and translucent. Remove from the heat and set aside.

Preheat the oven to 350°F.

Combine the potatoes, lentils, and onion. Mix well. Add the remaining ingredients and mix well. Shape into patties on 2 nonstick baking sheets. Bake for 20 minutes, then turn over and bake for an additional 20 minutes.

Serve in a whole wheat bun with all the trimmings, or try them stuffed into pita bread. They are also delicious as an open-face sandwich topped with a gravy or sauce.

Stuffed Twice-Baked Potatoes

SERVINGS: 5
PREPARATION TIME: 20 MINUTES
COOKING TIME: 2 HOURS FOR BAKED POTATOES,
15 MINUTES FOR STUFFED POTATOES

5 large baking potatoes
1 cup nonfat soy or rice milk
2 cups frozen mixed
   vegetables

Freshly ground pepper
(optional)
Paprika (optional)

Preheat the oven to 400°F.

Scrub the potatoes and wrap them in parchment paper and then in foil. Bake for 2 hours. Cool slightly, then remove from the wrapping. Slice the potatoes in half lengthwise. Carefully scoop out the centers, leaving a small amount of potato next to the skin. In a mixing bowl, mash the centers with the soy or rice milk, adding a small amount at a time.

Meanwhile, cook the vegetables until just tender, then drain. Mix the vegetables into the mashed potatoes, and add a few twists of freshly ground pepper, if desired.

Preheat the oven to 350°F.

Pile the potato mixture into the shells. Arrange on a baking sheet. Sprinkle with the paprika, if desired. Bake at 350°F. for 15 minutes, then turn the broiler on low for the last 2 to 3 minutes of baking time.

Serve plain or with a gravy or sauce.

Hint: These potatoes reheat well.

Lentil Sloppy Joes

SERVINGS: 8–10
PREPARATION TIME: 10 MINUTES
COOKING TIME: 30 MINUTES

2 **cups red lentils**
4 **cups water**
1 **onion, chopped**
1 **green bell pepper, chopped**
½ **cup ketchup**

2 **tablespoons prepared mustard**
2 **tablespoons cider vinegar**
2 **tablespoons soy sauce**
1 **tablespoon honey (optional)**
2 **teaspoons chili powder**

Place the lentils, water, onion, and green pepper in a medium saucepan. Bring to a boil, reduce the heat, cover, and simmer for 30 minutes, stirring occasionally. Remove from the heat. Add the remaining ingredients, mixing well. Serve hot over toast, rolls, or whole grains. This makes a wonderful sandwich spread when cold.

Hint: These sloppy joes freeze well. Use half and freeze the rest.

Potatoes Mexicali

SERVINGS: 6–8
PREPARATION TIME: 5 MINUTES
COOKING TIME: 30 MINUTES

6 **cups frozen chopped hash brown potatoes**
2⅔ **cups water**
1 **tablespoon canned chopped green chilies**

1 **tablespoon soy sauce**
1 **teaspoon chili powder**
1 **teaspoon ground cumin**
1 **teaspoon dried oregano**
1 **teaspoon parsley flakes**

Place all ingredients in a medium saucepan. Bring to a boil and cook uncovered for 25 minutes, until the potatoes are tender and the liquid has evaporated. The potatoes will be very mushy.

Serve with salsa and chopped green onions, stuffed into pita bread, or rolled up in a tortilla shell. It reheats well.

Holiday Stuffed Pumpkin

This makes a festive main dish for a holiday meal. Serve with mashed potatoes, gravy, assorted vegetables, salad, and bread or rolls.

SERVINGS: 6–8
PREPARATION TIME: 1 HOUR
COOKING TIME: 1½ HOURS

1 **loaf whole wheat bread, cut into cubes**	2 **teaspoons dried sage**
	1 **teaspoon dried marjoram**
3 **cups Vegetable Broth (page 308)**	1–2 **teaspoons poultry seasoning**
1 **onion, chopped**	½ **teaspoon dried rosemary**
2 **stalks celery, chopped**	**Several twists of freshly**
2–3 **tablespoons soy sauce**	**ground pepper to taste**
1 **tablespoon parsley flakes**	1 **medium pumpkin or**
2 **teaspoons dried thyme**	**large winter squash**

Preheat the oven to 300°F.

Place the bread on a baking sheet and bake for 15 minutes. In a medium saucepan, cook the broth, onion, celery, and seasonings over medium heat for 20 minutes.

Meanwhile, cut the top off the pumpkin or winter squash and save for a cover (as if you were going to make a jack-o'-lantern). Clean out the seeds and stringy portion, leaving plenty of the squash flesh along the sides. Rinse well and set aside.

Place the bread cubes in a large bowl, pour the cooked broth over the bread, and toss well until the bread is saturated with the liquid. Cover the bowl and allow the liquid to be absorbed for about 10 to 15 minutes. Taste and adjust seasonings, adding more poultry seasoning and ground pepper, if needed.

Preheat the oven to 350°F.

Place the stuffing in the cleaned pumpkin and cover with the pumpkin top. Place the pumpkin in a large baking dish. Add 1 inch of water to the bottom of the baking dish. Bake for 1½ hours or until a fork pierces the side of the pumpkin easily.

Hint: To save some time, cube the bread the night before and allow it to sit uncovered in a single layer overnight. This will eliminate the need to bake the bread cubes in the oven for 15 minutes.

Macaroni and Oaty Cheese

SERVINGS: 8
PREPARATION TIME: 15 MINUTES
COOKING TIME: 30 MINUTES

2 cups water
½ cup quick-cooking oatmeal flakes
¼ cup nutritional yeast
2 tablespoons cornstarch
2 tablespoons lemon juice
½ tablespoon onion powder
1½ teaspoons salt
1 4-ounce jar diced pimientos
1 pound uncooked elbow macaroni

Place all ingredients, except the macaroni, in a blender jar and process for several minutes until very smooth and well blended. Pour into a saucepan, cook, and stir until thickened.

Preheat the oven to 350°F.

Cook the macaroni until just tender, then drain. Place the macaroni in a covered baking dish, pour the cheese sauce over the top, and mix thoroughly. Bake, covered, for 30 minutes.

Macaroni and Tato Cheese

SERVINGS: 8
PREPARATION TIME: 15 MINUTES
COOKING TIME: 30 MINUTES

2 cups water
1 cup cooked potatoes
¼ cup nutritional yeast
2 tablespoons cornstarch
2 tablespoons lemon juice

½ tablespoon onion powder
1½ teaspoons salt
1 4-ounce jar diced
   pimientos
1 pound uncooked elbow
   macaroni

Place all ingredients, except the macaroni, in a blender jar and process for several minutes until very smooth and well blended. Pour into a saucepan, cook, and stir until thickened.

Preheat the oven to 350°F.

Cook the macaroni until just tender, then drain. Place the macaroni in a covered baking dish, pour the cheese sauce over the top, and mix thoroughly. Bake, covered, for 30 minutes.

Julie's Black Bean Torta

SERVINGS: 6
PREPARATION TIME: 30 MINUTES
COOKING TIME: 45 MINUTES

3 cups cooked black beans
⅓ cup Vegetable Broth
   (page 308) or water
2 cups finely chopped red
   onion
2 cups finely chopped mixed
   vegetables (zucchini, celery,
   bell peppers, etc)

2 cloves garlic, minced
1 cup frozen corn kernels,
   thawed and drained
1 teaspoon ground cumin
¼ teaspoon crushed red
   pepper
2 cups fresh salsa
6 8-inch corn tortillas

Place the beans and vegetable broth in a food processor and process until fairly smooth. Set aside. Sauté the onion, vegetables, and garlic in a small amount of water or vegetable broth for 10 minutes. Add the corn, cumin, and red pepper and cook for 3 more minutes. Remove from the heat and set aside.

Preheat the oven to 375°F.

Place 1 tortilla on the bottom of an 8-inch springform pan (or an 8-inch cake pan lined with parchment paper). Spread with ½ cup bean mixture, then 1 cup vegetable mixture, then ⅓ cup salsa. Continue to layer in the same order (tortilla, beans, vegetables, salsa).

Bake for 45 minutes. Let rest for 5 minutes before cutting into wedges.

Lima Bean Stew

SERVINGS: 8
PREPARATION TIME: 25 MINUTES
COOKING TIME: 35 MINUTES

½ cup water	1 teaspoon dried marjoram
1 onion, chopped	½ teaspoon dried sage
1 clove garlic, minced	¼ teaspoon dried rosemary
2 stalks celery, sliced	1 tablespoon soy sauce
3 medium red potatoes, diced	3 cups frozen lima beans
	2 cups frozen corn kernels
1 green bell pepper, chopped	3 tablespoons cornstarch
1 red bell pepper, chopped	mixed in ⅓ cup cold water
3½ cups vegetable broth or water	½ cup nonfat soy milk
	Freshly ground pepper

Place the water in a large pot with the onion, garlic, celery, potatoes, and bell peppers. Cook and stir for 3 to 4 minutes until the onion softens slightly. Add the vegetable broth, marjoram, sage, rosemary, and soy sauce. Bring to a boil, reduce the heat, cover, and cook for 15 minutes. Add the lima beans and corn. Cook an additional 15 minutes. Add the cornstarch mixture, cook, and stir until thickened. Stir in the soy milk, and season with pepper to taste. Heat through. Serve with whole grain bread.

Mexican Layered Casserole

SERVINGS: 8
PREPARATION TIME: 30 MINUTES
COOKING TIME: 40 MINUTES

¼ **cup water**
1 **onion, chopped**
1 **green bell pepper, chopped**
1 **clove garlic, minced**
1 **15-ounce can kidney beans, drained and rinsed**
1 **15-ounce can black beans, drained and rinsed**
1½ **cups frozen corn kernels**
1½ **cups cooked brown rice**

1½ **cups tomato sauce**
1 **4-ounce can chopped green chilies**
2 **teaspoons chili powder**
2 **teaspoons ground cumin**
4 **cups enchilada sauce**
12 **soft corn tortillas**
4 **green onions, finely chopped**

Place the water in a large pan with the onion, green pepper, and garlic. Cook over medium heat, stirring frequently, until softened, about 5 minutes. Add the beans, corn, rice, tomato sauce, chilies, chili powder, and cumin. Stir to mix, then cook over low heat until warmed through, about 10 minutes. Remove from the heat and set aside.

Preheat the oven to 350°F.

Pour about ½ cup of the enchilada sauce into the bottom of a 13 × 9-inch casserole dish and spread evenly over the bottom. Pour the rest of the enchilada sauce into a bowl. Dip 4 of the tortillas, one at a time, into the enchilada sauce, then layer them in the bottom of the casserole dish. Spread half of the bean mixture over the tortillas. Repeat with the next 4 tortillas and the remaining mixture. Finish with the last 4 tortillas. Pour the remaining enchilada sauce over the top and spread evenly. Sprinkle with the chopped green onion. Cover and bake for 40 minutes. Remove from the oven and let rest 5 minutes before serving. Serve with salsa to spoon over the top, if desired.

Garbanzos with Spinach

SERVINGS: 6
PREPARATION TIME: 20 MINUTES
COOKING TIME: 55 MINUTES

½ cup water
1 onion, chopped
2 cloves garlic, minced
1 15-ounce can chopped
  tomatoes, drained
1 bay leaf
1½ teaspoons paprika
2 15½-ounce cans
  garbanzo beans,
  undrained

1½ cups frozen chopped hash
  brown potatoes
2 tablespoons soy sauce
½ teaspoon dried oregano
2 cups packed chopped fresh
  spinach
Several twists of freshly
  ground pepper
Dash or two of Tabasco
  sauce (optional)

Place the water, onion, and garlic in a large pan. Cook, stirring occasionally, for 5 minutes. Add the tomatoes, bay leaf, and paprika. Cook for 2 minutes. Add the garbanzo beans, hash browns, soy sauce, and oregano. Cover and cook over medium-low heat for 45 minutes (covered for 30 minutes and uncovered for 15 minutes). Remove 1 cup of the mixture to a blender jar and process until smooth, then return to the pan. Remove the bay leaf. Add the spinach and mix well. Cook, covered, for 3 minutes. Add the pepper and Tabasco, if desired. Serve over rice or other grains.

Garbanzo à la King

SERVINGS: 8
PREPARATION TIME: 20 MINUTES
COOKING TIME: 30 MINUTES

1 medium onion, chopped
½ green bell pepper, chopped
½ yellow bell pepper,
  chopped
½ pound fresh mushrooms,
  sliced

½ cup sliced fresh oyster
  mushrooms
¾ cup water
⅓ cup unbleached white flour
3 cups nonfat soy or rice milk
1 tablespoon soy sauce

1 tablespoon parsley flakes
½ teaspoon paprika
¼ teaspoon freshly ground
   pepper
2 cups cooked garbanzo beans

1 4-ounce jar diced pimientos
2 tablespoons cornstarch or
   arrowroot mixed in ¼ cup
   cold water
1 tablespoon sherry (optional)

Place the onion, bell peppers, and mushrooms in a large pot with the water. Cook, stirring occasionally, for 10 minutes. Stir in the flour, and continue to cook and stir for about 2 to 3 minutes. Gradually add the soy or rice milk. Add the seasonings, garbanzo beans, and pimientos. Cook, stirring occasionally, over low heat for 10 minutes. Add the cornstarch mixture and the sherry, if desired. Cook and stir until the mixture boils and thickens. Serve over whole wheat toast, baked potatoes, or whole grains.

Cajun Red Beans

SERVINGS: 4–5
PREPARATION TIME: 20 MINUTES (need cooked beans)
COOKING TIME: 30 MINUTES

½ cup water
1 onion, chopped
1 green bell pepper, chopped
2 bunches green onions,
   chopped
2 cloves garlic, minced
1 8-ounce can tomato sauce
1 tablespoon Worcestershire
   sauce
1 teaspoon Dijon-style mustard

½ teaspoon ground oregano
1 bay leaf
1–2 pinches of cayenne
   pepper
½–1½ teaspoons Tabasco sauce
   Freshly ground pepper
   to taste
4 cups cooked small red
   beans (3 15-ounce cans,
   drained and rinsed)

Place the water in a large sauce pot with the onion, green pepper, scallions, and garlic. Cook, stirring occasionally, over low heat for 10 minutes. Add the remaining ingredients. Cook, covered, over low heat for 20 minutes. Remove the bay leaf. Serve over brown rice.

Hint: This is very spicy if you use the maximum amount of cayenne and Tabasco. Use the lesser amount to begin with and add more if your taste buds permit.

Lentil Vegetable Curry

SERVINGS: 8
PREPARATION TIME: 30 MINUTES
COOKING TIME: 30–40 MINUTES

⅓ cup sherry
1 onion, chopped
1 leek, thinly sliced
1 red bell pepper, chopped
1 sweet potato, peeled and
　chopped
2 carrots, grated

2 cups chopped broccoli
2½ cups red lentils
7 cups Vegetable Broth
　(page 308)
1½ teaspoons curry powder
½ teaspoon ground cumin
¼ teaspoon ground cinnamon

Place the sherry, onion, leek, and bell pepper in a large pot. Cook and stir for 1 minute. Add the potato and carrots. Cook and stir for another 2 minutes. Add the remaining ingredients. Bring to a boil, then reduce the heat to low, cover, and cook for 30 to 40 minutes, until the lentils are tender. Serve over long-grain brown rice.

Note: If you use brown lentils instead of red, the cooking time will increase by about 15 minutes.

Jazzy White Beans

SERVINGS: 4–6
PREPARATION TIME: 15 MINUTES (need cooked beans)
COOKING TIME: 20 MINUTES

½ cup water
1 onion, chopped
2–3 cloves garlic, minced
1 15-ounce can chopped
　tomatoes
1 teaspoon grated fresh
　gingerroot
½ teaspoon dried sage

½ teaspoon dried oregano
½ teaspoon dried basil
4 cups cooked white beans
　(3 15-ounce cans, drained
　and rinsed)
2 tablespoons soy sauce
　Lots of freshly ground
　pepper

Place the water in a large saucepan with the onion and garlic. Cook, stirring occasionally, for 3 minutes. Add the tomatoes and seasonings and cook for 2 minutes. Add the remaining ingredients and cook for an additional 15 minutes. Serve over rice or potatoes.

Monica's Burrito Filling

SERVINGS: 4
PREPARATION TIME: 10 MINUTES
COOKING TIME: 15 MINUTES

⅓ **cup water**
1 **small onion, chopped**
½ **green bell pepper, chopped**
½ **red bell pepper, chopped**
¼ **cup chopped green chilies**

½ **cup frozen corn kernels, thawed**
1 **15½-ounce can black beans, drained and rinsed**
½ **cup salsa**

Place the water in a saucepan with the onion and bell peppers. Cook, stirring occasionally, until the onion and peppers are tender, about 7 minutes. Add the remaining ingredients, mix, and continue to cook for another 8 minutes, stirring occasionally.

Roll up in a tortilla, adding some chopped green onions, tomatoes, and more salsa, if desired. This also makes a wonderful topping for baked potatoes.

Black Beans and Rice

SERVINGS: 6–8
PREPARATION TIME: 5 MINUTES (need cooked rice)
COOKING TIME: 10 MINUTES

1 **onion, chopped**
¼ **cup water**
1 **14½-ounce can stewed tomatoes**
1 **15-ounce can black beans, undrained**
1 **tablespoon canned chopped green chilies**

½ **teaspoon dried oregano**
½ **teaspoon garlic powder**
½ **teaspoon ground cumin**
1 **teaspoon balsamic vinegar**
1 **teaspoon prepared mustard (Dijon-style or regular)**
3 **cups cooked brown rice**

Place the onion and water in a medium pot. Cook, stirring occasionally, for 5 minutes. Add the remaining ingredients, mix well, and cook over low heat for an additional 5 minutes.

Easy Beans and Vegetables

SERVINGS: 6
PREPARATION TIME: 5 MINUTES
COOKING TIME: 18 MINUTES

⅓ cup water
1 onion, chopped
1 15½-ounce can Cajun- or Mexican-style stewed tomatoes
1 teaspoon chili powder
1 15½-ounce can black beans, drained and rinsed
1 15½-ounce can kidney beans, drained and rinsed

1 15½-ounce can white beans, drained and rinsed
1 10-ounce package frozen mixed vegetables, thawed
1 4-ounce can chopped green chilies
¼ cup barbecue sauce
½ cup water
¼ teaspoon ground cumin
Dash or two of Tabasco sauce (optional)

Place the ⅓ cup water and the onion in a large saucepan. Cook and stir for 3 minutes. Add the stewed tomatoes and chili powder. Reduce the heat and cook, stirring occasionally, for 5 minutes. Add the remaining ingredients. Cook, stirring occasionally, for 10 minutes. Serve in a bowl, on baked potatoes, over whole wheat toast, or stuffed into a pita bread.

Blanco Mexican Chili

SERVINGS: 6–8
PREPARATION TIME: 20 MINUTES
COOKING TIME: 3–4 HOURS

1 pound dried Great Northern Beans
2 medium onions, chopped
¼ cup water

2–3 cloves garlic, chopped
2 4-ounce cans chopped green chilies
1 tablespoon chili powder

1 tablespoon ground cumin
1 tablespoon dried
   oregano
8 cups Vegetable Broth
   (page 308)
2 12-ounce cans tomatillos,
   drained and chopped

2 bunches green onions,
   chopped
½ cup chopped fresh cilantro
½ tablespoon lime juice
   Salt
   Dash or two of Tabasco
   sauce (optional)

Soak the beans in water to cover overnight, or place them in a large pot with water to cover, bring to a boil, cook for 1 minute, turn off the heat, and let rest for 1 hour. Drain the beans and set aside. Place the onions and water in a large pot. Cook, stirring frequently, until the onions soften slightly, about 3 minutes. Add the garlic, chilies, chili powder, cumin, and oregano. Cook and stir for another 3 minutes. Add the soaked beans, broth, and tomatillos. Cover, bring to a boil, reduce the heat, and simmer for 2 to 3 hours, until the beans are fairly tender. Add the green onions and cilantro. Cook, uncovered, for an additional 1 hour until the chili is very thick. Stir in the lime juice and add salt to taste and Tabasco sauce, if desired.

Knock Out Chili

SERVINGS: 4–6
PREPARATION TIME: 10 MINUTES (cooked rice needed)
COOKING TIME: 45 MINUTES

1 onion, chopped
1–2 cloves garlic, chopped
¼ cup water
1 cup oil-free sun-dried
   tomatoes
1 26–28 ounce jar oil-free
   spaghetti sauce
1 16-ounce can black beans,
   drained and rinsed

1 16-ounce can kidney beans,
   drained and rinsed
1 cup cooked brown rice
½ cup water
¼ cup soy sauce
2 tablespoons chili powder
1 tablespoon ground cumin
½ tablespoon dried basil
⅛ teaspoon cayenne pepper

Sauté the onion and garlic in ¼ cup water until softened, about 3 to 5 minutes. Using a scissors, cut the sun-dried tomatoes into chunks. Add the tomatoes and the remaining ingredients to the onion mixture. Mix well, cover, and cook over low heat until the flavors are blended, about 40 minutes.

Variation: To make this into a rich chili that will fool all your meat-eating friends, replace the rice with textured vegetable protein (sold in most natural foods stores).

Sunny Bean Chili

SERVINGS: 6
PREPARATION TIME: 15 MINUTES
COOKING TIME: 4 HOURS

2 cups dried kidney beans
5 cups water
1 onion, coarsely chopped
1 green bell pepper, chopped
2 cloves garlic, minced
1 15½-ounce can tomato sauce
1 15½-ounce can Mexican- or Cajun-style stewed tomatoes

1 4-ounce can chopped green chilies
3 tablespoons chili powder
2 teaspoons ground cumin
⅓ cup chopped oil-free sun-dried tomatoes
1 cup frozen corn kernels

Place the beans and water in a large pot. Bring to a boil, cover, reduce the heat, and simmer for 2 hours. Add the remaining ingredients, except the corn, and cook an additional 2 hours. Add the corn about 10 minutes before the end of the cooking time.

Rainbow Chili

SERVINGS: 8–10
PREPARATION TIME: 30 MINUTES
COOKING TIME: 45 MINUTES

½ cup bulgur
½ cup water
1 28-ounce can chopped tomatoes

2 large onions, chopped
3 cloves garlic, crushed
½ cup water
1 green bell pepper, chopped

1 red bell pepper, chopped
2 cups frozen corn
1 15½-ounce can kidney beans, drained and rinsed
1 15½-ounce can pinto or black beans, drained and rinsed

1 15½-ounce can white beans, drained and rinsed
1 8-ounce can tomato sauce
1 tablespoon chili powder
1 teaspoon ground cumin
½–1 teaspoon Tabasco sauce

Place the bulgur and water in a small saucepan. Drain the tomatoes and add their liquid to the bulgur and water. Cook, uncovered, over low heat about 10 minutes, until the liquid is absorbed. Remove from the heat and set aside.

Place the onions, garlic, and water in a large soup pot. Cook, stirring frequently, until the onions soften, about 3 minutes. Add the bell peppers and cook an additional 7 minutes. Add the remaining ingredients and heat for 5 minutes. Add the cooked bulgur, mix thoroughly, and cook, covered, over very low heat for 30 minutes.

Black Bean Chili

SERVINGS: 6–8
PREPARATION TIME: 20 MINUTES
COOKING TIME: 1 HOUR

2 medium onions, chopped
2–3 cloves garlic, minced
½ cup sherry or water
1 small green bell pepper, chopped
1 small red bell pepper, chopped
1 stalk celery, chopped
3 15½-ounce cans black beans, drained and rinsed
2 cups Vegetable Broth (page 308)

1 15½-ounce can chopped tomatoes, undrained
4 teaspoons chili powder
2 teaspoons ground cumin
½ teaspoon dried oregano
   Several twists of freshly ground pepper
1 tablespoon honey
2 tablespoon tomato paste
¼ cup chopped fresh cilantro

Place the onions, garlic, and sherry in a large soup pot. Cook, stirring frequently, until the onion softens, about 3 minutes. Add the bell peppers and celery and cook 5 minutes, stirring frequently. Add the remaining ingredients, except the cilantro. Cook, covered, for 20 minutes, then uncover and cook for another 20 minutes. Add the cilantro and cook an additional 10 minutes.

Baked French Fries

SERVINGS: VARIABLE
PREPARATION TIME: 40 MINUTES
COOKING TIME: 30–40 MINUTES

Potatoes	**Pepper**
Salt	

Seasoning Mix (optional)

⅓ **cup Dijon-style mustard**	1 **teaspoon chili powder**
1 **teaspoon paprika**	1 **teaspoon ground cumin**

Preheat the oven to 450°F.

Scrub the potatoes, cut them into the desired shape (wedges, thick slices, or traditional "french fry" shape), and place them in a pot with cold water to cover. Soak for 30 minutes. Remove the potatoes from the water, and shake to remove excess water. Sprinkle with salt and pepper. Place on a nonstick baking tray. Bake for 30 to 40 minutes, until lightly browned.

Option: After removing the potatoes from the water, blot to remove excess water. Set aside. Mix the optional seasoning mix together in a small bowl. Spread a small amount of the mixture thinly on the surface of the potatoes. Bake as above.

Creamy Mashed Potatoes

SERVINGS: 6–8
PREPARATION TIME: 20 MINUTES
COOKING TIME: 45 MINUTES

10 medium potatoes, peeled   **Salt (optional)**
   Water to cover   **Pepper (optional)**

Cut the potatoes in half and place them in a large pot with the water. Cover and cook over low heat until the potatoes are very tender, about 45 minutes. Remove from the heat. Drain the potatoes, reserving the cooking liquid. Beat the potatoes with an electric mixer, adding small amounts of the cooking liquid to the potatoes while mashing. Beat until smooth and creamy. Season with a small amount of salt and pepper to taste, if desired.

Hint: To make the potatoes even more creamy, replace some or all of the reserved cooking liquid with nonfat soy or rice milk. Add the milk to the potatoes while mashing.

To make Garlic Mashed Potatoes, add several cloves of Roasted Garlic (page 306) while mashing.

REFERENCES

Chapter 1

Facts and figures on heart disease in America:

American Heart Association. *1992 Heart and Stroke Facts.*
Heart Disease: Public Enemy No. 1. Senate Subcommittee on Nutrition, May 22, 1979.

Cholesterol among Chinese:

Lang, Susan. The world's healthiest diet. *American Health*, Sept 1989, p. 105.
Campbell, T. Colin. Nutrition, Environment and Health Project, Chinese Academy of Preventive Medicine–Cornell–Oxford.
Brody, J. Huge study of diet indicts fat and meat. *New York Times*, May 8, 1990, p. C-1.

Japanese eat healthier and die less of heart disease:

Marmot, M. Why are the Japanese living longer? *Br Med J* 299:1547, 1989.

Migrating Asians develop heart disease:

Wandel, M. Nutrition-related diseases and dietary change among Third World immigrants in northern Europe. *Nutrition & Health* 9:117, 1993.

American youths have clogged arteries:

Pathobiological Determinants of Atherosclerosis in Youth (PDAY) Research Group. Natural history of aortic and coronary atherosclerotic lesions in youth: Findings from the PDAY study. *Arterioscler Thromb* 13:1291, 1993.

Joseph, A. Manifestations of coronary atherosclerosis in young trauma victims—an autopsy study. *J Am Coll Cardiol* 22:459, 1993.

Babies have the beginnings of atherosclerosis:

Lapinleimu, H. Prospective randomised trial in 1062 infants of diet low in saturated fat and cholesterol. *Lancet* 345:471, 1995.

Fuster, V. The pathogenesis of coronary artery disease and the acute coronary syndromes (first of two parts). *N Engl J Med* 326:242, 1992.

Pesonen, E. Intimal thickening in the coronary arteries of infants and children as an indicator of risk factors for coronary heart disease. *Eur Heart J* 11 (Suppl E):53, 1990.

Newman, W. Relation of serum lipoprotein levels and systolic blood pressure to early atherosclerosis: the Bogalusa Heart Study. *N Engl J Med* 314:138, 1986.

Holman, R. The natural history of atherosclerosis: the early aortic lesions as seen in New Orleans in the middle of the 20th century. *Am J Pathol* 34: 209, 1958.

Chapter 2

Exercise and collateral circulation:

McKirnan, M. Clinical significance of coronary vascular adaptions to exercise training. *Med Sci Sports Exercise* 26:1262, 1994.

Tomanek, R. Exercise-induced coronary angiogenesis: a review. *Med Sci Sports Exercise* 26:1245, 1994.

HDL and LDL cholesterol:

Austin, M. Epidemiology of triglycerides, small dense low-density lipoprotein, and lipoprotein(a) as risk factors for coronary heart disease. *Med Clin North Am* 78:99, 1994.

Oxidized cholesterol damages arteries:

Steinberg, D. Beyond cholesterol. Modifications of low-density lipoprotein that increase its atherogenicity. *N Engl J Med* 320:915, 1989.

Newborn infants and fatty streaks:

See "Babies have the beginnings of atherosclerosis" in references for Chapter 1.

The first stages of atherosclerosis—injury and plaque formation:

Fuster, V. The pathogenesis of coronary artery disease and the acute coronary syndromes (first of two parts). *N Engl J Med* 326:242, 1992.

Ulbricht, T. Coronary heart disease: seven dietary factors. *Lancet* 338:985, 1991.

The second stages of atherosclerosis—tiny plaques rupture and clots form, causing heart attacks:

Constantinides, P. Plaque fissures in human coronary thrombosis. *J Atheroscler Res* 6:1, 1966.

Oliva P. Pathophysiology of acute myocardial infarction, 1981. *Ann Intern Med* 94:236, 1981.

Davies, M. Plaque fissuring—the cause of acute myocardial infarction, sudden ischemic death, and crescendo angina. *Br Heart J* 53:363, 1985.

Epstein, S. Sounding board: sudden cardiac death without warning. Possible mechanisms and implications for screening asymptomatic populations. *N Engl J Med* 321:320, 1989.

Richardson, P. Influence of plaque configuration and stress distribution on fissuring of coronary atherosclerotic plaques. *Lancet* 2:941, 1989.

Fuster, V. The pathogenesis of coronary artery disease and the acute coronary syndromes (second of two parts). *N Engl J Med* 326:310, 1992.

Patterson, D. The culprit coronary artery lesion. *Lancet* 338:1379, 1991.

Brown, B. Regression of atherosclerosis—an ounce of prevention. *West J Med* 159:208, 1993.

Brown, B. Atherosclerosis regression, plaque disruption, and cardiovascular events: a rationale for lipid lowering in coronary artery disease. *Ann Rev Med* 44:365, 1993.

Artery disease is reversible:

See "Reversal of atherosclerosis" in references for Chapter 4.

Chapter 3

Vegetable fats cause the liver to excrete cholesterol:

Parfitt, V. Effects of high monounsaturated and polyunsaturated fat diets on plasma lipoproteins and lipid peroxidation in type 2 diabetes. *Diabet Med* 11:85, 1994.

Dietary fat causes the circulation to sludge:

Cullen, C. Intravascular aggregation and adhesiveness of the blood elements associated with alimentary lipemia and injections of large molecular substances. Effect on blood-brain barrier. *Circulation* 9:335, 1954.

Friedman, M. Serum lipids and conjunctival circulation after fat ingestion in men exhibiting type-A behavior patterns. *Circulation* 29:874, 1964.

Friedman, M. Effect of unsaturated fats upon lipemia and conjunctival circulation. A study of coronary-prone (pattern A) men. *JAMA* 193:882, 1965.

Dietary fat causes a 20 percent drop in oxygen concentration of the blood:

Kuo, P. The effect of lipemia upon coronary and peripheral arterial circulation in patients with essential hyperlipemia. *Am J Med* 26:68, 1959.

Dietary fat can cause angina and a low-fat diet relieves chest pain:

Kuo, P. Lipemia in patients with coronary heart disease. Treatment with low-fat diet. *JADA* 33:22, 1957.

Kuo, P. Angina pectoris induced by fat ingestion in patients with coronary artery disease. Ballistocardiographic and electrocardiographic findings. *JAMA* 158: 1008, 1955.

Kuo, P. The effect of lipemia upon coronary and peripheral arterial circulation in patients with essential hyperlipemia. *Am J Med* 26:68, 1959.

Williams, A. Increased blood cell agglutination following ingestion of fat, a factor contributing to cardiac ischemia, coronary insufficiency and anginal pain. *Angiology* 8:29, 1957.

Thuesen, L. Beneficial effect of a low-fat low-calorie diet on myocardial energy metabolism in patients with angina pectoris. *Lancet* 2:59, 1984.

Ribeiro, J. The effectiveness of a low lipid diet and exercise in the management of coronary artery disease. Clinical investigations. *Am Heart J* 108:1183, 1984.

Ellis, F. Angina and vegan diet. *Am Heart J* 93:803, 1977.

Ornish, D. Effects of stress management training and dietary changes in treating ischemic heart disease. *JAMA* 249:54, 1983.

Ornish, D. Can lifestyle changes reverse coronary heart disease? *Lancet* 336: 129, 1990.

Effects of dietary cholesterol and kinds of fat on blood cholesterol:

Hopkins, P. Effects of dietary cholesterol on serum cholesterol: a meta-analysis and review. *Am J Clin Nutr* 55:1060, 1992.

Anderson, J. The dependence of the effects of cholesterol and degree of saturation of the fat in the diet on serum cholesterol in man. *Am J Clin Nutr* 29:1784, 1976.

Jackson, R. Influence of polyunsaturated and saturated fats on plasma lipids and lipoproteins in man. *Am J Clin Nutr* 39:589, 1984.

Effects of various fats on cholesterol—omega-3 vs. other vegetable oils:

Simopoulos, A. Omega-3 fatty acids in health and disease and in growth and development. *Am J Clin Nutr* 54:438, 1991.

Animal fat raises cholesterol twice as much as vegetable fat lowers it:

Keys, A. Effect on serum cholesterol in man of mono-ene fatty acid (oleic acid) in the diet. *Proc Soc Exp Biol Med* 98:387, 1958.

Vegetable fat does not offset cholesterol-raising effects of animal fat:

Barr, S. Reducing total dietary fat without reducing saturated fatty acids does not significantly lower total plasma cholesterol concentrations in normal males. *Am J Clin Nutr* 55:675, 1992.

Healthy Tarahumara Indians with low HDL levels:

McMurray, M. Changes in lipid and lipoprotein levels and body weight in the Tarahumara Indians after consumption of an affluent diet. *N Engl J Med* 325:1704, 1991.

Worldwide, people with the lowest HDL have the lowest heart disease:

Knuiman, J. HDL-cholesterol in men from thirteen countries (letter). *Lancet* 2:367, 1981.

Olive oil has no special cholesterol-lowering effects over other vegetable oils:

Dreon, D. The effects of polyunsaturated fat vs monounsaturated fat on plasma lipoproteins. *JAMA* 263:2462, 1990.

Polyunsaturated fats promote artery disease as much as saturated fat:

Blankenhorn, D. The influence of diet on the appearance of new lesions in human coronary arteries. *JAMA* 263:1646, 1990.
Hennig, B. Linoleic acid and linolenic acid: effect on permeability properties of culture endothelial cell monolayers. *Am J Clin Nutr* 49:301, 1989.
Felton, C. Dietary polyunsaturated fatty acids and composition of human aortic plaques. *Lancet* 344:1195, 1994.

Fish oil does not lower total cholesterol, and raises LDL cholesterol:

Wilt, T. Fish oil supplementation does not lower plasma cholesterol in men with hypercholestrolemia—results of a randomized, placebo-controlled crossover study. *Ann Intern Med* 111:900, 1989.

Dart, A. Effects of Maxepa on serum lipids in hypercholesterolemic subjects. *Atherosclerosis* 80:119, 1989.

Demke, D. Effects of a fish oil concentrate in patients with hypercholesterolemia. *Atherosclerosis* 70:73, 1988.

Bilo, H. Fish oil in preventing coronary restenosis (letter). *Lancet* 2:693, 1989.

Harris, W. Effects of a low saturated fat, low cholesterol fish oil supplement in hypertriglyceridemic patients—a placebo-controlled trial. *Ann Intern Med* 109:465, 1988.

Weiner, M. Cholesterol in foods rich in omega-3 fatty acids (letter). *N Engl J Med* 315:833, 1986.

Simopoulos, A. Purslane: a terrestrial source of omega-3 fatty acids (letter). *N Engl J Med* 315:833, 1986.

Fish may or may not help heart patients—the current debate:

Prichard, B. Fish oils and cardiovascular disease. Beneficial effects on lipids and haemostatic system. *Br Med J* 310:819, 1995.

Ascherio, A. Dietary intake of marine n-3 fatty acids, fish intake, and the risk of coronary disease among men. *N Engl J Med* 332:977, 1995.

Fish oil does not slow progression of coronary artery disease:

Sacks, F. Controlled trial of fish oil for regression of human coronary atherosclerosis. *J Am Coll Cardiol* 25:1492, 1995.

Fish oil increases tendency to bleed:

Atkinson, P. Effects of a 4-week freshwater fish (trout) diet on platelet aggregation, platelet fatty acids, serum lipids, and coagulation factors. *Am J Hematol* 24:143, 1987.

Mortensen, J. The effect of n-6 and n-3 polyunsaturated fatty acids on hemostasis, blood lipids and blood pressure. *Thromb Haemost* 50:543, 1983.

Clarke, J. Increased incidence of epistaxis in adolescents with familial hypercholesterolemia treated with fish oil. *J Pediatr* 116:139, 1990.

Brox, J. Effects of cod liver oil on platelets and coagulation in familiar hypercholesterolemia (type IIa). *Acta Med Scand* 213:137, 1983.

The fat you eat is the fat you wear:

Danfourth, E. Diet and obesity. *Am J Clin Nutr* 41:1132, 1985.

Leo, T. Hydrogenated oils and fats: the presence of chemically-modified fatty acids in human adipose tissue. *Am J Clin Nutr* 34:877, 1981.

London, S. Fatty acid composition of subcutaneous adipose tissue and diet in postmenopausal US women. *Am J Clin Nutr* 54:340, 1991.

Western diet makes Tarahumara Indians fat:

McMurray, M. Changes in lipid and lipoprotein levels and body weight in the Tarahumara Indians after consumption of an affluent diet. *N Engl J Med* 325:1704, 1991.

Obese young men have three times the hypertension:

Egan, B. Comparative effects of overweight on cardiovascular risk in younger versus older men. *Am J Cardiol* 67:248, 1991.

Weight gain for women leads to heart disease increase comparable to smoking:

Willett, W. Weight, weight change, and coronary heart disease in women. Risk within the "normal" weight range. *JAMA* 273:461, 1995.

Adverse effects of vegetable fats: cancer, immunosuppression, gallbladder disease, diabetes, increased birthweight:

Reddy, B. Amount and type of dietary fat and colon cancer: animal model studies. *Prog Clin Biol Res* 222:295, 1986.

Zhao, L. Quantitative review of studies of dietary fat and rat colon carcinoma. *Nutr Cancer* 15:169, 1991.

Hopkins, G. Polyunsaturated fatty acids as promoters of mammary carcinogenesis induced in Sprague-Dawley rats by 7,12-dimethylbenz[a]anthracene. *JNCI* 66:517, 1981.

Endres, S. The effect of dietary supplementation with n-3 polyunsaturated fatty acids on the synthesis of interleukin-1 and tumor necrosis factor by mononuclear cells. *N Engl J Med* 320:265, 1989.

Weymen, C. Linoleic acid as an immunosuppressive agent. *Lancet* 2:33, 1975.

Fernandes, G. Dietary lipids and risk of autoimmune disease. *Clin Immunol Immunopathol* 72:193, 1994.

Vessby, B. Polyunsaturated fatty acids impair blood glucose in type 2 diabetic patients. *Diabet Med* 9:126, 1992.

Georgopoulos, A. Improved glycemic control lowers plasma apoprotein E and triglyceride levels following ingestion of a fat load in insulin-dependent diabetic subjects. *Metabolism* 37:837, 1988.

Lardinois, C. Effect of source of dietary fats on serum glucose, insulin, and gastric inhibitory polypeptide responses to mixed test meals in subjects with non-insulin-dependent diabetes mellitus. *J Am Coll Nutr* 7:129, 1988.

Glauber, H. Adverse metabolic effect of omega-3 fatty acids in non-insulin-dependent diabetes mellitus. *Ann Intern Med* 108:663, 1988.

Sturdervant, R. Increased prevalence of cholelithiasis in men ingesting a serum cholesterol-lowering diet. *N Engl J Med* 288:24, 1973.

LaMorte, W. Increased dietary fat content accelerates cholesterol gallstone formation in the cholesterol-fed prairie dog. *Hepatology* 18:1498, 1993.

Foran, J. Increased fish consumption may be risky (letter). *JAMA* 262:28, 1989.

Olsen, S. Intake of marine fat, rich in (n-3)-polyunsaturated fatty acids, may increase birthweight by prolonging gestation. *Lancet* 2:367, 1986.

Wilkinson, D. Psoriasis and dietary fat: the fatty acid composition of surface and scale (ether-soluble) lipids. *J Invest Dermatol* 47:185, 1966.

Switching from red meat to white meat makes little difference in cholesterol levels:

Flynn, M. Serum lipids in humans fed diets containing beef or fish and poultry. *Am J Clin Nutr* 34:2734, 1981.

Flynn, M. Dietary "meats" and serum lipids. *Am J Clin Nutr* 35:935, 1982.

O'Brien, B. Human plasma lipid responses to red meat, poultry, fish, and eggs. *Am J Clin Nutr* 33:2573, 1980.

Fehily, A. The effect of fatty fish on plasma lipid and lipoprotein concentrations. *Am J Clin Nutr* 38:349, 1983.

Kromhout, D. The inverse relation between fish consumption and 20-year mortality from coronary heart disease. *N Engl J Med* 312:1205, 1985.

Brown, A. A mixed Australian fish diet and fish-oil supplementation: impact on the plasma lipid profile of healthy men. *Am J Clin Nutr* 52:825, 1990.

A healthy diet relieves angina:

See "Dietary fat can cause angina and a low-fat diet relieves chest pain" above.

A healthy diet improves claudication time:

Kuo, P. The effect of lipemia upon coronary circulation and peripheral arterial circulation in patients with essential hyperlipemia. *Am J Med* 26:68, 1959.

Impotence is caused by an unhealthy diet:

Virag, R. Is impotence an arterial disorder? A study of arterial risk factors in 440 impotent men. *Lancet* 1:181, 1985.

Hearing loss caused by an unhealthy diet:

Rosen, S. Epidemiologic hearing studies in the USSR. *Arch Otolaryng* 91:424, 1970.

Rosen, S. Dietary prevention of hearing loss. *Acta Otolaryng* 70:242, 1970.

Spencer, J. Hyperlipoproteinemias in the etiology of inner ear disease. *Laryngoscope* 85:639, 1973.

Gates, G. The relation of hearing loss in the elderly to the presence of cardiovascular disease and cardiovascular risk factors. *Arch Otolaryngol Head Neck Surg* 119:156, 1993.

Chapter 4

Declining serum cholesterols in the United States:

Johnson, C. Declining serum total cholesterol levels among US adults. The National Health and Nutrition Examination Surveys. *JAMA* 269:3002, 1993.

Reversal of atherosclerosis:

Strom, A. Mortality from circulatory diseases in Norway 1940–1945. *Lancet* 1:126, 1951.

Wissler, R. Studies of regression of advanced atherosclerosis in experimental animals and man. *Ann NY Acad Sci* 275:363, 1976.

Armstrong, M. Regression of coronary atheromatosis in rhesus monkeys. *Circ Res* 27:59, 1970.

Duffield, R. Treatment of hyperlipidaemia retards progression of symptomatic femoral atherosclerosis. A randomised controlled trial. *Lancet* 2:639, 1983.

Nikkila, E. Prevention of progression of coronary atherosclerosis by treatment of hyperlipidaemia: a seven year prospective angiographic study. *Br Med J* 289:220, 1984.

Ost, C. Regression of peripheral atherosclerosis during therapy with high doses of nicotinic acid. *Scand J Clin Lab Invest* (Suppl) 99:241, 1967.

Barndt, R. Regression and progression of early femoral atherosclerosis in treated hyperlipoproteinemic patients. *Ann Intern Med* 86:139, 1977.

Hennerici, M. Spontaneous progression and regression of small carotid atheroma. *Lancet* 1:1415, 1985.

Basta, L. Regression of atherosclerotic stenosing lesions of the renal arteries and spontaneous cure of systemic hypertension through control of hyperlipidemia. *Am J Med* 61:420, 1976.

Bassler, T. Regression of athroma. *West J Med* 132:474, 1980.

Roth, D. Noninvasive and invasive demonstration of spontaneous regression of coronary artery disease. *Circulation* 62:888, 1980.

Hubbard, J. Nathan Pritikin's heart. *N Engl J Med* 313:52, 1985.

Brensike, J. Effects of therapy with cholestyramine on progression of coronary atherosclerosis: results of the NHLBI Type II Coronary Intervention Study. *Circulation* 69:313, 1984.

Cashin-Hemphill, L. Beneficial effects of colestipol-niacin on coronary atherosclerosis: a 4-year follow-up. *JAMA* 264:3013, 1990.

Arntzenius, A. Diet, lipoproteins, and the progression of coronary atherosclerosis: the Leiden Intervention Trial. *N Engl J Med* 312:805, 1985.

Blankenhorn, D. Beneficial effects of combined colestipol-niacin therapy on coronary atherosclerosis and coronary venous bypass grafts. *JAMA* 257: 3233, 1987.

Buchwald, H. Effect of partial ileal bypass surgery on mortality and morbidity from coronary heart disease in patients with hypercholesterolemia: Report of the Program on the Surgical Control of Hyperlipidemias (POSCH). *N Engl J Med* 323:946, 1990.

Brown, G. Regression of coronary artery disease as a result of intensive lipid-lowering therapy in men with high levels of apolipoprotein B. *N Engl J Med* 323: 1289, 1990.

Kane, J. Regression of coronary atherosclerosis during treatment of familial hypercholesterolemia with combined drug regimens. *JAMA* 264:3007, 1990.

Watts, G. Effects on coronary artery disease of lipid-lowering diet, or diet plus cholestyramine in the St. Thomas' Atherosclerosis Regression Study (STARS). *Lancet* 339:563, 1992.

Schuler, G. Regular physical exercise and low-fat diet. Effects on progression of coronary artery disease. *Circulation* 86:1, 1992.

Schuler, G. Myocardial perfusion and regression of coronary artery disease in patients on a regimen of physical exercise and low fat diet. *J. Am Coll Cardiol* 19:34, 1992.

Brown, B. Regression of atherosclerosis—an ounce of prevention. *West J Med* 159:208, 1993.

Haskell, W. Effects of intensive multiple risk factor reduction on coronary atherosclerosis and clinical cardiac events in men and women with coronary artery disease: the Stanford Coronary Risk Intervention Project (SCRIP). *Circulation* 89:975, 1994.

Blankenhorn, D. The influence of diet on the appearance of new lesions in human coronary artery disease. *JAMA* 263:1646, 1990.

Blankenhorn, D. Coronary angiographic changes with lovastatin therapy. The Monitored Atherosclerosis Regression Study (MARS). *Ann Intern Med* 119:969, 1993.

Ornish, D. Can lifestyle changes reverse coronary heart disease? *Lancet* 336: 129, 1990.

Levine, G. Cholesterol reduction in cardiovascular disease. *N Engl J Med* 332: 512, 1995.

Superko, H. Coronary artery disease regression. Convincing evidence for the benefit of aggressive lipoprotein management. *Circulation* 90:1056, 1994.

Thompson, G. Familial Hypercholesterolaemia Regression Study: a randomized trial of low-density-lipoprotein apheresis. *Lancet* 345:811, 1995.

Treasure, C. Beneficial effects of cholesterol-lowering therapy on the coronary endothelium in patients with coronary artery disease. *N Engl J Med* 332: 481, 1995.

Use of calcium channel blockers to reverse artery disease:

Lichtlen, P. Retardation of angiographic progression of coronary artery disease by nifedipine. *Lancet* 335:1109, 1990.

Loaldi, A. Comparison of nifedipine, propanalol and isosrobide dinitrate on angiographic progression and regression of coronary arterial narrowings in angina pectoris. *Am J Cardiol* 64:433, 1989.

Waters, D. A controlled clinical trial to assess the effect of a calcium channel blocker on progression of coronary atherosclerosis. *Circulation* 82:1940, 1990.

Rupture of the plaque causes the clot that closes the heart artery, causing the heart attack:

See "The second stages of atherosclerosis—tiny plaques rupture and clots form, causing heart attacks" in references for Chapter 2.

Reducing your cholesterol by diet and/or drugs reduces risk of plaque rupture:

Brown, B. Atherosclerosis regression, plaque disruption, and cardiovascular events: a rationale for lipid lowering in coronary artery disease. *Ann Rev Med* 44:365, 1993.

Brown, G. Regression of atherosclerosis—an ounce of prevention. *West J Med* 159:208, 1993.

Brown, B. Lipid lowering and plaque regression. New insights into prevention of plaque disruption and clinical events in coronary disease. *Circulation* 87:1781, 1993.

Levine, G. Cholesterol reduction in cardiovascular disease. Clinical benefits and possible mechanisms. *N Engl J Med* 332:512, 1995.

Diet changes the tendency for the blood to clot and form a coronary thrombosis:

Greig, H. Inhibition of fibrinolysis by alimentary lipemia. *Lancet* 2:16, 1956.

Mustard, J. Effect of different dietary fats on blood coagulation, platelet economy, and blood lipids. *Br Med J* 1:1651, 1962.

Hornstra, G. Influence of dietary fat on platelet function in men. *Lancet* 1:1155, 1973.

O'Brien, J. Acute platelet changes after large meals of saturated and unsaturated fats. *Lancet* 1:878, 1976.

Simpson, H. Hypertriglyceridaemia and hypercoagulability. *Lancet* 1:786, 1983.

Fuster, V. The pathogenesis of coronary artery disease and the acute coronary syndromes (second of two parts). *N Engl J Med* 326:310, 1992.

Report of a meeting of physicians and scientists, University of Texas Health Center at Houston and Texas Heart Institute, Houston. Platelet activation and arterial thrombosis. *Lancet* 344:991, 1994.

Hunt, B. The relation between abnormal hemostatic function and progression of coronary disease. *Curr Opin Cardiol* 5:758, 1990.

Barnard, R. Effects of a low-fat, low-cholesterol diet on serum lipids, platelet aggregation and thrombaxane formation. *Prostaglandins Leukot Med* 26: 241, 1987.

Saunders, T. Dietary fat and platelet function. *Clin Sci* 65:343, 1983.

Elkeles, R. Effects of treatment of hyperlipidemia on haemostatic variables. *Br Med J* 281:973, 1980.

Carvalho, S. Coagulation factor VII and plasma triglycerides. Decreased metabolism as a possible mechanism of factor VII hyperactivity. *Haemostasis* 19:125, 1989.

Renaud, S. Dietary fats and platelet functions in relation to atherosclerosis and coronary heart disease. *Haemostasis* 8:234, 1979.

Miller, G. Association between dietary fat intake and plasma factor VII coagulant activity—a predictor of cardiovascular mortality. *Atherosclerosis* 60: 269, 1986.

Ulbricht, T. Coronary heart disease: seven dietary factors. *Lancet* 338:985, 1991.

Thompson, S. Hemostatic factors and the risk of myocardial infarction or sudden death in patients with angina pectoris. *N Engl J Med* 332:635, 1995.

Prostaglandin release causes vasospasm:

Fuster, V. The pathogenesis of coronary artery disease and acute coronary syndromes (second of two parts). *N Engl J Med* 326:310, 1992.

Reduction of LDL cholesterol by 40 to 45 percent leads to reversal:

Kuo, P. Inducing regression of atherosclerosis. *Choices in Cardiology* 3:308, 1989.

Ideal cholesterol is less than 150 mg/dl:

Roberts, W. Atherosclerotic risk factors—are there ten or is there only one? *Am J Cardiol* 64:552, 1989.

Kannel, W. Is the serum total cholesterol an anachronism? *Lancet* 2:950, 1979.

Japanese eat healthier and die less of heart disease:

Marmot, M. Why are the Japanese living longer? *Br Med J* 299:1547, 1989.

Lewis, P. Japanese live longer, the U.N. finds. *New York Times*, April 26, 1992.

Drug therapy not as effective as diet:

Sacks, F. Effect on coronary atherosclerosis of decrease in plasma cholesterol concentrations in normocholesterolaemic patients. *Lancet* 344:1182, 1994.

Moser, M. Can dietary changes reverse or prevent the progression of coronary atherosclerosis? *Primary Cardiol* 17:10, 1991.

Diet without dairy lowers cholesterol best:

Sacks, F. Plasma lipoprotein levels in vegetarians. The effect of ingestion of fats from dairy products. *JAMA* 254:1337, 1985.

Sources of cholesterol variations:

Cooper, G. Blood lipid measurements. Variations and practical utility. *JAMA* 267:1652, 1992.

Chapter 5

Fruit (fructose) raises cholesterol and triglycerides in sensitive people:

Hollenbeck, C. Dietary fructose effects on lipoprotein metabolism and risk for coronary artery disease. *Am J Clin Nutr 58* (Suppl):800S, 1993.
Hallfrisch, J. Metabolic effects of fructose. *FASEB J* 4:2652, 1990.
Swanson, J. Metabolic effects of dietary fructose in healthy subjects. *Am J Clin Nutr* 55:851, 1992.

Artificial sweeteners increase appetite:

Rogers, P. Uncoupling sweet taste and calories: comparison of the effects of glucose and three intense sweeteners on hunger and food intake. *Physiol Behav* 43:547, 1988.
Tordoff, M. Oral stimulation with aspartame increases hunger. *Physiol Behav* 47:555, 1990.

Alcohol raises triglycerides:

Steinberg, D. Alcohol and atherosclerosis. *Ann Intern Med* 114:967, 1991.

Moderate alcohol consumption may increase longevity:

Klatsky, A. Alcohol and longevity. *Am J Public Health* 85:16, 1995.

Immune reactions with dietary protein found in severe cases of atherosclerosis:

Annand, J. Denatured bovine immunoglobulin pathogenic in atherosclerosis. *Atherosclerosis* 59:347, 1986.
Muscari, A. Serum IgA antibodies to apoproteins and milk-proteins in severe atherosclerosis. *Ann Ital Med Int* 7:7, 1992.

Muscari, A. Association of serum IgA antibodies to milk antigens in severe athero-sclerosis. *Atherosclerosis* 77:251, 1989.

Saturated and polyunsaturated oils cause blood sludging:

See "Dietary fat causes the circulation to sludge" in references for Chapter 3.

Food additives cause adverse reactions:

Opper, F. Food allergy and intolerance. *Gastroenterologist* 1:211, 1993.
Webber, R. Food additives and allergy. *Ann Allergy* 70:183, 1993.
Parker, S. Dietary aspects of adverse reactions to foods in adults. *Can Med Assoc J* 139:711, 1988.
Scopp, A. MSG and hydrolyzed vegetable protein induced headache: review and case studies. *Headache* 31:107, 1991.

Frequent meals encourage weight loss and reduction in cholesterol:

Southgate, D. Nibblers, gorgers, snackers, and grazers. Eating a little and (very) often is beneficial to health. *Br Med J* 300:136, 1990.
Jenkins, D. Nibbling versus gorging: metabolic advantages of increased meal frequency. *N Engl J Med* 321:929, 1989.

Chapter 6

Multiple benefits of exercise:

Pate, R. Physical activity and public health. A recommendation from Centers for Disease Control and Prevention and the American College of Sports Medicine. *JAMA* 273:402, 1995.
Fletcher, G. Exercise standards: a statement for healthcare professionals from the American Heart Association. *Circulation* 91:580, 1995.
Sady, S. Prolonged exercise augments plasma triglyceride clearance. *JAMA* 256:2552, 1986.
Margolis, S. Treatment of a low HDL cholesterol level. *JAMA* 264:3063, 1990.
Kokkinos, P. Miles run per week and high-density lipoprotein cholesterol levels in healthy, middle-aged men. *Arch Intern Med* 155:415, 1995.

Exercise, aging, and the immune system:

Mazzeo, R. The influence of exercise and aging on immune function. *Med Sci Sports Exerc* 26:586, 1994.
Nehlsen-Cannarella, S. The effects of moderate exercise on immune response. *Med Sci Sports Exerc* 23:64, 1991.

Mackinnon, L. Current challenges and future expectations in exercise immunology: back to the future. *Med Sci Sports Exerc* 26:191, 1994.

Nieman, D. Role of endurance exercise in immune senescence. *Med Sci Sports Exerc* 26:172, 1994.

Too much exercise increases risk of viral infections:

Nieman, D. Exercise, upper respiratory tract infection, and the immune system. *Med Sci Sports Exerc* 26:128, 1994.

Exercise lowers mortality:

Paffenbarger, R. Physical activity, all-cause mortality, and longevity of college alumni. *N Engl J Med* 314:605, 1986.

Blair, S. Physical fitness and all-cause mortality. A prospective study of healthy men and women. *JAMA* 262:2395, 1989.

Blair, S. Changes in physical fitness and all-cause mortality. A prospective study of healthy and unhealthy men. *JAMA* 273:1093, 1995.

Exercise improves your mood:

Daniel, M. Opiate receptor blockage by naltrexone and mood state after acute physical activity. *Br J Sports Med* 26:111, 1992.

Raglin, J. Exercise and mental health. Beneficial and detrimental effects. *Sports Med* 9:323, 1990.

Taylor, C. The relationship of physical activity and exercise to mental health. *Public Health Rep* 100:195, 1985.

King, A. Influence of regular aerobic exercise on psychological health: a randomized, controlled trial of healthy middle-aged adults. *Health Psychol* 8: 305, 1989.

Norris, R. The effects of aerobic and anaerobic training on fitness, blood pressure, and psychological stress and well-being. *J Psychosomatic Res* 34: 367, 1990.

Mersy, D. Health benefits of aerobic exercise. *Postgrad Med* 90:103, 1991.

Folkins, C. Physical fitness training and mental health. *Am Psychol* 36:373, 1981.

Carr, D. Physical conditioning facilitates the exercise-induced secretion of beta-endorphins and beta-lipotropin in women. *N Engl J Med* 90:103, 1981.

Chapter 7

Stress concentrates blood and raises cholesterol:

Muldoon, M. Effects of acute psychological stress on serum lipid levels, hemoconcentration, and blood viscosity. *Arch Intern Med* 155:615, 1995.

Food changes neurotransmitters:

Wurtman, J. Behavioral effects of nutrients. *Lancet* 1:1145, 1983.

Glaeser, B. Changes in brain levels of acidic, basic, and neutral amino acids after consumption of single meals containing various portions of protein. *J Neurochem* 41:1016, 1983.

Liberman, H. The effects of dietary neurotransmitter precursors on human behavior. *Am J Clin Nutr* 42:366, 1985.

Berkman, L. Social networks, host resistance, and mortality: a nine-year follow-up of Alameda county residents. *Am J Epidemiol* 109:186, 1979.

Williams, R. Prognostic importance of social and economic resources among medically treated patients with angiographically documented coronary artery disease. *JAMA* 267:520, 1992.

Chapter 8

Cigarette smokers have lower levels of antioxidants and greater clotting tendencies:

Brown, K. Vitamin E supplementation suppresses indexes of lipid peroxidation and platelet counts in blood of smokers and nonsmokers but plasma lipoprotein concentrations remain unchanged. *Am J Clin Nutr* 60:383, 1994.

Morrow, J. Increase in circulating products of lipid peroxidation (F2-isoprostanes) in smokers. Smoking as a cause of oxidative damage. *N Engl J Med* 332:1198, 1995.

Relationship between heart attacks and coffee:

Grobbee, D. Coffee, caffeine, and cardiovascular disease in men. *N Engl J Med* 323:1026, 1990.

LaCroix, A. Coffee consumption and the incidence of coronary heart disease. *N Engl J Med* 315:977, 1986.

Rosmarin, P. Coffee consumption and serum lipids: a randomized, crossover clinical trial. *Am J Med* 88:349, 1990.

Brewing method of coffee makes difference in cholesterol effects:

Zock, P. Effects of a lipid-rich fraction from boiled coffee on serum cholesterol. *Lancet* 335:1235, 1990.

Bak, A. The effect on serum cholesterol levels of coffee brewed by filtering or boiling. *N Engl J Med* 321:1432, 1989.

Decaffeinated coffee raises cholesterol:

Superko, H. Caffeinated and decaffeinated coffee effects on plasma lipoprotein cholesterol, apolipoproteins, and lipase activity: a controlled, randomized trial. *Am J Clin Nutr* 54:599, 1991.

Tea has antioxidants:

Imai, K. Cross sectional study of effects of drinking green tea on cardiovascular and liver disease. *Br Med J* 310:693, 1995.
Serafini, M. Red wine, tea, and antioxidants (letter). *Lancet* 344:626, 1994.

Cheese said to lower risk of heart disease over milk. Not!:

Gurr, M. Wine and coronary heart disease. *Lancet* 340:313, 1992.

Real difference is the French have only recently changed their diet:

Nestle, M. Wine and coronary heart disease. *Lancet* 340:314, 1992.
Criqui, M. Does diet or alcohol explain the French paradox? *Lancet* 344:1719, 1994.

Alcohol associated with less death from heart disease:

Lazarus, N. Change in alcohol consumption and risk of death from all causes and from ischaemic heart disease. *Br Med J* 303:553, 1991.
Rimm, E. Prospective study of alcohol consumption and risk of coronary disease in men. *Lancet* 338:464, 1991.

Alcohol raises HDL cholesterol of both types:

Steinberg, D. Alcohol and atherosclerosis. *Ann Intern Med* 114:967, 1991.

Wine has other benefits, like acting as an antioxidant and antithrombotic:

Langer, R. Lipoproteins and blood pressure as biological pathways for effect of moderate alcohol consumption on coronary heart disease. *Circulation* 85: 910, 1992.
Frankel, E. Inhibition of oxidation of human low-density lipoprotein by phenolic substances in red wine. *Lancet* 341:454, 1993.
Renaud, S. Wine, alcohol, platelets, and the French paradox for coronary heart disease. *Lancet* 339:1523, 1992.
Renaud, S. Alcohol and platelet aggregation: the Caerphilly Protective Heart Disease Study. *Am J Clin Nutr* 55:1012, 1992.
Fuhrman, B. Consumption of red wine with meals reduces the susceptibility of

human plasma and low-density lipoprotein to lipid peroxidation. *Am J Clin Nutr* 61:549, 1995.

Adverse effects of alcohol:

Steinberg, D. Alcohol and atherosclerosis. *Ann Intern Med* 114:967, 1991.
Regan, T. Alcohol and the cardiovascular system. *JAMA* 264:377, 1990.
Brewer, R. The risk of dying in alcohol-related automobile crashes among habitual drunk drivers. *N Engl J Med* 331:513, 1994.

Chapter 9

Gallup poll statistics:

January and February 1989 Gallup poll for the American Medical Association; reported in the *New York Times*, Feb 20, 1990.

Doctors fail to ask patients about nutrition:

Nutrition Information Center at New York Hospital–Cornell Medical Center. Reported in Sept/Oct 1993 issue of *Natural Health.*

Doctors don't believe lowering cholesterol can prevent heart disease:

Schucker, B. Change in physician perspective on cholesterol and heart disease. Results from two national surveys. *JAMA* 258:3521, 1987.
Schucker, B. Change in cholesterol awareness and action. Results from national physician and public surveys. *Arch Intern Med* 151:666, 1991.

Patient participation increases healing:

Spiegel, D. Effect of psychological treatment on survival of patients with metastatic breast cancer. *Lancet* 2:888, 1989.
Markman, M. Cancer survival and the mind (editorial). *J Ca Res Clin Oncol* 120:443, 1994.

Doctors can be rude:

Coleman, D. All too often the doctor isn't listening, studies show. *New York Times*, Nov 13, 1991.

Chapter 10

People die in hospitals after heart attacks:

American Heart Association. *1992 Heart and Stroke Facts.*

William C. Roberts editorial:

Roberts, W. Lipid lowering therapy after an atherosclerotic event. *Am J Cardiol* 64:693, 1989.

Rates of heart disease based on cholesterol levels:

National Cholesterol Education Program. "Report of the Expert Panel on Population Strategies for Blood Cholesterol Reduction," U.S. Department of Health and Human Services, Nov 1990.

Menu for low-fat, low-cholesterol diet:

The Marriott Corporation's "Fat/Cholesterol Controlled Diet" menu, provided to patients at the Cooley Dickenson Hospital in Northampton, Massachusetts.

American Heart Association diet is ineffective:

Roberts, W. The ineffectiveness of a commonly recommended lipid-lowering diet in significantly lowering the serum total and low-density lipoprotein cholesterol levels. *Am J Cardiol* 73:623, 1994.

Brown, B. Regression of coronary artery disease as a result of intensive lipid-lowering therapy in men with high levels of apolipoprotein B. *N Engl J Med* 323:1289, 1990.

Blankenhorn, D. Beneficial effects of combined colestipol-niacin therapy on coronary atherosclerosis and coronary venous bypass grafts. *JAMA* 257: 3233, 1987.

Cashin-Hemphill, L. Beneficial effects of colestipol-niacin on coronary atherosclerosis: a 4-year follow-up. *JAMA* 264:3013, 1990.

Kane, J. Regression of coronary atherosclerosis during treatment of familial hypercholesterolemia with combined drug regimens. *JAMA* 264:3007, 1990.

Watts, G. Effects on coronary artery disease of lipid-lowering diet, or diet plus cholestyramine in the St. Thomas' Atherosclerosis Regression Study (STARS). *Lancet* 339:563, 1992.

Blankenhorn, D. Coronary angiographic changes with lovastatin therapy. The Monitored Atherosclerosis Regression Study (MARS). *Ann Intern Med* 119:969, 1993.

Haskell, W. Effects of intensive multiple risk factor reduction on coronary atherosclerosis and clinical cardiac events in men and women with coronary artery disease: the Stanford Coronary Risk Intervention Project (SCRIP). *Circulation* 89:975, 1994.

Gould, K. Improved stenosis geometry by quantitative coronary arteriography after vigorous risk factor modification. *Am J Cardiol* 69:845, 1992.

Hunninghake, D. The efficacy of intensive dietary therapy alone or combined with lovastatin in outpatients with hypercholesterolemia. *N Engl J Med* 328: 1213, 1993.

Rupturing of plaques leads to the tragedy—a heart attack:

Brown, G. Regression of atherosclerosis—an ounce of prevention. *West J Med* 159:208, 1993.

Brown, B. Atherosclerosis regression, plaque disruption, and cardiovascular events: a rationale for lipid lowering in coronary artery disease. *Ann Rev Med* 44:365, 1993.

Effect of change to a near-vegetarian diet after heart attack:

Singh, R. Randomised controlled trial of cardioprotective diet in patients with recent acute myocardial infarction: results of one year follow up. *Br Med J* 304:1015, 1992.

Chapter 11

Increasing cholesterol means more chance of a heart attack:

The Expert Panel. Report of the National Cholesterol Education Program Expert Panel on Detection, Evaluation, and Treatment of High Blood Cholesterol in Adults. *Arch Intern Med* 148:36, 1988.

The National Cholesterol Education Program's Expert Panel. Population Strategies for Blood Cholesterol Reduction. U.S. Department of Health and Human Services, Nov 1990. NIH Publication No. 90-3046.

Low HDL cholesterol is a risk factor for heart disease:

National Institutes of Health Consensus Development Conference Statement: Triglyceride, High Density Lipoprotein, and Coronary Heart Disease. Feb 26–28, 1992.

Ratio of cholesterol to HDL predicts heart disease:

Kinosian, B. Cholesterol and coronary heart disease: predicting risks by levels and ratios. *Ann Intern Med* 121:641, 1994.

Role of elevated triglycerides:

Tenkanen, L. The triglyceride issue revisited. Findings from the Helsinki Heart Study. *Arch Intern Med* 154:2714, 1994.

Triglycerides less important than elevated cholesterol:

Garber, A. Triglyceride concentration and coronary heart disease (letter). *Br Med J* 310:259, 1995.

Too many unnecessary angiograms are performed:

Graboys, T. Results of a second-opinion trial among patients recommended for coronary angiography. *JAMA* 268:2537, 1992.

After a heart attack you don't always have to submit to an angiogram:

Cross, S. First myocardial infarction in patients under 60 years old: the role of exercise tests and symptoms in deciding whom to catheterise. *Br Heart J* 70:428, 1993.

Chapter 12

Antioxidants slow the progression of atherosclerosis:

Hoffman, R. Antioxidants and the prevention of coronary heart disease. *Arch Intern Med* 155:241, 1995.

Moris, D. Serum carotenoids and coronary heart disease. The Lipid Research Clinics Coronary Primary Prevention Trial and Follow-up Study. *JAMA* 272:1439, 1994.

Ames, B. Oxidants, antioxidants, and the degenerative diseases of aging. *Proc Natl Acad Sci, USA* 90:7915, 1993.

Frei, B. Ascorbate is an outstanding antioxidant in human blood plasma. *Proc Natl Acad Sci, USA* 86:6377, 1989.

Frei, B. Antioxidant defenses and lipid peroxidation in human blood plasma. *Proc Natl Acad Sci, USA* 85:9748, 1988.

Hertog, M. Dietary antioxidant flavonoids and risk of coronary heart disease: the Zutphen Elderly Study. *Lancet* 342:1007, 1993.

Pryor, W. The potential usefulness of the antioxidant vitamins as pharmoprotective agents. The use of oxidant stress status measurements. Biodynamics Institute, Louisiana State University, Baton Rouge, LA 70803-1800.

Supplementation with vitamin pills may not be the answer—more lung cancer, more colon adenomas:

The Alpha-Tocopherol, Beta Carotene Cancer Prevention Study Group. The effect of vitamin E and beta carotene on the incidence of lung cancer and other cancers in male smokers. *N Engl J Med* 330:1029, 1994.

Greenberg, E. A clinical trial in antioxidant vitamins to prevent colonrectal adenoma. *N Engl J Med* 331:141, 1994.

Free radicals are highly reactive substances and cause human diseases:

Halliwell, B. Reactive oxygen species in living systems: source, biochemistry, and role in human disease. *Am J Med* 91 (Supple3c): 3C:14S, 1991.

Free radicals damage DNA:

Ames, B. Oxidants, antioxidants, and the degenerative diseases of aging. *Proc Natl Acad Sci, USA* 90:7915, 1993.

Less heart disease with higher carotene levels in men and vitamin E intakes in men and women:

Rimm, E. Vitamin E consumption and the risk of coronary heart disease in men. *N Engl J Med* 328:1450, 1993.
Stampfer, M. Vitamin E consumption and the risk of coronary disease in women. *N Engl J Med* 328:1444, 1993.

Vitamin E slows progression of atherosclerosis:

Hodis, H. Serial coronary angiographic evidence that antioxidant vitamin intake reduces progression of coronary artery atherosclerosis. *JAMA* 273:1849, 1995

Low vitamin E level has stronger association with heart disease than high cholesterol:

Gey, K. Inverse correlation between plasma vitamin E and mortality from ischemic heart disease in cross-cultural epidemiology. *Am J Clin Nutr* 53: 326S, 1991.

Vegetarians have higher vitamin E levels than nonvegetarians:

Pronczuk, A. Vegetarians have higher plasma alpha-tocopherol relative to cholesterol than do nonvegetarians. *J Am Coll Nutr* 11:50, 1992.

Vitamin C (2 g) lowers cholesterol and platelet adhesiveness:

Bordia, A. The effect of vitamin C on blood lipids, fibrinolytic activity and platelet adhesiveness in patients with coronary artery disease. *Atherosclerosis* 35:181, 1980.
Turley, S. The role of ascorbic acid in the regulation of cholesterol metabolism and in the pathogenesis of atherosclerosis. *Atherosclerosis* 24:1, 1976.

Vitamin E supplements lower cholesterol:

Qureshi, A. Lowering of serum cholesterol in hypercholesterolemic humans by tocotrienols (palmvitee). *Am J Clin Nutr* 53:1021S, 1991.

Vitamin B₃ (niacin) supplements lower cholesterol, but long-acting forms cause hepatitis:

McKenney, J. A comparison of the efficacy and toxic effects of sustained- vs immediate-release niacin in hypercholesterolemic patients. *JAMA* 271: 672, 1994.
Henkin, Y. Niacin revisited: clinical observations on an important but underutilized drug. *Am J Med* 91:239, 1991.
Gray, D. Efficacy and safety of controlled-release niacin in dyslipoproteinemic veterans. *Ann Intern Med* 121:252, 1994.

Mineral supplements adversely affect heart patients:

Galloe, A. Influence of oral magnesium supplementation on cardiac events among survivors of an acute myocardial infarction. *Br Med J* 307:585, 1993.
Yusuf, S. Magnesium in acute myocardial infarction. ISIS 4 provides no grounds for its routine use. *Br Med J* 310:751, 1995.
Black, M. Zinc supplements and serum lipids in young adult white males. *Am J Clin Nutr* 47:970, 1988.
Burt, M. Iron and heart disease. Iron's role is undecided. *Br Med J* 307:575, 1993.
Danielian, P. Iron and coronary heart disease. Iron makes the myocardium vulnerable to ischemia (letter). *Br Med J* 307:1066, 1993.

Dietary fiber lowers cholesterol:

Salenius, J. Long term effects of guar gum on lipid metabolism after carotid endarterectomy. *Br Med J* 310:95, 1995.
Ripsin, C. Oat products and lipid lowering: a meta-analysis. *JAMA* 267:3317, 1992.
Davidson, M. The hypocholesterolemic effects of B-glucan in oatmeal and oat bran. A dose-controlled study. *JAMA* 265:1833, 1991.

Activated charcoal lowers cholesterol:

Neuvonen, P. The mechanism of the hypocholesterolaemic effect of activated charcoal. *Eur J Clin Invest* 19:251, 1989.
Kuusisto, P. Effect of activated charcoal on hypercholesterolaemia. *Lancet* 2:366, 1986.
Friedman, E. Reduction in hyperlipidemia in hemodialysis patients treated with charcoal and oxidized starch (oxystarch). *Am J Clin Nutr* 31:1903, 1978.
Neuvonen, P. Activated charcoal in the treatment of hypercholesterolaemia dose-response relationships and comparison with cholestyramine. *Eur J Clin Pharmacol* 37:225, 1989.

Numerous benefits of garlic:

Warshafsky, S. Effect of garlic on total serum cholesterol. A meta-analysis. *Ann Intern Med* 119:599, 1993.

Jain, A. Can garlic reduce levels of serum lipids? A controlled clinical study. *Am J Med* 94:632, 1993.

Kiesewetter, H. Effect of garlic on thrombocyte aggregation, microcirculation, and other risk factors. *Int J Clin Pharm* 29:151, 1991.

Mansell, P. Garlic. Effects on serum lipids, blood pressure, coagulation, platelet aggregation, and vasodilatation. *Br Med J* 303:379, 1991.

Brosche, T. Garlic (letter). *Br Med J* 303:785, 1991.

Odorless garlic also lowers cholesterol:

Lau, B. Effect of odor-modified garlic preparation on blood lipids. *Nutr Res* 7: 139, 1987.

Steiner, M. Cardiovascular and lipid changes in response to aged garlic extract ingestion. *J Am Coll Nutr* 13:524, 1994.

Powerful cholesterol-lowering effects of gugulipid:

Nityanand, S. Clinical trials with gugulipid. A new hyolipidaemic agent. *J Assoc Physicians India* 37:323, 1989.

Satyavati, G. Gum guggul (Commiphora mukul)—the success story of an ancient insight leading to a modern discovery. *Indian J Med Res* 87:327, 1988.

Verma, S. Effect of Commiphora mukul (gum guggulu) in patients of hyperlipidemia with special reference to HDL-cholesterol. *Indian J Med Res* 87: 356, 1988.

Ginko biloba for patients with blood vessel disease:

Kleijnen, J. Ginko biloba. *Lancet* 340:1136, 1992.

Capsaicin for patients with blood vessel disease:

Sambaiah, K. Hypocholesterolemic effect of red pepper & capsaicin. *Indian J Exp Biol* 18:898, 1980.

Wang, J. Antiplatelet effect of capsaicin. *Thrombosis Res* 36:497, 1984.

Simvastatin improves survival in heart patients:

Scandinavian Simvastatin Survival Study Group. Randomised trial of cholesterol lowering in 4444 patients with coronary heart disease: the Scandinavian Simvastatin Survival Study (4S). *Lancet* 344:1383, 1994.

Benefits of colestipol and lovastatin together in low doses:

Vega, G. Treatment of primary moderate hypercholesteremia with lovastatin (Mevinolin) and colestipol. *JAMA* 257:33, 1987.

Schrott, H. Enhanced low-density lipoprotein cholesterol reduction and cost-effectiveness by low-dose colestipol plus lovastatin combination therapy. *Am J Cardiol* 75:34, 1995.

Denke, M. Efficacy of low-dose cholesterol-lowering drug therapy in men with moderate hypercholesterolemia. *Arch Intern Med* 155:393, 1995.

Calcium channel blockers cause gingival hyperplasia and surgical bleeding:

See "Effects of calcium channel blockers" in references for Chapter 14.

Use of aspirin after an acute myocardial infarction:

Ridker, P. Are both aspirin and heparin justified as adjuncts to thrombolytic therapy for acute myocardial infarction? *Lancet* 341:1574, 1993.

Glynn, R. Adherence to aspirin in the prevention of myocardial infarction. The Physicians' Health Study. *Arch Intern Med* 154:2649, 1994.

Antiplatelet Trialists' Collaboration. Secondary prevention of vascular disease by prolonged antiplatelet treatment. *Br Med J* 296:320, 1988.

Orme, M. Aspirin all around? *Br Med J* 296:307, 1988.

Weil, J. Prophylactic aspirin and the risk of peptic ulcer bleeding. *Br Med J* 310:827, 1995.

Small doses of aspirin may be best:

Anonymous. A comparison of two doses of aspirin (30 mg vs. 283 mg a day) in patients after a transient ischemic attack or minor ischemic stroke. The Dutch TIA Trial Study Group. *N Engl J Med* 325:1261, 1991.

Foster, W. Superior prevention of reinfarction by 30 mg per day aspirin compared to 1000 mg: results of a two-year follow-up study in Cottbus. *Prog Clin Biol Res* 301:187, 1989.

Warfarin in prevention of recurrent heart attacks:

Van Berben, P. Costs and effects of long-term oral anticoagulant treatment after myocardial infarction. *JAMA* 273:925, 1995.

Aspirin is preferred over warfarin because of costs and safety:

Cairns, J. Editorial: Economics and efficacy in choosing oral anticoagulants or aspirin after myocardial infarction. *JAMA* 273:965, 1995.

Nitroglycerin in relief of chest pain:

Abrams, J. The role of nitrates in coronary heart disease. *Arch Intern Med* 155:357, 1995.

Chapter 13

As many as 80 percent of bypass surgeries gain no increase in life span:

Califano, J. A., Jr. The health-care chaos. *New York Times Magazine,* March 20, 1988.

Cleland, J., Dimmit, S., Friedman, H., and Hux, J. Effect of coronary artery bypass graft surgery on survival (letters). *Lancet* 344:1222, 1994.

Two indications for bypass surgery:

Kirklin, J. ACC/AHA guidelines and indications for coronary artery bypass graft surgery: a report of the American College of Cardiology/American Heart Association Task Force on Assessment of Diagnostic and Therapeutic Procedures (Subcommittee of Coronary Artery Bypass Graft Surgery). *Circulation* 83:1125, 1991.

Improved survival in left main coronary artery disease only seen with poor function of the left ventricle:

Caracciolo, E. Comparison of surgical and medical group survival in patients with left main coronary artery disease. Long-term CASS experience. *Circulation* 91:2325, 1995.

Caracciolo, E. Comparison of surgical and medical group survival in patients with left main equivalent coronary artery disease. Long-term CASS experience. *Circulation* 91:2335, 1995.

Survival rates from the CASS study:

Alderman, E. Ten-year follow-up of survival and myocardial infarction in the randomized Coronary Artery Surgery Study. *Circulation* 82:1629, 1990.

Early closure of grafts after bypass surgery and return of symptoms:

Grodin, C. Coronary artery bypass grafting with saphenous vein. *Circulation* 79 (suppl I):24, 1989.

Campeau, L. Atherosclerosis and late closure of aortocoronary saphenous vein grafts: sequential angiographic studies at 2 weeks, 1 year, 5 to 7 years, and 10 to 12 years after surgery. *Circulation* 68 (Suppl II): 1, 1983.

A low-fat diet relieves chest pain (angina) and improves blood oxygen, almost overnight:

See "Dietary fat can cause angina and a low-fat diet relieves chest pain" in references for Chapter 3.

Studies that compare surgery vs. medical treatment:

The Veterans Administration Coronary Artery Bypass Surgery Cooperative Study Group. Eleven-year survival in the Veterans Administration Randomized Trial of Coronary Bypass Surgery for Stable Angina. *N Engl J Med* 311:1333, 1984.

Alderman, E. Ten-year follow-up of survival and myocardial infarction in the Randomized Coronary Artery Surgery Study. *Circulation* 82:1629, 1990.

Varnauskas, E. The European Coronary Surgery Study Group: twelve-year follow-up in the randomized European Coronary Surgery Study. *N Engl J Med* 319:332, 1988.

Outcomes of patients who refused bypass surgery:

Hueb, W. Two- to eight-year survival rates in patients who refused coronary artery bypass grafting. *Am J Cardiol* 63:155, 1989.

Mortality from bypass surgery varies and rates are higher than told to patient:

O'Connor, G. A regional prospective study of in-hospital mortality associated with coronary artery bypass grafting. *JAMA* 266:803, 1991.

Hannan, E. The decline in coronary artery bypass graft surgery mortality in New York state. The role of surgeon volume. *JAMA* 273:209, 1995.

Williams, S. Differences in mortality from coronary artery bypass surgery at five teaching hospitals. *JAMA* 266:810, 1991.

McDonald, C. CABG surgical mortality in different centers (letter). *JAMA* 267:932, 1992.

Steinbrook, R. Hospital death rates for five surgeries vary. *Los Angeles Times,* March 27, 1988.

Shortell, S. The effects of regulation, competition, and ownership on mortality rates among hospital inpatients. *N Engl J Med* 318:1100, 1988.

Kirklin, J. Summary of a consensus concerning death and ischemic events after coronary artery bypass grafting. *Circulation* 79 (Suppl I):81, 1989.

Green, J. Sounding Board: report cards on cardiac surgeons. Assessing New York State's Approach. *N Engl J Med* 332:1229, 1995.

Odds of having bypass surgery vary with sex and race:

Loop, F. Coronary artery surgery in women compared with men: analysis of risks and long-term results. *J Am Coll Cardiol* 1:383, 1983.

Ayanian, J. Racial differences in the use of revascularization procedures after coronary angiography. *JAMA* 269:2642, 1993.

Brain damage from bypass surgery:

Orenstein, J. Microemboli observed in deaths following cardiopulmonary bypass surgery: silicone antifoam agents and polyvinyl chloride tubing as sources of emboli. *Hum Path* 13:1082, 1982.

Hill, J. Neuropathological manifestations of cardiac surgery. *Ann Thorac Surg* 7:409, 1969.

Editorial: Brain damage after open-heart surgery. *Lancet* 1:1161, 1982.

Henriksen, L. Evidence suggestive of diffuse brain damage following cardiac operations. *Lancet* 1:816, 1984.

Aberg, T. Release of adenylate kinase into cerebrospinal fluid during open-heart surgery and its relation to postoperative intellectual function. *Lancet* 1:1139, 1982.

Henriksen, L. Brain hyperfusion during cardiac operations: cerebral blood flow measured in man by intra-arterial injection of xenon 133: evidence suggestive of intraoperative microembolism. *J Thorac Cardiovasc Surg* 86:202, 1983.

Taylor, K. Brain damage during open-heart surgery (editorial). *Thorax* 37:873, 1982.

Savageau, J. Neuropsychological dysfunction following elective cardiac operation. *J Thorac Cardiovasc Surg* 84:585, 1982.

Kornfeld, D. Delirium after coronary artery bypass surgery. *J Thorac Cardiovasc Surg* 76:93, 1978.

Barash, P. Cardiopulmonary bypass and postoperative neurologic dysfunction. *Am Heart J* 99:675, 1980.

Orr, W. Sleep disturbances after open heart surgery. *Am J Cardiol* 39:196, 1977.

Blauth, C. Retinal microembolism during cardiopulmonary bypass demonstrated by fluorescein angiography. *Lancet* 2:837, 1986.

Shaw, P. Neurological complications of coronary artery bypass graft surgery: six month follow-up study. *Br Med J* 293:165, 1986.

Henriksen, L. Evidence suggestive of diffuse brain damage following cardiac operations. *Lancet* 1:816, 1984.

Editorial: Brain damage and open heart surgery. *Lancet* 2:364, 1989.

Townes, B. Neurobehavioral outcome in cardiac operations. *J Thorac Cardiovasc Surg* 98:774, 1989.

Pugsley, W. Microemboli and cerebral impairment during cardiac surgery. *Vasc Surg* 24:34, 1990.

Harrison, M. Detection of middle cerebral emboli during coronary artery bypass using transcranial doppler sonography (letter). *Stroke* 21:1512, 1990.

Van der Linden, J. When do cerebral emboli appear during open heart operations? A transcranial doppler study. *Ann Thorac Surg* 51:237, 1991.

Murkin, J. Anesthesia, the brain, and cardiopulmonary bypass. *Ann Thorac Surg* 56:1461, 1993.

Complications from bypass surgery:

Kuan, P. Coronary artery bypass surgery morbidity. *J Am Coll Cardiol* 3:1391, 1984.

Mohan, R. Coronary artery bypass grafting in the elderly—a review of studies on patients older than 64, 69, or 74 years. *Cardiology* 80:215, 1992.

Ivert, T. Coronary artery operations. Early and late results in 101 patients. *Scand J Thor Cardiovasc Surg* 22:111, 1988.

Heart surgery can be done for inappropriate reasons:

Winslow, C. The appropriateness of performing coronary artery bypass surgery. *JAMA* 260:505, 1988.

Schoenbaum, S. Toward fewer procedures and better outcomes (editorial). *JAMA* 269:794, 1993.

Graboys, T. Results of a second-opinion program for coronary artery bypass graft surgery. *JAMA* 258:1611, 1987.

Graboys, T. Results of a second-opinion trial among patients recommended for coronary angiography. *JAMA* 268:2537, 1992.

Change your diet even after the surgery to stay alive:

Coronary bypasses 10 years on. About two in five will occlude. *Br Med J* 303: 661, 1991.

Angioplasty therapy:

Landau, C. Percutaneous transluminal coronary angioplasty. *N Engl J Med* 330: 981, 1994.

Editorial: Mechanical coronary artherectomy. *Lancet* 340:1509, 1992.

Baim, D. Angioplasty as a treatment for coronary artery disease. *N Engl J Med* 326:56, 1992.

Hilborne, L. The appropriateness of use of percutaneous transluminal coronary angioplasty in New York state. *JAMA* 269:761, 1993.

Complications of angioplasty:

Kent, K. Percutaneous transluminal coronary angioplasty: report from the Registry of the National Heart, Lung, and Blood Institute. *Am J Cardiol* 49: 2011, 1982.

Editorial: The expanding scope of coronary angioplasty. *Lancet* 1:1307, 1985.

Wyman, R. Current complications of diagnostic and therapeutic cardiac cathe-
    terization. *J Am Coll Cardiol* 12:1400, 1988.
Plante, S. Acute complications of percutaneous transluminal angioplasty for
    total occlusion. *Am Heart J* 121:417, 1991.

Angioplasty does not save lives:

Parisi, A. A comparison of angioplasty with medical treatment of single vessel
    coronary artery disease. *N Engl J Med* 326:10, 1992.
Graboys, T. Results of a second-opinion trial among patients recommended for
    coronary angiography. *JAMA* 268:2537, 1992.
Graboys, T. Second-opinion trial in patients recommended for coronary angiog-
    raphy (letter). *JAMA* 269:1504, 1993.
McGivney, S. Angioplasty versus medical therapy for single-vessel coronary
    artery disease (letter). *N Engl J Med* 326:1632, 1992.

Angioplasty less traumatic and costly relief of angina than bypass surgery:

Goy, J. Coronary angioplasty versus left internal mammary grafting for isolated
    proximal left anterior descending artery stenosis. *Lancet* 343:1449, 1994.
Sculper, M. Health service costs of coronary angioplasty and coronary artery
    bypass surgery: the Randomised Intervention Treatment of Angina (RITA)
    trial. *Lancet* 344:927, 1994.
Hillis, L. Coronary angioplasty compared with bypass grafting (editorial). *N Engl
    J Med* 331:1086, 1994.

Chapter 14

*Hypertension varies around the world and is rare among people living on starch-
    based, low-salt diets:*

Freis, E. Salt, volume and the prevention of hypertension. *Circulation* 53:589,
    1976.
Finn, R. Blood pressure and salt intake: an intra-population study. *Lancet* 1:
    1097, 1981.

Diet and lifestyle changes lower blood pressure:

The Treatment of Mild Hypertension Research Group. The treatment of mild
    hypertension study. A randomized, placebo-controlled trial of a nutritional-
    hygenic regimen with various drug monotherapies. *Arch Intern Med* 151:
    1413, 1991.
The Trials of Hypertension Prevention Collaborative Research Group. The ef-
    fects of nonpharmacologic intervention on blood pressure of persons with

high normal levels. Results of the Trials of Hypertension Prevention, phase I. *JAMA* 267:1213, 1992.

Beilin, L. Non-pharmacological control of blood pressure. *Clin Exp Pharmacol Physiol* 15:215, 1988.

Swales, J. Non-pharmacological antihypertensive therapy. *Eur Heart J* 9 (Suppl G):45, 1988.

Cappiccio, F. Non-pharmacological treatment of hypertension (letter). *Lancet* 344:884, 1994.

Blood pressure at home more accurate than in the doctor's office:

White, W. Average daily blood pressure, not office blood pressure, determines cardiac function in patients with hypertension. *JAMA* 261:873, 1989.

Coffee raises blood pressure:

Sung, B. Prolonged increase in blood pressure by a single dose of caffeine in mildly hypertensive men. *Am J Hypertens* 7:755, 1994.

Superko, R. Effects of cessation of caffeinated-coffee consumption on ambulatory and resting blood pressure in men. *Am J Cardiol* 73:780, 1994.

30 percent of people are salt sensitive and reducing salt lowers blood pressure:

Muntzel, M. A comprehensive review of salt and blood pressure relationship. *Am J Hypertens* 5 (Suppl):1S, 1992.

Little, P. A controlled trial of a low sodium, low fat, high fibre diet in treated hypertensive patients: effect on antihypertensive drug requirement in clinical practice. *J Hum Hypertens* 5:175, 1991.

Sodium restriction lowers blood pressure:

MacGregor, G. Double-blind study of three sodium intakes and long-term effects of sodium restriction in essential hypertension. *Lancet* 2:1244, 1989.

Vegetarians on high-salt diets have low blood pressure:

Sacks, F. Blood pressure in vegetarians. *Am J Epidemiol* 100:390, 1974.

Armstrong, B. Urinary sodium and blood pressure in vegetarians. *Am J Clin Nutr* 32:2472, 1979.

40 percent of people with cholesterols over 240 mg/dl have high blood pressure:

Working Group on Management of Patients with Hypertension and High Blood Cholesterol. National Education Programs Working Group Report on the management of patients with hypertension and high cholesterol. *Ann Intern Med* 114:224, 1991.

Fat causes the blood to sludge, increasing peripheral resistance:

Friedman, M. Serum lipids and conjunctival circulation after fat ingestion in men exhibiting type-A behavior pattern. *Circulation* 29:874, 1964.

Friedman, M. Effects of unsaturated fats upon lipemia and conjunctival circulation. A study of coronary-prone (pattern A) men. *JAMA* 193:110, 1965.

Freis, E. Hemodynamics of hypertension. *Physiol Rev* 40:27, 1960.

Frohlich, E. Re-examination of the hemodynamics of hypertension. *Am J Med Sci* 257:9, 1969.

Malhotra, S. Dietary factors causing hypertension in India. *Am J Clin Nutr* 23: 1353, 1970.

Clumping of platelets and release of prostaglandins cause spasm:

Hamberg, M. Thromboxanes: a new group of biologically active compounds derived from prostaglandins endoperoxides. *Proc Nat l Acad Sci, USA* 72: 2994, 1975.

O'Brien, J. Acute platelet changes after large meals of saturated and unsaturated fats. *Lancet* 1:878, 1976.

Vegetarian diet normalizes blood pressure:

Rouse, I. Nutrient intake, blood pressure, serum and urinary prostaglandins and serum thrombaxane B_2 in a controlled trial with a lacto-ovo-vegetarian diet. *J Hypertens* 4:241, 1986.

Magetts, B. Vegetarian diet in mild hypertension. A randomized controlled trial. *Br Med J* 293:1468, 1986.

Sanders, T. Blood pressure, plasma renin activity and aldosterone concentrations in vegans and omnivore controls. *Hum Nutr Appl Nutr* 41A:204, 1987.

Lindahl, O. A vegan regimen with reduced medication in the treatment of hypertension. *Br J Nutr* 52:11, 1984.

British scientists find low fat, low sodium, high fiber work well together:

Little, P. A controlled trial of a low sodium, low fat, high fibre diet in treated hypertensive patients: effect on antihypertensive drug requirement in clinical practice. *J Hum Hypertens* 5:175, 1991.

Weight loss reduces blood pressure:

Applegate, W. Nonpharmacologic intervention to reduce blood pressure in older patients with mild hypertension. *Arch Intern Med* 152:1162, 1992.

The Trials of Hypertension Prevention Collaborative Research Group. The effects of nonpharmacologic interventions on blood pressure of persons with high normal levels. Results of the Trials of Hypertension Prevention, phase I. *JAMA* 267:1213, 1992.

Exercise lowers blood pressure:

Arroll, B. Does physical activity lower blood pressure: a critical review of the clinical trials. *J Clin Epidemiol* 45:439, 1992.

Nelson, L. Effect of changing levels of physical activity on blood-pressure and haemodynamics in essential hypertension. *Lancet* 2:473, 1986.

Cleroux, J. Aftereffects of exercise on regional and systemic hemodynamics in hypertension. *Hypertension* 19:183, 1992.

Complications of diabetes:

Diabetes: 1991 Vita Statistics; Diabetes Complications. The American Diabetes Association.

Quote on aggressive treatment of hypertension by British physician:

Hart, J. The practitioner's view. In Gross, F., and Strasser, Y., eds. *Mild hypertension: recent advances.* New York: Raven Press, 1983, p. 365.

Quote from Normal Kaplan, M.D., on ineffectiveness of drug therapy:

Braunwald, E., ed. *Heart disease: a textbook of cardiovascular medicine,* 4th edit. Philadelphia: W. B. Saunders Co., 1992, p. 852.

Review of drug studies fails to show survival benefits for treating mild hypertension:

Wilcox, R. Treatment of high blood pressure: should clinical practice be based on results of clinical trials? *Br Med J* 293:433, 1986.

Campbell, B. Treating hypertension in elderly patients (letter). *Br Med J* 306: 396, 1993.

Aggressive treatment kills—the J-shaped curve of mortality:

Alderman, M. Treatment-induced blood pressure reduction and the risk of myocardial infarction. *JAMA* 262:920, 1989.

Cruickshank, J. Benefits and potential harm of lowering blood pressure. *Lancet* 1:581, 1987.

Farnett, L. The J-curve phenomenon and the treatment of hypertension. Is there a point beyond which pressure reduction is dangerous? *JAMA* 265:489, 1991.

Cruickshank, J. Coronary flow reserve and the J curve relation between diastolic blood pressure and myocardial infarction. *Br Med J* 297:1227, 1988.

Kuller, L. Unexpected effects of treating hypertension in men with electrocardiographic abnormalities: a critical analysis. *Circulation* 73:114, 1986.

Cooper, S. The relation between degree of blood pressure reduction and mortality among hypertensives in the Hypertensive Detection and Follow-up Program. *Am J Epidemiol* 127:387, 1988.

Berglund, G. Goals of antihypertensive therapy. Is there a point beyond which pressure reduction is dangerous? *Am J Hypertens* 2:586, 1989.

McCloskey, L. Level of blood pressure and risk of myocardial infarction among treated hypertensive patients. *Arch Intern Med* 152:513, 1992.

Weinberger, M. Do no harm. Antihypertensive therapy and the 'J' curve (editorial). *Arch Intern Med* 152:473, 1992.

Samuelsson, O. The J-shaped relationship between coronary heart disease and achieved blood pressure level in treated hypertension: further analysis of 12 years of follow-up of treated hypertensives in Primary Prevention Trial in Gothenberg, Sweden. *J Hypertens* 8:547, 1990.

Lindblad, U. Control of blood pressure and risk of first acute myocardial infarction: Skaraborg hypertensive project. *Br Med J* 308:681, 1994.

Diabetics have a very high death rate from blood pressure treatment:

Warram, J. Excess mortality associated with diuretic therapy in diabetics. *Arch Intern Med* 151:1350, 1991.

Effects of beta receptor blockers:

Stone, R. Proximal myopathy during beta-blockade. *Br Med J* 2:1583, 1979.

Leren, P. Effect of propranolol and prazosin on blood lipids: the Oslo study. *Lancet* 2:4, 1980.

Editorial: Antihypertensive drugs, plasma lipids, and coronary disease. *Lancet* 2:19, 1980.

Norman Kaplan's quote on diuretic-induced biochemical derangements:

Braunwald, E, ed. *Heart disease: a textbook of cardiovascular medicine,* 4th edit. Philadelphia: W. B. Saunders Co., 1992, p. 853.

Effects of diuretics:

Ballantyne, D. Long-term effects of antihypertensives on blood lipids. J Hum Hypertens 4 (Suppl 2):35, 1990.

Multiple Risk Factor Intervention Trial Research Group. Multiple Risk Factor Intervention Trial. Risk factor changes and mortality results. *JAMA* 248:1465, 1982.

Holme, I. Treatment of mild hypertension with diuretics. The importance of ECG abnormalities in the Oslo study and in MRFIT. *JAMA* 251:1298, 1984.

Kannel, W. Sudden death: lessons from subsets in population studies. Lessons from epidemiology. *J Am Coll Cardiol* 5:141B, 1985.

Anti-HT therapy seems to add to sudden death risk in some. *Int Med News* 18: 60, 1985.

Higher death rates in hypertensive patients treated with diuretics raise many questions. *Cardiovascular News,* Oct 1984, p. 12.

Grimm, R. Effects of thiazide diuretics on plasma lipids and lipoproteins in mildly hypertensive patients. A double-blind controlled trial. *Ann Intern Med* 94:7, 1981.

Ames, R. Serum cholesterol during treatment of hypertension with diuretic drugs. *Arch Intern Med* 144:710, 1984.

Editorial: Diuretics, hyperuricaemia, and tienilic acid. *Lancet* 2:681, 1980.

Murphy, M. Glucose intolerance in hypertensive patients treated with diuretics; a fourteen-year follow-up. *Lancet* 2:1293, 1982.

Holland, O. Diuretic-induced ventricular ectopic activity. *Am J Med* 70:762, 1981.

Editorial: Intellectual performance in hypertensive patients. *Lancet* 1:87, 1984.

Beta blockers vs. diuretics fail to show any advantage:

Wilhelmsen, L. Beta-blockers versus diuretics in hypertensive men: main results of the HAPPY trial. *J Hypertens* 5:561, 1987.

Collins, R. Blood pressure, stroke, and coronary heart disease. Part 2, short-term reductions in blood pressure: overview of randomised drug trials in their epidemiological content. *Lancet* 335:827, 1990.

Effects of calcium channel antagonists:

Steele, R. Calcium antagonist-induced gingival hyperplasia. *Ann Intern Med* 120: 663, 1994.

Psaty, B. The risk of myocardial infarction associated with antihypertensive drug therapies. *JAMA* 274:620, 1995.

Wagenknecht, L. Surgical bleeding: unexpected effect of a calcium antagonist. *Br Med J* 310:776, 1995.

Held, P. Calcium channel blockers in acute myocardial infarction and unstable angina: an overview. *Br Med J* 299:1187, 1989.

Effects of ACE inhibitors:

Armario, P. Adverse effects of direct-acting vasodilators. *Drug Safety* 11:80, 1994.

Schnaper, H. Angiotensin-coverting enzyme inhibitors for systemic hypertension in young and elderly patients. *Am J Cardiol* 69:54C, 1992.

Parish, R. Adverse effects of angiotension-converting enzyme (ACE) inhibitors. An update. *Drug Safety* 7:14, 1992.

General side effects of blood pressure medications often cause people to stop taking them:

Curb, J. Long-term surveillance for adverse effects of antihypertensive drugs. *JAMA* 253:3263, 1985.

Curb, J. Antihypertensive drug side effects in the hypertensive detection and follow-up program. Hypertension 11(Suppl II):II-51, 1988.

Sackett, D. Randomised clinical trial of strategies for improving medication compliance in primary hypertension. *Lancet* 1:1205, 1975.

Kasiske, B. Effects of antihypertensive therapy on serum lipids. *Ann Intern Med* 122:133, 1995.

WHO urges three to six months of blood pressure observation because BP often drops without treatment:

WHO/ISH Mild Hypertension Liaison Committee. 1989 guidelines for the management of mild hypertension: memorandum from WHO/ISH meeting. *J Hypertens.* 7:689, 1989.

Report by the Management Committee: The Australian therapeutic trial in mild hypertension. *Lancet* 1:1261, 1980.

Stopping blood pressure medications:

Schmieder, R. Antihypertensive therapy. To stop or not to stop? *JAMA* 265: 1566, 1991.

Van den Bosch, W. Withdrawal of antihypertensive drugs in selected patients (letter). *Lancet* 343:1157, 1994.

Smoking raises blood pressure:

Mann, S. Elevation of ambulatory blood pressure in hypertensive smokers. A case-control study. *JAMA* 265:2226, 1991.

Alcohol raises blood pressure:

Moore, R. Alcohol consumption and blood pressure in the 1982 Maryland hypertension survey. *Am J Hypertens* 3:1, 1990.

Potter, J. Pressor effect of alcohol in hypertension. *Lancet* 1:119, 1984.

Marmiot, M. Alcohol and blood pressure: the INTERSALT study. *Br Med J* 308:1263, 1994.

Caffeine raises blood pressure:

Sung, B. Prolonged increase in blood pressure by a single dose of caffeine in mildly hypertensive men. *Am J Hypertens* 7:755, 1994.

Superko, R. Effects of cessation of caffeinated-coffee consumption on ambulatory and resting blood pressure in men. *Am J Cardiol* 73:780, 1994.

Curatolo, P. The health consequences of caffeine: a review. *Ann Intern Med* 98:641, 1983.

Freestone, S. Effect of coffee and cigarette smoking on the blood pressure of untreated and diuretic-treated hypertensive patients. *Am J Med* 73:348, 1982.

Potassium lowers blood pressure:

Geleijnse, J. Sodium and potassium intake and blood pressure change in childhood. *Br Med J* 300:899, 1990.

Krishna, G. Potassium depletion exacerbates essential hypertension. *Ann Intern Med* 115:77, 1991.

Siani, A. Increasing the dietary potassium intake reduces the need for antihypertensive medication. *Ann Intern Med* 115:753, 1991.

Garlic lowers blood pressure:

Silagy, C. A meta-analysis of the effect of garlic on blood pressure. *J Hypertens* 12:463, 1994.

McMahon, F. Can garlic lower blood pressure? A pilot study. *Pharmacotherapy* 13:406, 1993.

Chapter 15

After menopause women have more heart disease:

Mathews, K. Menopause and risk factors for coronary heart disease. *N Engl J Med* 321:641, 1989.

Women are not given the same treatments as men for heart disease:

Jackson, G. Coronary artery disease and women. Justifies equal opportunity management. *Br Med J* 309:555, 1994.

Clarke, K. Do women with acute myocardial infarction receive the same treatment as men? *Br Med J* 309:563, 1994.

Wilkinson, P. Acute myocardial infarction in women: survival analysis in first six months. *Br Med J* 309:566, 1994.

Becker, R. Comparison of clinical outcomes for men and women after acute myocardial infarction. *Ann Intern Med* 120:638, 1994.

Karlson, B. Prognosis in myocardial infarction in relation to gender. *Am Heart J* 128:477, 1994.

Hormone replacement therapy decreases your risk of osteoporosis and heart disease, but increases your risk of uterine and breast cancer:

The Writing Group for the PEPI Trial. Effects of estrogen or estrogen/progestin regimens on heart disease risk factors in postmenopausal women. The Post-menopausal Estrogen/Progestin Interventions (PEPI) Trial. *JAMA* 273: 199, 1995.

Gorsky, R. Relative risks and benefits of long-term estrogen replacement therapy: a decision analysis. *Obstet Gynecol* 83:161, 1994.

Harlap, S. The benefits and risks of hormone replacement therapy: an epidemiologic overview. *Am J Obstet Gynecol* 166:1986, 1992.

Gambrell, R. Changes in lipids and lipoproteins with long-term estrogen deficiency and hormone replacement therapy. *Am J Obstet Gynecol* 165:307, 1991.

Adding progestins to the therapy may increase the risk of heart disease and breast cancer:

Lobo, R. The role of progestins in hormone replacement therapy. *Am J Obstet Gynecol* 166:1997, 1992.

Hirvonen, E. Effects of different progestogens on lipoproteins during postmenopausal replacement therapy. *N Engl J Med* 304:560, 1981.

Ernster, V. Benefits and risks of menopausal estrogen and/or progestin hormone use. *Prev Med* 17:201, 1988.

Bergkvist, L. The risk of breast cancer after estrogen and estrogen-progestin replacement. *N Engl J Med* 321:293, 1989.

Appropriate use of hormone supplements is needed:

Rosenberg, L. Hormone replacement therapy: the need for reconsideration. *Am J Public Health* 83:1670, 1993.

Heart disease takes 500,000 women yearly and other statistics:

The American Heart Association. *Silent epidemic: the truth about women and heart disease.* AHA National Center, 7320 Greenville Avenue, Dallas, Texas, 75231.

Diet raises a woman's hormone levels:

Rose, D. High-fiber diet reduces serum estrogen concentrations in premenopausal women. *Am J Clin Nutr* 54:520, 1991.

Heber, D. Reduction of serum estradiol in postmenopausal women given free access to low-fat high-carbohydrate diet. *Nutrition* 7:137, 1991.

Adlercreutz, H. Diet and plasma androgens in postmenopausal vegetarian and omnivorous women and postmenopausal women with breast cancer. *Am J Clin Nutr* 49:433, 1989.

Woods, M. Low-fat, high-fiber diet and serum estrone sulfate in premenopausal women. *Am J Clin Nutr* 49:1179, 1989.

Rose, D. Effect of a low-fat diet on hormone levels in women with cystic breast disease. I. Serum steroids and gonadotropins. *J Natl Cancer Inst* 78:623, 1987.

Rose, D. Effect of a low-fat diet on hormone levels in women with cystic breast disease. II. Serum radioimmunoassayable prolactin and growth hormone and bioactive lactogenic hormones. *J Natl Cancer Inst* 78:627, 1987.

Hill, P. Diet, lifestyle and menstrual activity. *Am J Clin Nutr* 33:1192, 1980.

Hill, P. Diet and prolactin release. *Lancet* 2:806, 1976.

Ingram, D. Effect of low-fat diet on female sex hormone levels. *J Natl Cancer Inst* 79:1225, 1987.

Gorbach, S. Estrogens, breast cancer, and intestinal flora. *Rev Infect Dis 6* (Suppl 1):S85, 1984.

Goldin, B. Estrogen excretion patterns and plasma levels in vegetarian and omnivorous women. *N Engl J Med* 307:1542, 1982.

Goldin, B. Effect of diet on excretion of estrogens in pre- and postmenopausal women. *Ca Res* 41:3771, 1981.

Men also have a rise in hormone levels with a rich diet:

Hill, P. Plasma hormones and lipids in men at different risk of coronary artery disease. *Am J Clin Nutr* 33:1010, 1980.

Hamalainen, E. Diet and serum sex hormones in healthy men. *J Steroid Biochem* 20:459, 1984.

Risk of uterine cancer increased with estrogens:

Voigt, L. Progestagens supplementation of exogenous oestrogens and risk of endometrial cancer. *Lancet* 338:274, 1991.

Zeil, H. Increased risk of endometrial carcinoma among users of conjugated estrogens. *N Engl J Med* 293:1167, 1975.

Smith, D. Association of exogenous estrogen and endometrial carcinoma. *N Engl J Med* 293:1164, 1975.

Mack, T. Estrogens and endometrial cancer in a retirement community. *N Engl J Med* 294:1262, 1976.

Ljunghall, S. Postmenopausal osteoporosis. *Br Med J* 285:1504, 1982.

Asian women have lower estrogen levels and less breast cancer:

Adams, J. Human breast cancer: concerted role of diet, prolactin and adrenal C19-delta 5-steroids in tumorigenesis. *Int J Cancer* 50:854, 1992.

Hill, P. Plasma hormone levels in different ethnic populations of women. *Cancer Res* 36:2297, 1976.

Other health problems from estrogens:

Boston Collaborative Drug Surveillance Program. Surgically confirmed gall-bladder disease, venous thromboembolism, and breast tumors in relation to postmenopausal estrogen therapy. *N Engl J Med* 290:15, 1974.

Ajabor, L. Effect of exogenous estrogen on carbohydrate metabolism on postmenopausal women. *Am J Obstet Gynecol* 113:383, 1972.

Pfeffer, R. Estrogen use and stroke risk in postmenopausal women. *Am J Epidemiol* 103:445, 1976.

Judd, H. Estrogen replacement therapy: indications and complications. *Ann Intern Med* 98:195, 1983.

A 17 percent reduction in estrogen (estradiol) could mean much less breast cancer:

Rose, D. Plasma estrogens, diet, and breast cancer (editorial). *Nutrition* 7:139, 1991.

Reduction in estrogen levels reduces the risk of breast cancer, and cuts levels in half:

Heber, D. Reduction of serum estradiol in postmenopausal women given free access to low-fat high-carbohydrate diet. *Nutrition* 7:137, 1991.

Benefits of HRT on heart disease are overrated:

Posthuma, W. Cardioprotective effect of hormone replacement therapy in postmenopausal women: is the evidence biased? *Br Med J* 308:1268, 1994.

Rate of bone loss in women:

Smith, D. Age and activity effects on rate of bone mineral loss. *J Clin Invest* 58:716, 1976.

Raisz, L. Osteoporosis. *J Am Geriatrics Soc* 30:127, 1982.

Excess protein causes calcium loss, resulting in osteoporosis:

Hu, J. Dietary intakes and urinary excretion of calcium and acids: a cross-sectional study of women in China. *Am J Clin Nutr* 58:398, 1993.

Abelow, B. Cross-cultural association between dietary animal protein and hip fracture: a hypothesis. *Calcific Tissue Int* 50:14, 1992.

Acidification from animal protein dissolves the bones—plants are usually alkaline:

Sabastian, A. Improved mineral balance and skeletal metabolism in postmenopausal women treated with potassium bicarbonate. *N Engl J Med* 330:1776, 1994.

Sebastian, A. Improved mineral balance and skeletal metabolism in post-menopausal women treated with potassium bicarbonate (letter). *N Engl J Med* 331:279, 1994.

Worldwide, the more animal protein consumed the more osteoporosis:

Abelow, B. Cross-cultural association between dietary animal protein and hip fracture: a hypothesis. *Calcific Tissue Int* 50:14, 1992.
Walker, A. The human requirement of calcium: should low intakes be supplemented? *Am J Clin Nutr* 25:518, 1972.

Doubling the protein increases calcium loss by 50 percent:

Hegsted, M. Urinary calcium and calcium balance in young men as affected by level of protein and phosphorous intake. *J Nutr* 111:553, 1981.

Wide variations for recommendations of calcium intake:

McDougall, J. *McDougall's medicine: a challenging second opinion.* Clinton, N.J. New Win Publishing, 1985, p. 67.

Gut regulates calcium absorption:

Spencer, H. Influence of dietary calcium intake on Ca 47 absorption in man. *Am J Med* 46:197, 1969.

Actual calcium requirements of people are quite small:

Heaney, R. Calcium nutrition and bone health in the elderly. *Am J Clin Nutr* 36:986, 1982.
Paterson, C. Calcium requirements in man: a critical review. *Postgrad Med J* 54:244, 1978.

Dairy protein from skim milk causes calcium loss and a negative calcium balance:

Recker, R. The effect of milk supplements on calcium metabolism, bone metabolism and calcium balance. *Am J Clin Nutr* 41:254, 1985.

Calcium inhibits iron absorption:

Hallberg, L. Calcium: effect of different amounts of nonheme- and heme-iron absorption in humans. *Am J Clin Nutr* 53:112, 1991.
Cook, J. Calcium supplementation: effect on iron absorption. *Am J Clin Nutr* 53:106, 1991.

Phytoestrogens help relieve menopausal symptoms:

Adlercreutz, H. Dietary phyto-estrogens and the menopause in Japan (letter). *Lancet* 339:1233, 1992.

Conjugated estrogens are less cancer-promoting than synthetic estrogens:

Bergkvist, L. The risk of breast cancer after estrogen and estrogen-progestin replacement. *N Engl J Med* 321:293, 1989.

Use of topical estrogens for vaginal dryness:

Intern Med News, June 1, 1989, p. 28.

Chapter 16

Lecithin lowers cholesterol no more than other vegetable oils:

Knuiman, J. Lecithin intake and serum cholesterol. *Am J Clin Nutr* 49:266, 1989.

Recipe Index

General Index